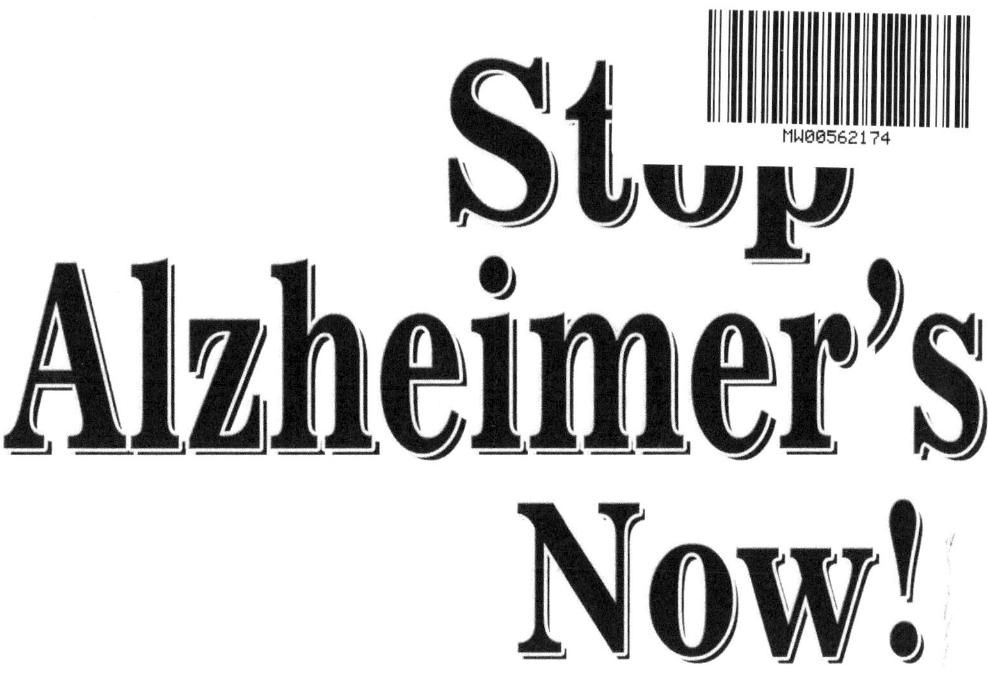

How to Prevent and Reverse Dementia, Parkinson's, ALS, Multiple Sclerosis, and Other Neurodegenerative Disorders

Second Edition

Bruce Fife, ND

Foreword by
Russell L. Blaylock, MD

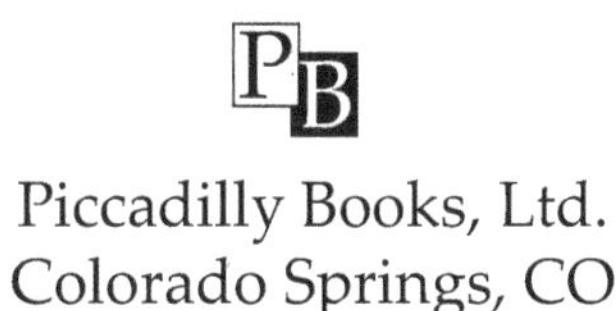

Piccadilly Books, Ltd.
Colorado Springs, CO

Grateful acknowledgment is given to Wikimedia Commons for the use of photographs on pages 20, 22, 25, 26, 32, 35, 38, 39, 42, 46, 70, 90, 91, 111, 119, 130, 133, and to Mary Newport, MD for the photos on pages 173 and 174.

Second Edition

Piccadilly Books, Ltd.
P.O. Box 25203
Colorado Springs, CO 80936, USA
info@piccadillybooks.com
www.piccadillybooks.com

Library of Congress Cataloging-in-Publication Data

Fife, Bruce, 1952-
Stop Alzheimer's now!: how to prevent and reverse dementia, Parkinson's, ALS, multiple sclerosis, and other neurodegenerative disorders / by Bruce Fife ; foreword by Russell L. Blaylock.
p. cm.
Includes bibliographical references and index.
ISBN 978-0-936709-12-0
1. Alzheimer's disease—Prevention—Popular works. 2. Alzheimer's disease—Diet therapy—Popular works. 3. Nervous system—Diseases—Prevention—Popular works. 4. Nervous system—Diseases—Diet therapy—Popular works. 5. Nervous system—Degeneration—Prevention—Popular works. 6. Nervous system—Degeneration—Nutritional aspects—Popular works. 7. Ketonic acids—Therapeutic use—Popular works. I. Title.

RC523.2.F53 2011
616.8'31—dc22

2010037444

Published in the USA

Table of Contents

"*Stop Alzheimer's Now!* by Dr. Bruce Fife offers a diet strategy based on metabolic understanding that will not only be beneficial for Alzheimer's but also for a wide variety of other diseases. I strongly recommend reading this book!"

Sofie Hexeberg, MD, PhD

"This is an important book which describes fundamental biochemical and physiologic processes that occur within us in a very readable fashion. As such, it demythologizes much current belief about causality of most degenerative diseases. Of particular importance is the discussion of fats, a much maligned source of sustenance, as well as correctly challenging the notion that the cause of many conditions is the lack of a pharmaceutical agent."

Jean R. Eckerly, MD

"The book *Stop Alzheimer's Now!* by Dr. Bruce Fife is a must read for everyone concerned with Alzheimer's disease. After a comprehensive review of the factors contributing to the actual Alzheimer's epidemic, the author explains how diet modifications and the addition of coconut oil can drastically change the course of the disease."

Edmond Devroey, MD, The Longevity Institute, www.longevinst.org

"*Stop Alzheimer's Now!* represents a major step forward in Alzheimer's disease, exposing the reality that Alzheimer's and other brain diseases are inflammation-related disorders and therefore can be effectively treated and potentially completely prevented by reversing inflammation through better nutrition and healthy lifestyles. Thank you Dr. Fife for writing a book that can inspire people to take a second look at what they eat."

Catherine Shanahan, MD
Author of *Deep Nutrition: Why Your Genes Need Traditional Food*

"Dr. Fife has written a superlative treatise on the subject of medium chain triglycerides and the treatment of neurodegenerative diseases including: Alzheimer's disease (dementia), amyotrophic lateral sclerosis (ALS), and Parkinson's disease. This seminal work is a 'must read' for any and all health care professionals, as well as any family members or friends of those stricken by these maladies. The meticulous research contained in Dr. Fife's manuscript is nothing short of 'miraculous.'"

Jeffrey Grill, MD

This book describes, clearly and in a plain language, the mechanisms by which nutritional deficiencies damage the body. It also helps to understand the links between hypoxia, imbalances of carbohydrate turnover, environmental toxicity, and neurodegeneration. The author's dietary recommendations are a valuable aid to nutritional therapy of chronic neurodegenerative diseases. I recommend this enlightening book to both physicians and those who simply want to better understand how our brain functions.

Igor Bondarenko, MD, PhD
Deputy Director of Research Oceania University of Medicine

In this book *Stop Alzheimer's Now!*, Dr. Bruce Fife has assembled the disparate facts of neurodegeneration, environmental toxins, inflammation, fats and cholesterol into a new understanding of mental health built on solid science. With the depth and breadth of his knowledge, Dr. Fife has made the fearful topic of Alzheimer's disease understandable and has provided us with evidence for an equally accessible cure—the coconut. I encourage you to read this book and follow his advice!

Fabian M. Dayrit, PhD
Dean, School of Science & Engineering
Department of Chemistry, Ateneo de Manila University

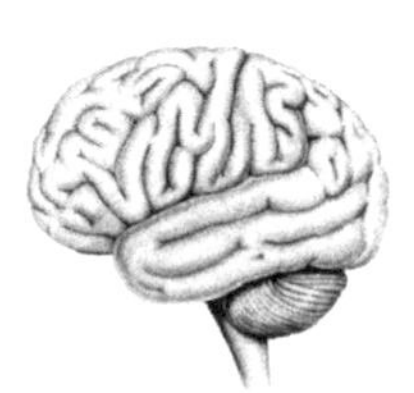

Foreword

I am often asked to write forwards to new books and have tried to be rather discerning in agreeing to do so. When Dr. Fife asked me to write a forward to his book *Stop Alzheimer's Now*, I told him I would have to read the manuscript first to see if I agreed with what he was saying. He sent it without hesitation.

As I began to read through the various chapters I was pleased to see that Dr. Fife had not only read a great deal of scientific and medical literature concerning degeneration of the human brain, but that he had a real understanding of the mechanisms that were leading up to these devastating disorders, such as Alzheimer's dementia, Parkinson's disease, and Lou Gehrig's disease (ALS).

For many years neuroscientists were puzzled by the occurrence of such neurodegenerative diseases as Alzheimer's dementia and Parkinson's disease. These diseases seemed to resist all efforts to understand why a select number of people developed either focal or widespread degeneration of their brains and why it occurred with increased frequency with aging.

It seemed that a great many things were associated with these disorders, such as exposure to heavy metals (mercury and lead), certain light metals (aluminum, cadmium), pesticides/herbicides, fungicides, head injury, infections, and inheritance of certain genes (APOE4). Despite massive amounts of data and pathological examination of thousands of affected brains, neuroscientists still had little to explain the phenomenon.

While they knew that certain microscopic pathological changes were frequently found with each of the neurodegenerative diseases, they understood little of how and why these changes were taking place. They knew, for example, that an abnormal constructed protein called beta-amyloid accumulated in certain areas of the Alzheimer's brain and that the neurotubules within dendrites were abnormal (called neurofibrillary tangles—composed of hyperphosphorylated tau proteins). But, what is causing these changes?

Despite tens of millions of dollars of research money being spent on studying the biochemistry of beta-amyloid and tau proteins, few answers are forthcoming. Meanwhile, millions of cases of neurodegenerative diseases are being diagnosed each year and, of great concern, these diseases are increasing in incidence and are rapidly moving into younger age groups—that is, younger people, even in their forties, are developing dementing diseases that were once thought to be limited to the elderly.

In this book, you will learn why this growth in devastating neurological disorders is occurring. Over the past decade neuroscientists have discovered a number of surprising findings. Most important is that as we age our brains become increasingly inflamed and for some, this increase is tremendous. It is these individuals who are at the highest risk for developing one of the neurodegenerative diseases.

Dr. Fife's book will lead you through this tangle of information in a way that is understandable and makes logical sense. The human brain is an incredibly complex structure, one that still defies a full understanding. Unlike many organs, brain function is dependent on a miraculous interplay of trillions of connections, tens of thousands of biochemical reactions, biophysical structures of incredible complexity and an interplay of neurons, glia cells, neurotransmitters, neuromodulators, and neuropeptides, most of which are changing constantly.

Central to our understanding of the cause of these neurodegenerative diseases is an understanding of the brain's unique immune system, which is controlled by an interplay of intrinsic brain immune cells, microglia and astrocytes, and immune cells from the body, macrophages, monocytes, and T-cells.

Normally, these brain immune cells are in a quiescence, resting state until the brain is disturbed, and when disturbed, for any reason, these immune cells leap into action. When active they can pour out very destructive immune cytokines, excitotoxins, and massive amounts of free radicals and lipid peroxidation products—some pretty nasty customers. Their purpose is to kill bacteria, viruses, or fungi invading the brain. Under normal conditions, this attack is quickly contained and the microglial cells then switch to a mode that tries to repair the damage it had to do to kill the invaders—that is, it cleans up the collateral damage (called bystander injury).

It is now evident that a similar process is occurring with neurodegenerative diseases of many types, including Alzheimer's dementia, frontotemporal degeneration, dementia with Lewy bodies, vascular dementia, Huntington's disease, ALS, multiple sclerosis, and even age-related memory loss. For a number of reasons, the brain's immune system is activated, but rather than shutting off, as it should, it continues to release the destructive cytokines, excitotoxins and free radicals. This can continue for decades.

In Dr. Fife's book you will learn of the vital importance of brain energy production in this process. Most cell energy, including neurons, is generated by the mitochondria. The mitochondria are also the source for most of the free radicals and lipid peroxidation products as well. It is now known that a loss of mitochondrial energy production occurs decades before any neurological symptoms occur—that is, before memory problems, disorientation, or confusion present themselves.

One study of men of an average age of 55 having the APOE4 gene found significant suppression of their mitochondrial energy production in the same areas of the brain affected in Alzheimer's dementia. This was decades before the onset of the disease. An even more startling study examined brain metabolism in APOE4 carrier young men, average age 30.7 years, and found that even at this young age their brain mitochondrial energy production was significantly impaired in these same regions. So, it is firmly established that brain energy metabolism begins to fail decades before any symptom surfaces. The big question is—what is causing our mitochondria to fail?

We now live in a sea of toxic chemicals in our environment, that is, in our drinking water, the air we breathe, and the foods we eat. Compelling evidence indicates that many of these chemicals impair the ability of mitochondria to make energy. It is also known that many of these chemicals interact in a way that enhances each other's toxicity; that is they are synergistic. What this means is that when neurotoxic chemicals in doses below what normally causes toxicity are mixed they become fully toxic. The EPA and FDA rarely consider or check for chemical synergism in their evaluations.

Mercury, lead, cadmium, fluoride, aluminum, many pesticides, herbicides and fungicides are toxic to mitochondria. We are all exposed to all of these toxins. No one can escape them. There is also compelling evidence that all of these toxins also cause brain inflammation by chronically activating microglia. The resulting neurological disorder depends on which group of microglia is activated. The highest concentration of microglia is seen in the substantia nigra area of the midbrain (Parkinson's disease) and the areas affected by Alzheimer's disease.

Ironically, it has also been shown that triggering inflammation, as by vaccination, can increase the neurotoxicity of a number of these environmental toxins—especially pesticides. It is also known that the receptors for excitatory neurotransmitters and inflammatory cytokines crosstalk (interact) to enhance excitotoxicity. I have coined the name immunoexcitotoxicity to describe this destructive interaction between brain inflammation and excitotoxicity. There is compelling evidence that immunoexcitotoxicity is playing a central role in a great many neurological diseases and disorders, including neurodegenerative diseases, strokes, MS, head injury, and brain infections. This explains why so many things can be associated with these conditions.

There is also a link to mitochondrial dysfunction as well. It is known that excitotoxicity itself impairs mitochondrial function, dramatically increases oxidative stress and lipid peroxidation and impairs the essential migration of mitochondria from the neuron cell body to the synapse. Interestingly, brain inflammation has the same effect. Immunoexcitotoxicity has also been shown to produce all of the characteristics of the neurodegenerative diseases themselves, including beta-amyloid accumulation and neurofibrillary tangles.

It is also well established that mitochondrial suppression, no matter the cause, greatly enhances excitotoxicity. It may well be that mitochondrial dysfunction precedes the immunoexcitotoxic process itself and magnifies it once it occurs. This explains why people with mitochondrial abnormalities can have normal brain function for such a long time before the symptoms of dementia set in. Studies have shown that moderate reduction of mitochondrial function by itself rarely impairs brain function. But, over time, oxidative stress and lipid peroxidation triggered by mitochondrial dysfunction can damage the connections and dendrites to a degree that it begins to impair brain function. At this stage, the microglia are activated and perpetuate the pathological process by immunoexcitotoxicity.

As this book explains, by causing the body to produce more ketones and by supplying ketones from medium-chain triglycerides, one not only dramatically improves mitochondrial energy production, but also, as shown in several studies, at the same time causes the mitochondria to produce fewer free radicals. It has also been shown that ketones have strong anti-inflammatory properties and strongly protect the brain from excitotoxicity.

While increasing ketones is key to correcting the metabolic and immunoexcitotoxic problems, even more protection is provided by combining certain dietary changes and the use of special supplements, as described in this book. For example, curcumin has been shown to protect against excitotoxicity, reduce brain inflammation and offer powerful protection against some of the most harmful brain reactive oxygen and nitrogen species, something that vitamin antioxidants are powerless to do. A number of plant flavonoids have shown similar effects, including apigenin, luteolin, hesperidin, ellagic acid, and tea catachins.

I was particularly impressed by the book not only by the quality of its overall scholarship, but also because of the detailed discussion of the importance of controlling chronic infections, especially oral infections. These infections are major players in initiating and driving brain immunoexcitotoxicity. As Dr. Fife has shown, coconut oil has been shown to significantly reduce oral infections as well as systemic infections. Another major player in our protection is vitamin D3. His discussion of the antimicrobial peptides generated by vitamin D3 is one of the best I have read.

Finally, this book is more than a scientific treatise on the neuropathological causation of neurodegenerative disease, Dr. Fife outlines a specific battle plan to combat these disorders, one that fits very nicely with what we know of these disorders and is easy to follow. I would encourage everyone faced with the possibility of encountering neurodegenerative disease, which now includes most of us, to read this book carefully. It is a treasure trove of invaluable information and practical advice.

Russell L. Blaylock, M.D., CCN
Theoretical Neurosciences Research, LLC
Visiting Professor of Biology.
Belhaven University, Jackson, MS
www.blaylockwellness.com
www.russellblaylockmd.com

Russell L. Blaylock, MD is a board certified neurosurgeon and formerly a clinical assistant professor of neurosurgery at the University of Mississippi. He has written three books, *Excitotoxins: The Taste That Kills*, *Health, Nutrition Secrets That Can Save Your Life*, and *Natural Strategies for Cancer Patients*, and co-authored the book *Cellular and Molecular Biology of Autism Spectrum Disorders*. Dr Blaylock serves on the editorial staff of the *Journal of the American Nutraceutical Association* and the *Journal of American Physicians and Surgeons*. He is currently a visiting professor of biology at Behnaven University in Jackson, Mississippi and is the president of Theoretical Neurosciences Research, LLC.

1 Is There a Cure for Alzheimer's?

IT'S ALL IN THE HEAD

Alzheimer's is a frightening disease that robs people not only of their memories, but also of their ability to think, reason, care for themselves, and function in society. It is a disease that respects no person, afflicting the rich and the poor, the educated and the uneducated, celebrities and non-celebrities. All are alike.

Former President Ronald Reagan died after a ten-year battle with the mind-deteriorating effects of Alzheimer's disease. On November 5, 1994, in a handwritten letter, Reagan announced that he had entered the early stages of Alzheimer's disease. "I now begin the journey," he wrote, "that will lead me into the sunset of my life...I only wish there was some way I could spare Nancy from this painful experience."

Later, Nancy Reagan spoke of her anguish as her husband's health deteriorated: "Ronnie's long journey has finally taken him to a distant place where I can no longer reach him. We can't share the wonderful memories of our 52 years together. And I think that's the hardest part."

Sarah Harris knows all too well the grief associated with Alzheimer's disease. Her husband Ernie is only 56 years old, but three years into the disease she does everything for him: she feeds him, washes him, dresses him, even brushes his teeth. "One day he woke up and he looked at me and said 'Who are you?'" says Harris. "That was probably the most devastating thing that could happen to a person."

For millions of people, the twilight years have become a debilitating walk through darkness. There is no cure, and current treatments can only offer the hope of slowing down the disease.

Currently, drug therapy is the only option readily available. Antonio Vasquez was 60 when Alzheimer's disease began to affect his life. He lost his job at a bakery because he kept burning chocolate chip cookies, forgetting he had put them in the oven. Then he got lost going to job interviews, walking in circles around his neighborhood. Antonio takes a drug widely prescribed for Alzheimer's called Aricept, which is believed to ease symptoms but does nothing to stop the disease or even slow it down. Side effects often include nausea, vomiting, diarrhea, headache, insomnia, generalized pain, and dizziness, and less frequently may involve muscle cramps, fatigue, depression, arthritis, skin discoloration, and fainting. In recent studies the drug was also shown to increase the risk of death. The reported benefits to the drug are very slight and generally unnoticeable since it cannot reverse or even stop the progression of the disease. The drawbacks seem overwhelming. What else can be done?

Drug therapy didn't appeal to Sue and Don Miller. Don was diagnosed at age 55. "Previous to Alzheimer's I had a very sharp mind," says Don. "I had a high IQ which basically sort of took a large dive."

Don built a career as a financial manager only to find that he could no longer make change or pay bills. The doctor's diagnosis was a shock.

"I remember going to the second visit and he looked at us and said, 'have you two considered Alzheimer's?' and I think you could have picked us up off the floor," says Sue Miller. "That's a disease of the elderly!"

While most people are diagnosed after age 70, Alzheimer's disease also strikes in middle age. Faced with a long, drawn-out loss of memory and mind, the Millers are considering a new form of treatment—gene therapy. The procedure involves injecting certain growth proteins deep into the brain. Scientists believe nerve growth factors have the potential to revive dying brain cells and slow the aging process.

The experiment means drilling holes into Don's brain, risking pain, bleeding, permanent brain damage, and even death. "I don't know that I'm a risk taker," says Sue Miller. "But on the other hand, there's nothing else, and that's what's so frustrating here, there's nothing."

For the Millers, it's an agonizing choice between subjecting Don to the certain slow march of Alzheimer's or the uncertain and risky race of medical exploration. Neither offers comfort.

Take heart! If you have a friend or a loved one who is headed toward Alzheimer's or if you want to protect yourself from ever developing this devastating disease, there is hope! You need not take drugs or undergo risky brain surgeries. The solution revolves around diet and certain brain-enhancing medicinal foods that can stop the disease dead in its tracks and, in most cases, bring about significant improvement, which is something no drug or therapy has yet been able to do.

Many Alzheimer's sufferers are now using this program with phenomenal success.

"It was like a light being turned on in my head."

"I feel like a different person."

"I've got my life back."

These are some of the comments people have made after following the program outlined in this book. These people are reclaiming lost cognitive skills and memory, experiencing improved social skills, increasing their interaction with others, showing improved ability to make conversation, recapturing their sense of humor, resuming favorite activities, and are enjoying life again. Many have reported improved eyesight even from conditions as serious as glaucoma and macular degeneration. This makes sense because the eyes are extensions of the brain; in many cases, as the brain heals, so do the eyes.

A WORLDWIDE EPIDEMIC

More than 35 million people have dementia today. Each year 260,000 new cases are diagnosed in the United States, and 4.6 million new cases occur worldwide, or one new case every 7 seconds. The number of people affected is expected to double to about 70 million by the year 2030.

Alzheimer's disease is the most common form of dementia. In the United States, one in eight persons over the age of 65 and as many as half the population age 85 and over have Alzheimer's disease. At least one member out of every three families is affected by Alzheimer's disease. Half of the elderly in long-term care facilities are reported to have Alzheimer's disease or some other form of dementia.

Next to Alzheimer's, Parkinson's disease, a neuromuscular disorder, is the most common neurodegenerative disease, affecting about 4 million people worldwide. Millions more are affected by amyotrophic lateral sclerosis, Huntington's disease, and other neurodegenerative disorders.

Age is the biggest risk factor for these neurodegenerative diseases. As life expectancy increases and as the population ages, the number of people affected is expected to rise dramatically. The baby boomer generation (those born between 1946 and 1964 when the birth rate was at its peak) are now entering their golden years, the age at which neurodegenerative disease usually begins to manifest itself.

Recent newspaper headlines have called it an impending "epidemic." "We are facing an emergency," says Daisy Acosta, MD, director of Alzheimer's Disease International (ADI). Alzheimer's, as well as Parkinson's and other neurodegenerative diseases, are rising even more than expected. The incidence of Alzheimer's is 10 percent higher today than what scientists had predicted just five years ago. If this keeps up, it will far outpace the already dire predictions.

Alarmed by the rising rates, ADI is urging the World Health Organization to declare dementia a health priority and for national governments to follow suit. It recommends major new investments in research to uncover what causes dementia and how to slow, if not stop, the creeping brain disease that gradually robs sufferers of their memories and ability to care for themselves, eventually killing them. There is no known cure; today's drugs only temporarily alleviate symptoms. Scientists aren't even sure what causes Alzheimer's. The US Alzheimer's Association is pushing for an increase in research funding to one billion dollars annually.

While more research is definitely needed, we don't have to wait another 10, 20, or 30 years for an effective treatment. The treatment already exists. What is needed is to get the word out to all those who can benefit from this treatment. That is the purpose of this book. In this book, you will discover the primary factors that lead to the development of neurodegeneration, which factors are the most important and the most common, but more importantly, you will learn what can be done to both prevent the disease and even reverse it.

A REVOLUTIONARY BREAKTHROUGH

Steve Newport, an accountant in his mid 50s, began experiencing problems at work. As the months went by he became increasingly disorganized, error prone, frustrated, and depressed. "I didn't know what was happening to me, I was confused," says Steve. He eventually consulted a neurologist who diagnosed him with early-onset Alzheimer's. He was prescribed Aricept, the first of several drugs he would eventually take. The drugs didn't seem to do much good, and the disease continued to get worse. He eventually developed hand and face tremors and began to have difficulty keeping his balance and walking.

His wife, Mary Newport, MD, was constantly on the lookout for new therapies that might help. She came across a notice seeking volunteers for a clinical study on a new Alzheimer's drug. Preliminary studies had produced unbelievable results. It not only stopped the progression of the disease but also produced actual memory improvement, which was something no other drug had ever done.

She tried to enroll Steve into the study but he was rejected because his condition was too severe. He was considered hopeless and beyond help, even for this new miracle drug. "We were devastated," she said.

While researching the new drug, Dr. Newport discovered that the active ingredient was a special type of oil known as medium chain triglyceride oil or MCT oil. MCT oil is derived from coconut oil, which is composed of 60 percent medium chain triglycerides. "And then it hit me," she said. "Why don't we just try coconut oil as a dietary supplement? What have we got to lose?" So she went to the health food store, picked up some coconut oil, and began giving it to Steve every day. Miraculously, it seemed to "lift the fog." By the fifth day, there was tremendous improvement.

"He said it was like someone had turned on a light bulb," says Dr. Newport. "He was alert, smiling, joking. He was Steve again. He was back!"

Over the following months his tremors subsided, the visual disturbances that prevented him from reading disappeared, and he became more social and interested in those around him. He still speaks in halting sentences, but he is reading again, volunteering at his wife's hospital, and mowing the lawn. Before the dietary intervention, he would dismantle the mower, pour oil in the gas tank, and forget about the lawn.

Steve Newport was diagnosed with severe Alzheimer's disease two years ago. Today, after dietary intervention, much of his cognitive skills and memory have been restored. Steve was fortunate enough to be married to a physician who was able to lead him in the right direction.

"I've got living proof that this will help people," says Dr. Newport. "I want to just tell everybody about this. It may help them improve, too."

KETONE THERAPY

The secret behind Steve's remarkable success can be attributed to ketone therapy. Ketones are a special type of high-energy fuel produced in the liver specifically to nourish the brain. Under normal conditions, we have very few ketones circulating in our blood, but under special circumstances ketone levels can rise. When they do, they provide the brain with a burst of energy and supply the building blocks to form new brain tissue.

In Alzheimer's disease, brain cells have difficulty metabolizing glucose, the brain's principal source of energy. Without adequate fuel, brain cells die. Ketones supply the brain with the energy it needs to not only survive, but thrive.

"We know that if we give patients ketones, we can bypass this glucose block," says Theodore VanItallie, MD, professor emeritus at the College of Physicians and Surgeons at Columbia University in New York City. He has been researching ketones for more than 35 years. "Ketones are a high-energy fuel that nourish the brain," VanItallie says.

When a person does not eat foods that supply glucose, such as during starvation or severe calorie restriction, the body produces ketones from dissolved body fat to supply the brain the energy it needs to survive. Ketones can also be made directly from MCTs without being in a state of starvation. The liver converts MCTs into ketones. One place where MCTs are found naturally is human breast milk. MCTs are essential for the proper growth and development of the brain and spinal cord in newborns.

MCTs are used in medicine to provide energy for premature infants, patients recovering from surgery, and those with malnutrition and absorption problems. They are used by athletes to improve performance and endurance and by dieters to control appetite and stimulate fat burning. Studies suggest that they also enhance heart function and immune health. Much of the benefit derived from MCTs comes after they have been converted by the liver into ketones.

Ketones have a potent therapeutic effect on the brain, normalizing brain function and bringing about homeostasis. Ketone therapy has been used successfully in the treatment of epilepsy for more than 90 years. It is the only known treatment that can actually cure epilepsy.

In 2005 Dr. VanItallie applied ketone therapy in the treatment of five Parkinson's patients. After 28 days the participants' tremors, stiffness, and ability to walk improved by as much as 81 percent. "Our study was very successful," says VanItallie.[1] It demonstrated that ketone therapy has the potential to treat a number of neurodegenerative conditions, not just Alzheimer's or epilepsy.

Ketone therapy is proving useful in various applications. The United States army put out a call to research institutions for a way to keep soldiers in the battlefield for several days with little or no food while maintaining physical and cognitive function. Kieran Clarke, PhD, professor of physiological biochemistry at the University of Oxford, England, answered the call. Dr. Clarke heads the Cardiac Metabolism Research Group at Oxford. "We've developed this diet that is based on ketone bodies," says Dr. Clarke. "Ketone bodies are actually the most efficient fuel you could have." Ketones produce 28 percent more energy than glucose, and they can improve endurance and cognitive function under extreme conditions, such as on the battlefield.

"We'd been studying ketone bodies for years and looking at the effect on heart function and things like that," says Dr. Clarke. "Then the US army put out a call for a way to send what they call 'war fighters' into a battlefield without giving them anything to eat for five days and they wanted them to maintain cognitive function. We said, well, you can't actually do that, it's not possible, but we can invent a food for you to give them that will make them far more efficient than they normally are and will help them to think better." The US army responded by investing 12 million dollars in Clarke's research.

Ketone therapy has applications beyond the battlefield. "We're hoping that we will be able to use this for treatment of Alzheimer's and Parkinson's disease," she says. "By providing an alternative form of energy for the brain that circumvents their metabolic defect, then you may be able to rescue the brain."

"Ketones are a superfuel for the brain," says Richard Veech, MD, senior research scientist at the National Institutes of Health in Bethesda, Maryland. Dr. Veech has been working with ketones for more than 40 years and has published numerous research articles on the subject. Dr. Veech says ketones can be therapeutic any time cells are threatened by energy deprivation, which covers a broad array of diseases.

VanItallie, Clarke, Veech, and others have been suggesting for years that ketone therapy could help treat Alzheimer's disease, Parkinson's disease, amyotrophic lateral sclerosis (Lou Gehrig's disease), Huntington's disease, epilepsy, multiple sclerosis (MS), autism, type 1 and type 2 diabetes, stroke, heart failure, head trauma, depression, various forms of dementia, Rett syndrome, Tourette's syndrome, Meniere's disease, and several metabolic disorders caused by rare mutations, as well as other conditions.

"These diseases appear wildly different," Veech says. Treating "all these different things with some magic substance sounds improbable," he adds. Yet doctors who've experimented with ketone-based therapies are seeing results and the idea no longer seems so outlandish.

Ketone therapy is so new that most doctors know little, if anything, about it. They may have heard of the ketogenic diet used in the treatment of epilepsy, but this is different. Consequently, doctors treat neurodegenerative diseases using the standard drugs that they have been using for years, even though they do little, if any, good. You don't have to wait for your doctor to catch up on the latest developments in ketone science. You can start ketone therapy right now with products readily available at your local health food or grocery store. Many people already have, and are experiencing incredible results.

In Sandy Hook, Connecticut, 83-year-old Mary Hurst started dressing herself again. Before using the oil, she was never out of her nightgown and robe. She would sit in a chair all day, incommunicative, "like a vegetable," says her daughter Diane Standish.

"Recently, Hurst walked into the kitchen and opened the refrigerator, something she hadn't done in years," Standish says. "I asked what she was doing." Hurst retorted: "Getting myself a piece of cake, do you mind?"

"She remembered that I had brought her a cake the day before," Standish says. "Miraculous!"

Robert Condap of San Leandro, California, talks more after taking coconut and MCT oils. When his wife, Gwen, was blow-drying his hair recently, he even cracked an off-color joke. "I was excited," she says. "That was an old part of him coming back."

"I started checking into coconut oil," says Roxie Long, "because I saw on the news that Alzheimer's patients were dramatically improving after taking this oil. I bought some for my father who had recently been diagnosed with Alzheimer's. He now thinks the Alzheimer's has gone away! I'm using it too and I feel so good, physically and mentally better!"

Retired computer tech, Dick Kerstiens of Westcliff, Colorado began taking the oil after seeing what it had done for his wife Betty. Betty began experiencing signs of Alzheimer's five years earlier at the age of 71. The disease progressed to the point that she required full-time care from her husband.

After reading an article by Dr. Julian Whitaker about the success of ketone therapy, Dick began giving her the oil twice daily. "In eight days," says Dick, "she went from speaking gibberish to articulate speech!" He was amazed. Two weeks later they had friends over for the evening and he heard his wife laugh for the first time in nearly three years.

"This powerful natural therapy and possible cure for some of our most devastating diseases has been hiding in plain sight for years, recognized by nobody except a drug company and a handful of researchers," says Julian Whitaker, MD, Director of the Whitaker Wellness Institute, Newport Beach, California. "I'm now recommending ketone therapy for all of my patients with Alzheimer's disease, Parkinson's disease, dementia, multiple sclerosis, ALS (Lou Gehrig's disease), and other neurodegenerative disorders. There is evidence to suggest that it may also be beneficial for individuals with Down syndrome, autism, and diabetes."

AN OUNCE OF PREVENTION

This book is written not only for those who are suffering from neurodegenerative diseases, but for those who want to save themselves from ever encountering one or more of these devastating afflictions. Alzheimer's and Parkinson's don't just happen overnight. They take years, often decades, to develop. In the case of Alzheimer's disease, for example, approximately 70 percent of the brain cells responsible for memory are destroyed *before* symptoms become noticeable. Once symptoms surface, the brain is already in an advanced stage of degeneration, and full recovery is impossible.

You do not want to wait until most of your brain is dead before you start to do something about it. The old saying "an ounce of prevention is worth a pound of cure" is definitely true when it comes to neurodegeneration. You can stop Alzheimer's and Parkinson's and other neurodegenerative diseases before they take over your life, but you must start now. Keeping what you have now is far easier than trying to recapture what has been lost.

Fortunately, complete restoration is not necessary in order to recapture "normal" function. The brain has an amazing ability to adapt and rewire itself. If brain cells in one area die, then others can take over their function. This is why many stroke and accident victims who experience brain damage can still function normally, without any loss of intelligence. The brain also contains stem cells that can create new nerve tissue.

Ketone therapy can stop the progression of the disease and even aid in rebuilding damaged or lost cells. But ketone therapy alone is not the complete answer. A proper diet is also needed to supply adequate nutrition, balance blood sugar, and to reduce exposure to harmful substances that promote neurodegeneration.

In this book you will learn about the Alzheimer's Battle Plan, a program that combines ketone therapy with a brain regenerative diet to stop the disease dead in its tracks and regain lost function. Although it's called the "Alzheimer's Battle Plan", it could just as well be titled the Parkinson's Battle Plan or the ALS Battle Plan or the Huntington's Battle Plan because the program works equally well for a variety of neurodegenerative conditions.

Although inherited factors may influence some cases of neurodegeneration, diet, lifestyle, and environment are the major factors involved. Those who have parents, grandparents, or siblings who are affected by neurodegeneration are at increased risk themselves, not necessarily because of genetics, but due to a shared environment or learned habits that promote the disease.

A study of elderly couples has found that where one partner has dementia, the other is six times more likely to develop the condition themselves.[2] This suggests that something in the couple's shared environment, rather than genetics, is the primary cause of the disease in these cases. If you have a family member who has neurodegenerative disorder, you are at increased risk.

Dementia and other forms of neurodegeneration are *not* a part of the normal aging process. You should not expect to develop dementia as you grow older. The mind is fully capable of functioning normally for a lifetime, regardless of how long a person might live. While aging is a risk factor for neurodegeneration, it is not the cause! Dementia and other neurological conditions are disease processes that can be prevented and treated. This book will show you how you can hold on to your mental faculties for your entire life.

I encourage you to read this book from cover to cover. However, there is a lot of information contained in these pages, if you are too anxious and want to get to the meat of the program as quickly as possible, the most important information about the program is contained in Chapters 12 though 19. Nevertheless greater appreciation and understanding of the program will be gained by reading the entire book.

As a preview, Chapter 2 provides basic information about the structure of the brain. Chapter 3 briefly describes the major neurodegenerative diseases. Chapters 4 through 11 describe the major factors that can lead to neurodegeneration. Chapters 12 through 15 discuss the role fat and cholesterol play in brain health and explains how dietary fat can either harm or heal the brain. In these chapters the miracle of ketone therapy is introduced. Chapters 16 through 18 look at the effects of diet on brain health. Chapter 19 brings all the pertinent information in the previous chapters together and distills it into the Alzheimer's Battle Plan. Finally, Chapter 20 provides several recipe ideas to assist you in achieving success with the program.

2 The Human Brain

A SUPER COMPUTER

Nearly every animal on earth has a brain—birds, fish, frogs and even the tiniest insects. The only exceptions are some very primitive animals like jellyfish and sponges. The brain is like a powerful computer that coordinates a complex array of data with a multitude of feedback mechanisms and a continuing stream of incoming data. But even the most advanced supercomputers are no match for the human brain. While a computer can perform calculations or retrieve data in a fraction of a second, it cannot use this data to think, reason, make decisions, process emotions, or be creative. Your brain can do all of this and much more. Yet, it is only about the size of a small head of cauliflower, weighing about three pounds on average.

Your nervous system consists of the brain, spinal cord and peripheral nerves, making up a complex, integrated information processing and control network. At the center of this network are the brain and spinal cord, which function as the control center for the body and together are referred to as the central nervous system.

The brain is continually active. It coordinates innumerable functions both when alert and asleep. This requires a great deal of energy and a constant need for oxygen and nutrients. Consequently, the brain has one of the body's richest networks of blood vessels. Even though it accounts for only about 2 percent of an adult's body weight, with every heartbeat arteries carry 20-25 percent of your blood to your brain, consuming almost one-quarter of the body's available oxygen.

BRAIN CELLS

The brain consists of several thousand miles of interconnected nerve cells (about 100 billion in all) with innumerable extensions that control every movement, sensation, thought, and emotion that encompasses the human experience. Nerve cells come in different varieties with varying functions. Some relay sensory information from peripheral nerves throughout the body to the brain, others deliver commands from the brain to the rest of the body, and still others function as scaffolding for the support of other nerves. Despite being composed entirely of nerve cells, the brain does not feel pain. The nerves there have no pain receptors. A headache is felt because of sensory impulses coming chiefly from the tissues surrounding the skull.

The brain contains two types of nerve cells: glia and neurons. Glia (Latin for "glue") are the most numerous of the brain's cells and provide the structural support, the glue, so to speak, that holds all the brain cells together. There are a number of different types of glial cells, each of which performs different critical functions, including nutritional support, insulating neurons from one another, fighting off pathogens, removing dead neurons, and regulating the environment of the cerebrospinal fluid surrounding the brain. Glia, however, do not relay signals; that is the function of the neurons. Neurons transmit signals by means of electrochemical impulses which allow us to think, act, and perceive our environment. Nerve cells vary greatly in size. A single nerve cell in your fingertip can extend up the entire length of your arm, while neurons in the brain may reach only a few millimeters. A single neuron can be directly linked to tens of thousands of other neurons, creating a totality of more than a 100 trillion connections, each capable of performing hundreds of calculations per second. This forms the basis of your brain's capacity for memory and thinking.

Neurons consist of three basic parts: (1) the cell body, which contains most of the cell's organelles (cell organs), including the nucleus, mitochondria (which make energy), ribosomes (for building proteins), etc., (2) the axon, a long cable-like projection of the cell that carries electrochemical messages (nerve impulses) along the length of the cell, and (3) dendrites or nerve endings that branch out like a tree to make connections to other cells and allow the neurons to "talk" with each other or sense the environment.

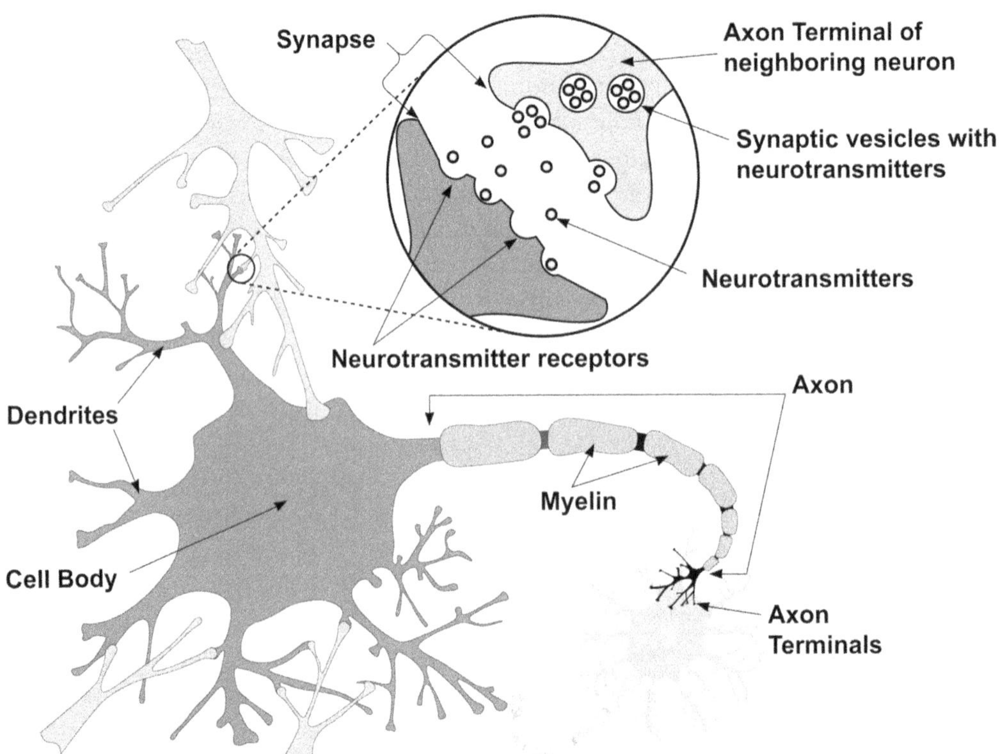

Structure of a neuron and the synaptic juncture between two neurons.

Neurons send messages at lightning speed in the form of electrochemical pulses. There is no partial pulse—that is, they either fire a transmission or remain silent. Intensity is expressed by how many neurons fire and how rapidly. A strong reaction results from many neurons firing in rapid succession. Neurons fire pulses whenever instructed to do so. This can be triggered by sensations from peripheral nerves or commands or thoughts in the brain. Neurons relay electrochemical signals from one nerve cell to the next. The signals are sent in only one direction. They are picked up by the dendrites and transported along the cell through the axon, then branch out to the many axon terminals and are passed to the dendrites of connecting neurons.

The axon terminals do not actually touch the dendrites of neighboring neurons. The electrochemical signal must "jump" from one cell to the next. The gap between an axon terminal and a dendrite is called the synapse. Each neuron typically has between 1,000 to 10,000 synapses. The synapse is an incredibly narrow space—only about two millionths of a centimeter in width. When a nerve impulse reaches the end of an axon, it transfers the signal to the next neuron by releasing chemicals called *neurotransmitters*, into this fluid-filled space. These neurotransmitters cross the synapse to the next neuron, triggering an electrochemical impulse that is passed along in a like manner to the next neuron.

Neurotransmitters are the means by which neurons communicate with each other. There are a number of different neurotransmitters. Endorphins, epinephrine, melatonin, glutamine, and dopamine are some of the more recognizable ones. Specific neurotransmitters are used by specific neurons in different parts of the brain. Psychoactive drugs exert their effects by activating neurotransmitter receptors in neurons. For example, addictive drugs such as cocaine, amphetamine, and heroin trigger neurons sensitive to dopamine.

STRUCTURE OF THE BRAIN

Axons take up most of the space in the brain. Many axons are wrapped in thick sheaths of a white fatty substance called myelin, which serves to greatly increase the speed of the impulse through the nerve. Myelin-covered axons form an area called the *white matter* in the brain. Nerve cell bodies, which are not covered by myelin, form the *gray matter*. The neurons in the brain are structurally supported by hair-like glial cells.

Compared to other cells in the body, nerves contain a disproportionately high amount of lipids (fat and cholesterol). Ignoring the water content, the brain consists of about 60 percent fat. This gives the brain a soft consistency similar to gelatin. Because it is a delicate and vital organ, it is encased within the hard protective shield of the skull, wrapped in a tough fibrous membrane called the dura mater (Latin for "hard mother"), and surrounded with a liquid filling called the cerebrospinal fluid to act as a cushion to absorb traumatic shocks. This design protects the brain from most bumps and falls.

Blood vessels in the brain provide another form of protection. The brain is very sensitive to chemical and microbial insults. Toxins and microorganisms which are often carried in the blood could cause a great deal of harm to sensitive brain tissues.

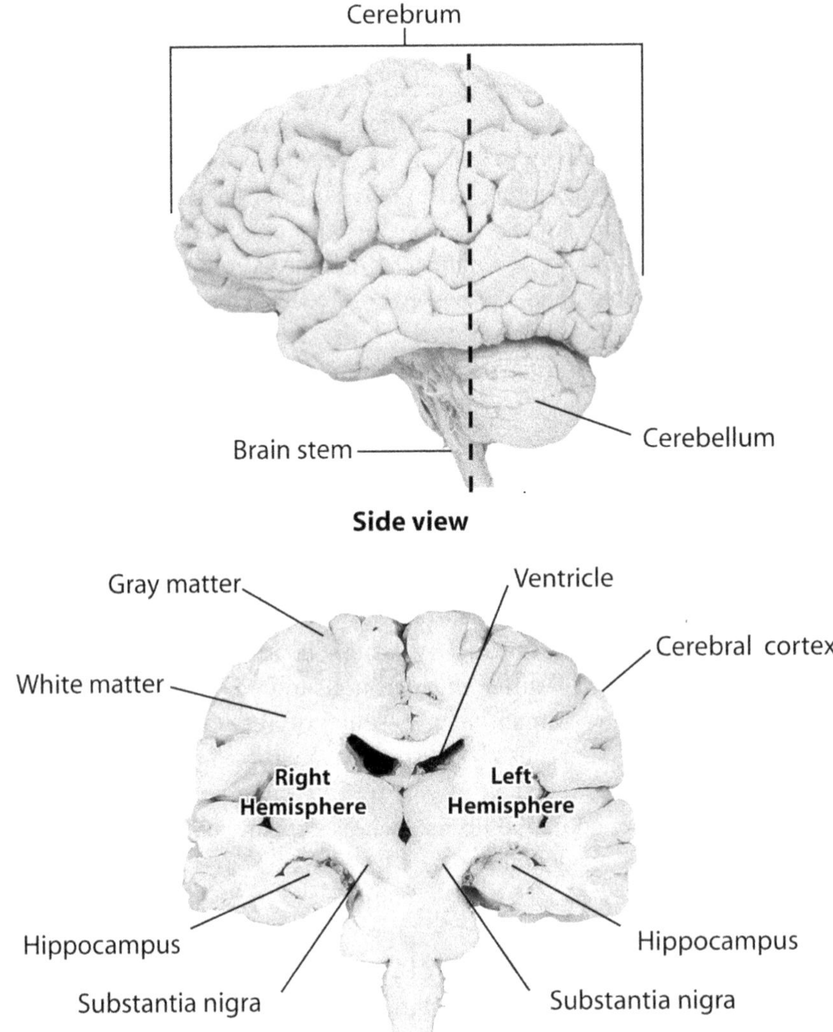

To screen out harmful substances, the cells in the blood vessel walls of the brain are joined tightly, forming what is called the *blood-brain barrier*. This barrier keeps out most unwanted substances and, for the most part, allows only the passage of hormones, oxygen, glucose, ketones, amino acids, and other nutrients.

The three main structures of the brain are the brain stem, the cerebellum and the cerebrum. Every area in the brain has an associated function, although many functions may involve a number of different areas. The brain stem is an extension of the spinal cord and monitors involuntary activities such as breathing and digestion. The cerebellum coordinates muscular movements and monitors posture and balance. The cerebrum, which occupies the topmost portion of the brain, is by far the largest of the three, comprising 70 percent of the weight of the entire nervous system. Its appearance is that of being convoluted and folded. Its outer surface, which consists of gray matter, is called the *cerebral cortex* and contains most of the master controls of the body. In the cortex, sensory data is analyzed; we think, remember and reason; and impulses originate that control the entire spectrum of muscle and gland activity. Beneath the cerebral cortex and deep within the cerebrum is the seat of emotions and learning. The cerebrum is split vertically by a deep fissure into left and right hemispheres. For reasons that are unclear, the connections are crossed; the left half of the cerebrum controls the right side of the body and the right half controls the left side. For example, the left hemisphere controls the actions of the right hand and the right hemisphere the actions of the left hand.

When serious injury occurs, the cells of the cerebral cortex are able to gradually adopt new functions. And because the two hemispheres duplicate each other to a certain extent, one can take over some of the functions of the other.

BRAIN DEGENERATION

Excessive injury or death of neurons within different areas of the brain cause the symptoms associated with the various neurodegenerative diseases.

A stroke cuts off the delivery of oxygen to brain cells and causes the affected areas of the brain to die. A stroke in the left hemisphere of the cerebral cortex can cause loss of function on the right side of the body. The left hemisphere in most people controls language skills, so a stroke in this area may also cause a loss in the ability to speak or understand speech.

Amyotrophic lateral sclerosis (ALS) comes about by the destruction of cells in the cerebral cortex which control voluntary muscle movement.

Underneath the cerebral cortex, within the body of the cerebrum, is the white matter that contains a few islands of gray matter known as the basal ganglia. The basal ganglia control voluntary movement. Disruption of the normal function of the basal ganglia gives rise to Parkinson's or Huntington's disease.

Myelin is an important substance that surrounds the axons of the nerve cells. It is concentrated in the white matter of the brain but is found throughout the brain and spinal cord. If this protective sheath of myelin breaks down, nerve cell communication is disrupted, causing symptoms that are characteristic of multiple sclerosis.

At the heart of the cerebrum lies a structure called the hippocampus. This is the center for short term memory and thought. It is here, as well as in the cerebral cortex, that dysfunctional cells lead to Alzheimer's disease and dementia. Arteries that feed this portion of the brain that become clogged by plaque or suffer numerous tiny strokes can lead to vascular dementia.

As we grow older, all of our organs become less efficient; that's just a part of the aging process. Our minds too, become less efficient. Yet we can live well into old age without ever developing the crippling effects of neurodegenerative disease. There are striking differences between the brains of those who are affected by Alzheimer's disease, for instance, and those who have simply aged normally. The deterioration that happens as a normal process of aging occurs uniformly throughout the brain; in Alzheimer's or Parkinson's disease, it occurs in selected areas of the brain. Aging shows minimal physical and chemical change in brain tissue. In neurodegenerative disease there are significant physical, chemical, and degenerative changes present.

Dementia and other forms of neurodegeneration are not normal consequences of aging. They are disease conditions with a cause and a solution. You can live your entire life, even into very old age, without suffering from any neurodegenerative disease. People have and do. Age is not an excuse.

Hendrikje van Andel-Schipper of Hoogeveen, Netherlands, is a good example. Hendrikje was the oldest person in the world when she died at the age of 115 in 2005. She appeared sharp right up to the end, joking that eating pickled herring was the secret to her longevity. Always ready with a quick response, when asked what advice she would give to people who want to live a long time, she quipped. "Keep breathing." Scientists say that Henrikje's mind was as good as it seemed: a postmortem analysis of her brain revealed few signs of degeneration associated with declining mental ability.

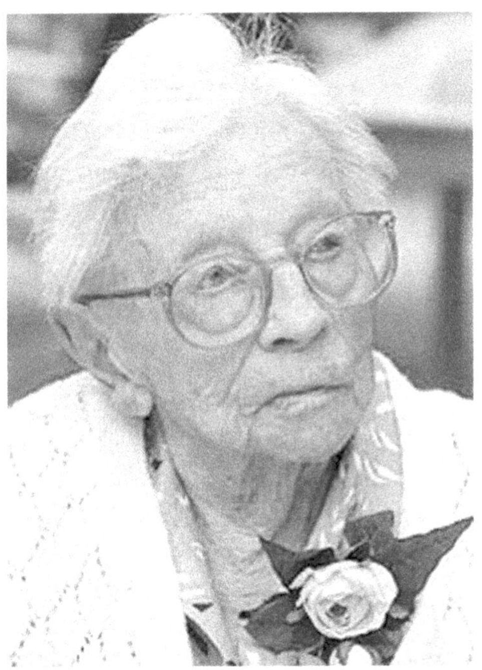

Van Andel-Schipper at the age of 113.

In 1972, when she was 82 years old, Hendrikje called the University of Groningen in order to donate her body to science. She called again at age 111 because she worried she might no longer be of interest. Researchers recognized a rare opportunity to study someone who was very old. They began testing her cognitive abilities almost immediately. Although she had problems with her eyesight, she was alert and performing better than the average 60- or 70-year-old. Hendrikje's health wasn't perfect. She had survived breast cancer for 15 years and eventually succumbed to stomach cancer. Despite these problems, her mind was clear and sharp to the end. Hendrikje demonstrated that growing old is not a prescription for neurodegenerative disease. A person can live to a very old age without suffering significant mental decline.

Neurons are the longest-living cells in the body. Most other cells die and are replaced every few weeks or months. Some, such as those along the lining of the digestive tract, only last a few days. Bone cells, which are among the most durable, are replaced every few years. Nerve cells, however, can last a lifetime. This is why it is so important to take care of them. The brain cells you have now, for the most part, are the ones you were born with. As we age, brain cells gradually die. Injury and disease also cause a loss of brain cells. For these reasons, you could have fewer brain cells now than when you were born. Neurodegenerative diseases accelerate the loss of brain cells, hastening mental decline.

BRAIN REGENERATION

Three-year-old Nico suffered with severe life-threatening epileptic seizures. Drug therapy had proven useless. His only hope was a radical form of surgery that could leave him permanently retarded and physically disabled. The potential for relief from otherwise untreatable seizures outweighed the risks. Doctors removed the entire right side of Nico's brain. The seizures stopped.

The operation was successful, but how could Nico function with only half a brain? Despite some minor problems with motor skills, Nico is quite normal. Eight years after the surgery, he runs and plays with only a slight limp. Nico's right-hemisphere skills—mathematics, visual arts, and music—have migrated to the left hemisphere. Nico performs well above average verbally, a left-brain skill. At school, he performs as a child of his age in arithmetic and music; only his draftsmanship and handwriting are poor for his age, but he has no cognitive handicap. He is mastering written language with a computer and is showing talent in graphic design. Nico's remarkable story is told by his doctor Antonio Battro, MD, PhD, in the book *Half A Brain is Enough.*

Nico isn't the only one who has had a large portion of his brain removed and survived without suffering any major mental defects. Many others have had similar experiences. In 1987, 14-year-old high school student Ahad Israfil was shot in the head at work when his employer accidentally knocked a firearm to the floor. The injury destroyed much of the right side of Ahad's skull and brain. After a five-hour operation to save his life, doctors were stunned when he attempted to speak.

The operation left a large void on the side of Ahad's head. Eventually the void was filled with a silicone block and covered by a flap of skin which regrew hair, giving him a fairly normal appearance. Although Ahad uses a wheelchair to get around, he has regained most of his cognitive abilities and graduated with honors from his local junior college.

While the brain cannot reconstruct a missing hemisphere, it can compensate for it. If half a brain can function as well as the whole, then a brain that is damaged by injury, disease, or aging also has the potential to function normally. The brain has an amazing ability to rewire itself. If one portion stops working, the remaining neurons can take over the function.

The brain, however, can do more than just rewire itself. It has the ability to repair and regenerate new brain cells. For many, this is a shocking revelation. For almost a century, conventional medical wisdom has held to the belief that all 100 billion of our brain cells existed at the time of birth and that the adult human brain was unable to grow new cells. The brain cells we were born with had to last us for a lifetime, it was believed. As brain cells died due to injury, disease, or age, they were gone for good. There was no hope for those people who had suffered significant brain cell loss. However, evidence over the past several years has shown that this is not the case. Neurons are continually being replaced throughout most of our lives,

Neurogenesis or cell regeneration occurs in the human brain even into old age.

indicating that it is possible for brain cells destroyed by injury or neurodegenerative diseases such as Alzheimer's and Parkinson's to be restored. Neurodegenerative disease is not a hopeless condition.

Scientists have observed brain cell regeneration (known as neurogenesis) in birds and rats for many years, but assumed that as evolution advanced and mental capacities increased, the brain supported less and less neurogenesis. In 1999, researchers at Princeton observed brain cell regeneration in adult macaque monkeys, which strongly implied that the same process occurs in humans.[1]

The Princeton scientists found that the new neurons were formed in the lining of the cerebral ventricles, large fluid-filled structures deep in the center of the brain, and then migrated a considerable distance to various parts of the cerebral cortex of the brain, and established synapses with older cells in the frontal lobes (where personality, planning, decision making, and working memory are located) and in the parietal lobes (where visual recognition memory exists).

In cancer treatment, doctors sometimes inject patients with a chemical tracer known as bromodeoxyuridine, or BrdU, to monitor the development of tumors. BrdU is incorporated into the DNA of newly formed cells. BrdU allows doctors to locate new areas of uncontrolled cell growth in cancer patients. The chemical shows up not only in the DNA of cancer cells but any cell that has formed around the time of the injection. When examining the brains of deceased cancer patients, doctors discovered BrdU in the cells, indicating new brain cell growth in adult humans.

Further research has shown new cell growth in various parts of the human brain, including the olfactory system (responsible for sense of smell) and the hippocampus (a primary center for memory).[2] Researchers also discovered that the fluid-filled ventricles contain a reservoir of brain stem cells, which are capable of transforming into any of the various types of brain cells. It is now evident that neurogenesis occurs in the adult human brain even into old age. This recent discovery offers hope for those currently suffering from neurodegenerative conditions as well as for those who hope to prevent them.

3 The Many Faces of Neurodegeneration

There are numerous neurodegenerative disorders. In this chapter we will discuss some of the most common. Each of those mentioned here, as well as many others, can be treated using the techniques described later in this book.

ALZHEIMER'S DISEASE

In 2002, actor Charlton Heston, who portrayed such notable characters as Moses in *The Ten Commandments* and Judah Ben-Hur in *Ben-Hur,* announced that he was suffering from Alzheimer's disease. Often cast as a fearless and unconquerable hero in his movie roles, he declared in a burst of eloquence, "I must reconcile courage and surrender in equal measure." He accepted his fate with courage and yet was resolved to the inevitable end. Alzheimer's disease affects people of all walks of life; even a movie hero could not overcome the grip of this devastating disease. Other celebrities who struggled with Alzheimer's disease include former US President Ronald Reagan, actors Charles Bronson, James Doohan, and Rita Hayworth, singer Perry Como, and boxing champion Sugar Ray Robinson.

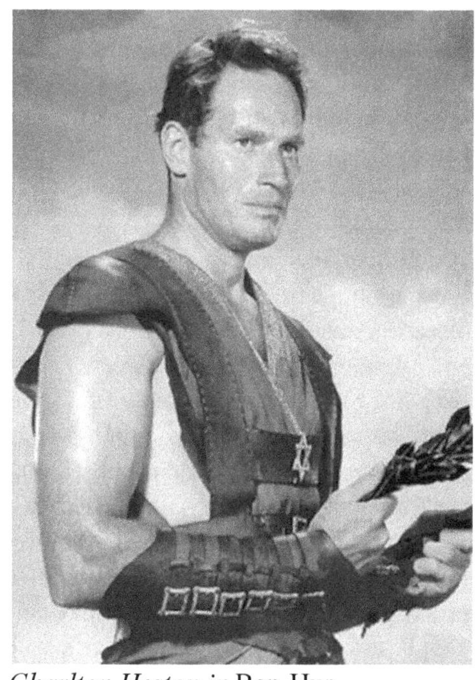
Charlton Heston in Ben-Hur.

Alzheimer's disease was first described in 1906 by Alois Alzheimer (1864-1915) a German neuropathologist and psychiatrist. Today, Alzheimer's disease is the most common form of dementia in Western countries and Japan. As many as 5.3 million Americans are living with Alzheimer's disease. Alzheimer's destroys brain cells, causing memory loss and problems with thinking and behavior severe enough to interfere with normal activities of daily living.

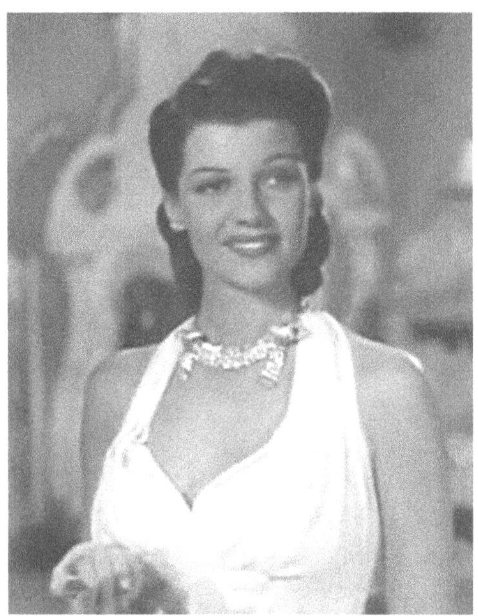
Actress Rita Hayworth.

The disease gets worse over time, and it is fatal. Today it is the seventh leading cause of death in the United States.

Currently there is no recognized medical cure. Treatments focus on reducing the severity of the symptoms, combined with providing services and support to make living with the disease more manageable.

Alzheimer's usually surfaces after the age of 60 and is marked by a decline in cognitive functions such as remembering, reasoning, and planning. There is a gradual decline in mental function, beginning with barely noticeable lapses in memory followed by losses in the ability to plan and execute familiar tasks, and to reason and exercise judgment. Eventually, memory loss increases in severity until it is incapacitating. The ability to articulate words correctly and changes in mood and personality may also be evident. Emotional problems such as easy agitation, poor judgment, mental confusion, feelings of withdrawal, disorientation, and hallucinations are common. Affected individuals may also develop seizures, hypertonicity (increased muscle movements), and incontinence.

People with Alzheimer's disease live an average of eight years from the time of diagnosis, but that interval can be as short as one year or as long as 20. The duration of the disease depends, in part, on age at diagnosis and the presence of other health problems.

Alzheimer's disease doesn't appear suddenly; it is a progressive disease that begins decades before the first symptoms become manifest. The mild to moderate stages of Alzheimer's generally last 2 to 10 years. Severe Alzheimer's may last 1 to 5 years.

While Alzheimer's disease usually affects the elderly, in 10 percent of the cases it occurs in people who are in their 40s or 50s. This is called early-onset Alzheimer's disease. Alzheimer's disease affects 3 percent of all people between the ages of 65 and 74, about 19 percent between 75 and 84, and 47 percent, or nearly half, of those over 85. Slightly more women than men are affected.

The incidence of Alzheimer's is growing rapidly. In 1979 the disease affected only about 0.2 people for every 100,000. By 2006 that number had shot up to 20 per 100,000.[1] Incidence is expected to double over the next 20 years.

Some have suggested that Alzheimer's is increasing because people are living longer than they used to. This is not so. Alzheimer's disease is not a normal process of aging; it is an abnormal condition—a disease. In fact, the age at which people are developing Alzheimer's is growing younger over time. Ten percent of all Alzheimer's patients get it early (usually in their 40s and 50s): the youngest on record was only 17. So the increase in incidence is not due solely to an aging

Stages of Alzheimer's

Stage 1: No Impairment

No detectable memory problems or changes in mood or personality are evident.

Stage 2: Very Mild Cognitive Decline

Some memory loss, especially in forgetting familiar words or names or the location of keys, eyeglasses, or other everyday objects. But these problems are not evident during a medical examination or apparent to friends, family, or coworkers.

Stage 3: Mild Cognitive Decline

Alzheimer's can be diagnosed in some, but not all, individuals at this point. Friends, family, or coworkers begin to notice problems with memory or concentration. It may be measurable in clinical testing or a detailed medical interview. Symptoms include decreased ability to remember names when introduced to new people, noticeable decline in performance, retaining little of reading material, losing or misplacing valuable objects, and a decline in the ability to plan or organize.

Stage 4: Moderate Cognitive Decline

Can be detected by a careful medical interview. Decreased knowledge of recent personal and current events; impaired ability to perform basic, but challenging, arithmetic (e.g., counting backward from 100 by 3); decreased ability to perform tasks, such as planning dinner for guests, paying bills, and managing finances; reduced memory of personal history; and may become withdrawn, especially in social situations.

Stage 5: Moderately Severe Decline

Major problems with memory and cognitive function become noticeable. Unable to recall important details such as address, telephone number, or name of high school attended; confusion about where they are, the date, day of the week, or season; trouble working simple arithmetic; need help choosing proper clothing. Still capable of remembering personal knowledge such as their own name and names of their spouse and children; and usually require no assistance with eating or using the toilet.

Stage 6: Severe Decline

Quickly forgetting recent experiences; difficulty recalling personal history, although their own name is still recognizable; forgetting the name of their spouse, children, and close friends but still capable of distinguishing familiar from unfamiliar faces; needing help getting dressed properly, may make such errors as putting pajamas over daytime clothes or shoes on wrong feet; disruption in normal sleep-awake cycle; needing help using the toilet; episodes of urinary or fecal incontinence; significant personality and behavioral changes, including suspiciousness and delusions (for example, believing that their caregiver is an impostor), hallucinations, or compulsive, repetitive behaviors such as hand-wringing or tissue shredding; and tendency to wander and become lost.

Stage 7: Very Severe Decline

Inability to speak coherently, although some words or phrases may occasionally be understood; needing help with eating and toileting along with general bladder incontinence; being unable to walk without assistance, progressing to inability to sit without support, smile, and hold head up; and reflexes become abnormal, muscles grow rigid, and swallowing becomes impaired.

Source: Alzheimer's Association, www.alz.org.

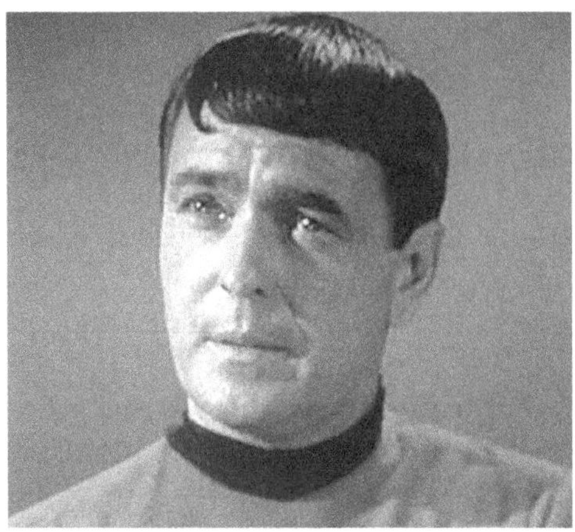

James Doohan as "Scotty" in the TV series Star Trek. *Later in life Doohan suffered from diabetes, Parkinson's, and Alzheimer's disease.*

population. Environmental conditions are apparently strongly involved.

The best time to treat Alzheimer's is before it progresses to the point that symptoms become easily recognizable. As with any neurological condition, once the disease has progressed to the point that symptoms become evident, a great deal of damage has already been done. The earlier a problem is identified, the more effective the treatment.

Doctors use the mini mental state exam (MMSE) to screen for dementia. This exam tests memory skills and evaluates the severity of mental decline. The test has 30 questions. The number of incorrectly answered questions indicates the level of cogitative impairment: the greater the number of incorrect answers, the greater the impairment. The MMSE can be administered repeatedly over the course of the disease to monitor an individual's response to treatment and identify rate of disease progression.

The MMSE is a copyrighted test, so it can't be reproduced here, but some older versions of the test can be found online. Appendix A: Mental Status Test is a 30-question exam that is similar to the MMSE. You can take this test yourself or administer it to another person to get an estimate of mental status.

VASCULAR DEMENTIA

Vascular dementia is considered the second most common form of dementia after Alzheimer's disease, accounting for about 20 percent of all cases of dementia. The term "vascular" refers to conditions related to the circulatory system. It develops when the flow of blood-carrying nutrients and oxygen to the brain is interrupted. This can occur when arteries that feed the brain become clogged by plaque and blood clots (atherosclerosis) or when one or more of these arteries rupture (aneurysm) and bleeds into surrounding tissues. When blood flow through an artery to the brain is interrupted by blockage or rupture, a stroke occurs. Clogged arteries cause what is called *ischemic* strokes. Those caused by blood vessel ruptures are called *hemorrhagic* strokes. Ischemic stroke accounts for about 85 percent of all diagnosed cases. Hemorrhagic stroke accounts for about 15 percent. Stroke is the third-leading cause of death in the North America. Strokes can be mild and nearly unnoticeable, severe and crippling, or deadly. Survivable strokes can lead to dementia.

Diagnosis is clearest when symptoms appear soon after a single major stroke. This is sometimes called "post-stroke dementia." Statistics show that up to one third of those who have a stroke will develop vascular dementia within six months. Vascular dementia can also arise due to multiple small strokes. Individually, these mini-strokes do not cause major symptoms and generally go unnoticed, but over time their accumulative effect becomes apparent. Mini-strokes cause damage to the cortex of the brain in areas associated with learning, memory, and language.

Vascular dementia and Alzheimer's disease can occur simultaneously. This is called *mixed dementia*. Brain autopsies have shown that up to 45 percent of people with dementia have signs of both Alzheimer's and vascular dementia.

Symptoms of vascular dementia can vary, depending on the specific areas of the brain involved. Memory loss may or may not be the most prominent symptom, depending on whether the brain regions involved in memory are affected. Besides memory and language difficulties, decreased motor skills, failure to recognize or identify objects, and inability to plan or think abstractly may be manifest. Mental decline may occur in noticeable steps, rather than the slow, steady decline usually seen in Alzheimer's disease.

Advancing age is one of the major risk factors for vascular dementia. A history of past heart attacks, strokes, high blood pressure, atherosclerosis (hardening of the arteries), diabetes, or other risk factors for heart disease are often present in those who suffer from vascular dementia.

Symptoms may include confusion, which may get worse at night; difficulty concentrating, planning, communicating, and following instructions; reduced ability to carry out daily activities; changes in behavior; and physical symptoms associated with strokes such as difficulty speaking and sudden muscular weakness, especially on one side of the body. The condition may be diagnosed by magnetic resonance imaging (MRI) of the brain showing characteristic abnormalities associated with vascular damage.

Most of us might experience incidental lapses in memory such as forgetting where we put the car keys or in what part of the parking lot we parked the car. As we age, some forgetfulness is normal. A screening tool to help differentiate between ordinary forgetfulness and the earliest stages of dementia or Alzheimer's disease has been developed: a questionnaire called "Everyday Cognition" or ECog. This checklist consists of 39 questions based on a person's ability to complete common tasks, such as following a conversation, shopping for a few items without a list, or reading a map to find a new location. The test is completed by a family member or close friend who lives with or has known the patient well for a number of years and can compare the patient's current state of mind to previous years.

There is no recognized cure for vascular dementia. Treatment consists of reducing risk of suffering further strokes by lowering blood pressure, getting regular exercise, adequate nutrition, improving blood sugar control, and addressing cardiovascular issues associated with heart disease. Drugs are also prescribed to ease symptoms, although they may do more harm than good.

If the patient is obese, weight reduction is also recommended. Central body obesity (the size of the waistline) is related to dementia: the larger the waistline, the greater the risk. People with larger stomachs in their 40s are more likely to have dementia when they reach their 70s. Researchers at Johns Hopkins Bloomberg School of Public Health found that obesity increases the risk of developing Alzheimer's later in life by 80 percent, and vascular dementia by 73 percent.[2] These findings were based on 10 previous studies examining the relationships between dementia and body weight. The senior author of the study, Youfa Wang, MD, PhD, stated that "Preventing or treating obesity at a younger age could play a major role in reducing the number of dementia patients and those with other commonly associated illnesses, such as Alzheimer's disease, by up to 20 percent."

Being underweight also affects risk. Another study found that older people who are underweight or who have lost weight quickly are at a higher risk of developing dementia, especially if they started out overweight or obese.[3] It should be noted that weight loss in this case is not the result of improving health through sensible dieting or exercise but from happenstance. Weight loss that occurs without conscious effort is most likely a result of altered glucose metabolism. The lead researcher, Tiffany Hughes, PhD, MPH, noted that rapid weight loss in the elderly may be a sign of emerging brain disease. "In middle age," says Hughes, "obesity may be a risk factor for dementia, while declining weight in later life may be considered one of the first changes from the disease that occurs before it actually affects a person's memory." In yet another study, researchers discovered that women who have dementia start losing weight at least 10 years before the disease is diagnosed.[4]

Alzheimer's disease is by far the most common form of dementia, followed by vascular dementia and dementia with Lewy bodies; the latter includes Parkinson's disease dementia. The reported percentage of those with each of the different forms of dementia varies from study to study. The Rotterdam Study gives a general idea of the percentages of each. This study was conducted in Europe and involved 7,528 participants aged 55-106 years. There were 474 cases of dementia, giving an overall prevalence of 6.3 percent. In this group, Alzheimer's disease accounted for 72 percent, vascular dementia 16 percent, Parkinson's disease dementia 6 percent, and other dementias 5 percent.[5]

DEMENTIA WITH LEWY BODIES

Dementia with Lewy bodies, also known as *Lewy body dementia*, is a progressive brain disease characterized by the accumulation of abnormal microscopic protein deposits in regions of the brain involved in thinking and movement. These protein deposits, called *Lewy bodies*, are named after Dr. Frederich Heinrich Lewy (1885-1950), who first described them in 1912 while working with brain samples from patients who had died with Parkinson's disease.

Dementia with Lewy bodies includes Parkinson's disease dementia and a closely related condition called *diffuse Lewy body disease*. In Parkinson's disease, Lewy bodies occur most frequently in an area of the brain (substantia nigra) that controls voluntary movement. In diffuse Lewy body disease, the Lewy bodies are diffused throughout the brain and are found in the substantia nigra as well as in the cerebral cortex, where they may affect regions controlling emotion, behavior, judgment, and awareness.

Because Lewy bodies are distributed throughout the brain, people with Lewy body dementia usually have some symptoms commonly associated with Parkinson's, such as stooped posture, shuffling walk, slow movements, and involuntary tremors.

They also usually share some symptoms associated with Alzheimer's disease such as memory loss, mental confusion, and emotional problems. The defining symptoms of the disease include a decline in mental abilities (dementia), fluctuating attention and alertness, vivid visual hallucinations, and motor skill difficulties. The most striking symptom may be its visual hallucinations, which can be one of the first signs of the disorder. Hallucinations may range from abstract shapes or colors to conversations with deceased loved ones. In many cases, but not all, Lewy body dementia affects memory.

The disease usually progresses slowly over several years, but the way it progresses can vary significantly from person to person. For example, it may begin with signs of dementia, with loss of motor skills later. Or the disease may start with movement difficulties, with signs of dementia emerging some time later. Most people with Lewy body dementia experience the onset of dementia and the onset of motor skill difficulties within one to two years of each other. As the disease progresses, all symptoms usually become more severe.

Currently, there is no cure and no specific therapy to stop or slow the progression of the disease. However, symptoms can be tempered somewhat to improve patients' ability to function and their quality of life. Medications designed for those with Parkinson's and Alzheimer's disease are often used. Drug therapy needs to be monitored carefully because of undesirable side effects which can worsen symptoms such as hallucinations, muscle rigidity, and tremors.

Lewy body dementia is estimated to affect less than 1 percent of the population over the age of 65. Risk increases with age. It is believed that at least 5 percent of noninstitutionalized adults 85 years and older have the disease.

PARKINSON'S DISEASE

In 1984 three-time world heavyweight boxing champion Muhammad Ali was diagnosed with Parkinson's disease. He was only 42 years old at the time. Symptoms such as slurred speech, loss of hand-eye coordination, and reduced muscle strength began to surface soon after his retirement from the ring in 1981. Doctors speculated that he developed the disease, in part, as a result of taking numerous punches to the head and face over the course of his boxing career. Indeed, studies do show that boxers have a higher rate of Parkinson's disease than average. But you don't need to be a professional fighter to develop Parkinson's disease. Even mild-mannered individuals who have never suffered any serious head injury can fall victim. Some of the most notable people with this disease include Michael J. Fox, Billy Graham, Pope John Paul II, Deborah Kerr, and Vincent Price.

It's hard to imagine asking a doctor to destroy a part of your brain. However, that is exactly what actor Michael J. Fox did. Ordinarily, drugs can ease the involuntary tremors characteristic of the disease, but when drugs cease to work, surgery becomes an option. The irreversible procedure involves drilling a hole in the patient's skull and inserting an electrode into the brain to kill tremor-causing neurons. The target area is deep within the brain. The patient's head must be clamped to an unmovable metal frame. The surgeon, relying on magnetic resonance imaging, inserts

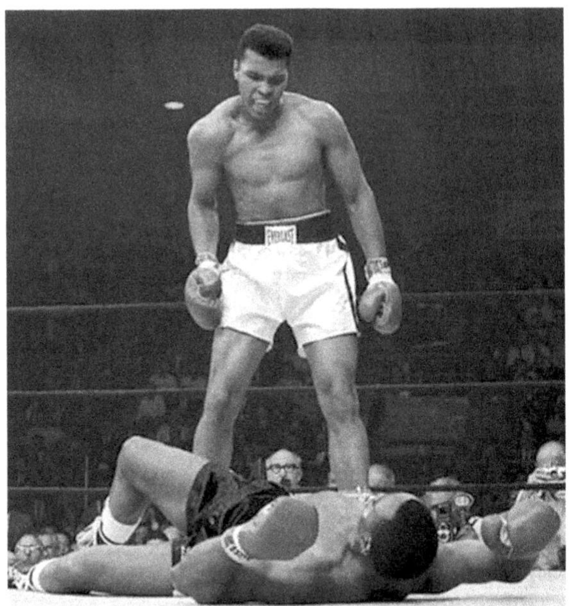

Muhammad Ali standing over defeated world heavyweight champion Sonny Liston.

the electrode into the brain, being very careful of the exact position and depth—a mere millimeter too deep will destroy vision, while a millimeter to the side could cause paralysis. The patient remains awake during the entire operation so the surgeon can be sure no harm is being done. Despite the operation, Fox still suffers from uncontrollable tremors and stiffness. While drastic procedures such as destroying brain cells may provide some help, none of the current treatments for Parkinson's disease can remotely be called a cure.

Parkinson's disease is a progressive brain disorder that affects more than 1.5 million people in the United States, 120,000 in the UK, and 4 million worldwide. Most people who develop this disease are over the age of 60, but it can affect people in their 40s or younger. Michael J. Fox was diagnosed with the disease at the age of 30. When the disease occurs before the age of 60 it is referred to as early-onset Parkinson's disease. Like all neurodegenerative diseases, brain cell deterioration occurs over a long period of time and 80 percent of the cells in the affected area of the brain have already died before symptoms become evident.

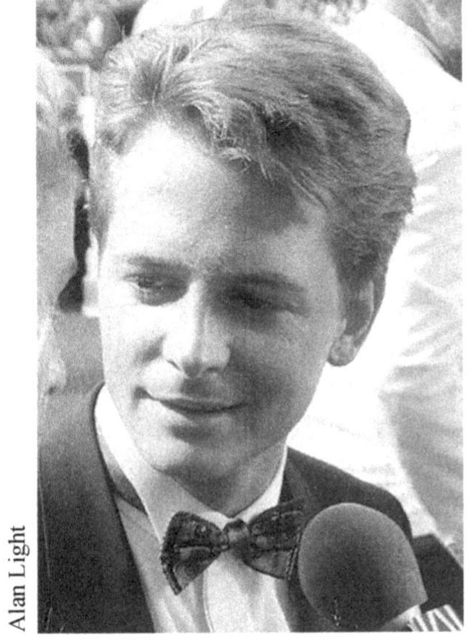

Alan Light

Michael J. Fox.

Although not commonly thought of as a fatal illness, the Centers for Disease Control and Prevention (CDC), ranks Parkinson's disease as the 14th leading cause of death in the United States.

The characteristic feature of Parkinson's disease is the accumulation of Lewy bodies in the substantia nigra—an area in the midbrain that controls voluntary movement. Affected neurons are unable to produce the neurotransmitter dopamine, which is needed to activate the nerves that control movement, including automatic movements.

The most common symptoms of Parkinson's disease are tremor (shaking or trembling) of the hands, arms, jaw, and face; rigidity (stiffness) of the trunk and limbs; bradykinesia (slowness of movement); and loss of balance and coordination. Other symptoms include walking by shuffling the feet, speaking difficulties (or speaking very softly), facial masking (expressionless, mask-like face), swallowing problems, and stooped posture.

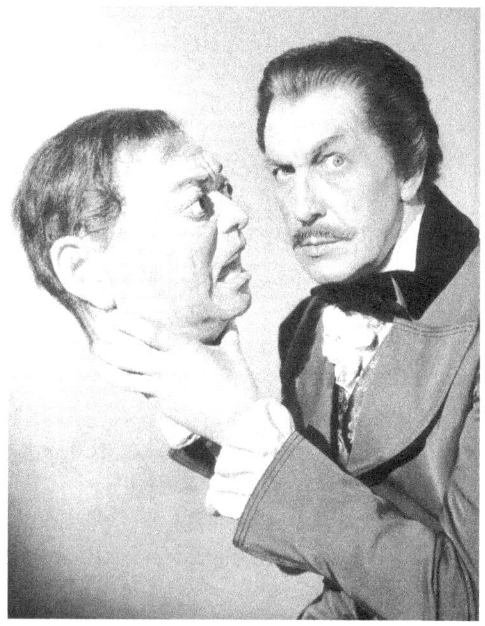

Vincent Price, who suffered from Parkinson's disease later in life, was famous for his horror and suspense films.

The onset of Parkinson's disease is very gradual, usually beginning as a slight tremor in the hands when at rest and involuntary nodding of the head. The facial muscles react slowly, so that the expression tends to become masklike and the eyes fixed and unblinking. As the disease advances, muscular tremors may affect the whole body. Because shaking or tremors are common symptoms of Parkinson's disease, it is also called "shaking palsy." There may be some speech impairment and involuntary rolling of the eyes. Walking becomes slow with shuffling steps, the body bends forward, and occasionally the affected person may break into a run or trot in an attempt to maintain balance. Fatigue or emotional stress tends to make the symptoms worse.

Most of the symptoms of the disease involve disruption of motor functions (muscle and movement). However, lack of energy, depression, anxiety, personality and behavior changes, sleep disturbances, memory loss, and pain can also occur as part of the disease. Symptoms gradually worsen over time. Not everyone with the disease experiences all of the symptoms and the progression of the disease is different from one person to the next.

In many cases, Parkinson's disease does not affect a person's ability to think, reason, learn, or remember. In some patients, however, one or more cognitive processes eventually become impaired. Parkinson's patients who experience hallucinations and more severe motor control problems are at greater risk for developing dementia. When this happens it is called Parkinson's disease dementia. Parkinson's disease often overlaps with other degenerative brain disorders that can cause dementia, such as vascular dementia and dementia with Lewy bodies. Approximately half of those with Parkinson's disease have some mild cognitive impairment.[6] Between 20 to 40 percent may develop more severe symptoms of dementia. Regardless of age at the onset of the disease, dementia symptoms tend to appear approximately 10 to 15 years later in the course of the disease.

Technically, the term Parkinson's disease dementia is used to refer to dementia that develops at least two years after the diagnosis of Parkinson's disease. If dementia develops before or within two years after the onset of motor symptoms, then the

Symptoms of Parkinson's Disease

Primary Symptoms

Bradykinesia. Voluntary movements such as standing up, walking, and sitting down are accomplished in slow motion. This is caused by delayed transmission signals from the brain to the muscles. May lead to difficulty initiating walking and can cause "freezing episodes" while walking.

Tremors. Uncontrollable, shaking movement in the hands, fingers, forearms, feet, mouth, and chin. Typically, tremors take place when the muscles are at rest, rather than during conscious movement.

Rigidity. Muscle stiffness, often produces muscle pain that increases during movement.

Poor balance. Loss of reflexes that help control balance and posture.

Secondary Symptoms

Anxiety, depression, isolation
Choking, coughing, or drooling
Constipation
Difficulty swallowing
Excessive salivation
Excessive sweating
Hallucinations
Loss of bowel and/or bladder control
Loss of memory and intellectual capacity
Scaling, dry skin on the face or scalp
Slow response to questions
Small cramped handwriting
Soft, whispery voice

criteria are met for the related condition—dementia with Lewy bodies. The cognitive profile is similar to that of Alzheimer's disease, but patients with Parkinson's disease dementia generally have more severe visuospatial deficits, large fluctuations in attention, frequent visual hallucinations, and less severe memory problems.

There is no recognized cure for Parkinson's disease. Treatment consists of exercise, physical therapy, and drug therapy. None of the medications stop the progress of the disease, but are meant to ease the symptoms.

Parkinson's disease involves the slow loss of dopamine-producing neurons. Dopamine injection into the bloodstream is not an effective treatment because dopamine cannot cross the blood-brain barrier. A breakthrough in treatment of Parkinson's disease came when the drug levodopa or L-dopa was found to increase the dopamine levels in afflicted patients. Neurons use L-dopa, which can cross the blood-brain barrier, to make dopamine. For some reason, L-dopa does not always have the desired effects in individual patients, so a number of alternate treatments have been developed. One option that is being explored is surgical grafting of normal dopamine-secreting neurons into the brains of individuals with Parkinson's disease.

Another drug used in the treatment of Parkinson's disease is Sinement, which consists of a combination of levodopa and carbidopa (a chemical that helps the levodopa reach the brain). It works well for controlling symptoms for most patients but can cause some side effects, especially after several years of use. Its effectiveness tends to decrease as the disease progresses and more dopamine-producing neurons die.

Side effects reported for levodopa include uncontrolled movements, muscle twitching, seizures, nausea, vomiting, diarrhea, irregular heartbeat, unusual changes in mood or behavior, depression, constipation, dry mouth, blurred vision, dizziness, insomnia, fatigue, mental confusion, and hallucinations. Some of the existing symptoms associated may be intensified and may go unrecognized because they are believed to be simply part of the progression of the disease.

An alternative to levodopa are medications that stimulate the brain cells to produce more dopamine. Two common drugs are ropinorole (Requip) and paramipaxole (Mirapex). They do not have as much risk of long-term side effects as levodopa. However, they can cause dizziness and hallucinations, especially in the elderly or in patients with dementia, so they are better tolerated by younger patients.

How can you tell if someone is developing Parkinson's disease? Doctors use a tool called the Unified Parkinson Disease Rating Scale (UPDRS) as an aid in diagnosis, to assess severity of Parkinson's symptoms, and to monitor the course of the disease. A modified version of this rating tool is reproduced in Appendix B.

HUNTINGTON'S DISEASE

The celebrated folk singer/songwriter Woody Guthrie is perhaps the most recognized sufferer of this disorder. One day in the 1950s Guthrie's wife, Marjorie, noticed her husband walking lopsidedly, which seemed very odd. Later, she began to notice that his speech was becoming slurred. Despite these telltale signs she didn't suspect anything to be seriously wrong until he began to fly into major rages, which was uncharacteristic of him. Eventually, he lost all ability to talk, read, or walk. The only way he could communicate with his wife and children was by waving his arm at cards printed with the words "Yes" and "No." Nine years after his death in 1967 Marjorie Guthrie founded The Huntington's Disease Society of America to help people with Huntington's disease and their families better their lives, encourage research, and educate the public and medical community about the disease.

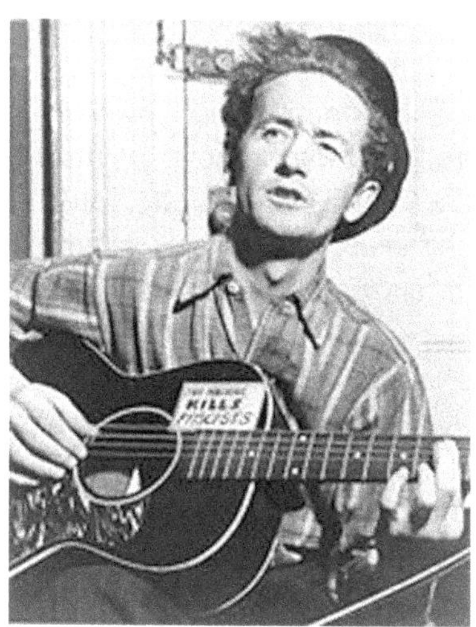

Woody Guthrie.

Huntington's disease is believed to be primarily an inherited condition in which nerve cells in the brain waste away leading to uncontrolled movements, loss of intellectual ability, and emotional disturbances. It is named after Dr. George Huntington (1850-1916), a New York physician, who first described the disorder in 1872. Children who have a parent with the disease are at high risk of also developing the disease. However, in some cases, there appears to be no genetic link because no history of the disease can be found in parents or other family members.

Huntington's disease affects both women and men of all ethnic groups. Symptoms typically appear between the ages of 30 and 50, but may appear earlier or later. When the disease is diagnosed in adulthood, usually in middle age, it is referred to as adult-onset Huntington's disease. If it develops in adolescence, it is called early-onset or juvenile Huntington's disease. Adult-onset Huntington's disease is by far the more common of the two.

About 30,000 people (10 in every 100,000 people) in the United States have been diagnosed with Huntington's disease, and another 150,000 are believed to be at risk of possibly developing the disease at some point in their lives. In the UK it affects about 4,800 people, about 8 out of every 100,000. The highest prevalence of this disorder in the world is near Lake Maracaibo in Venezuela, where it affects around 700 people out of every 100,000.

The gene tied to Huntington's disease controls the production of a protein called huntingtin protein (note the ending is spelled "tin" rather than "ton"). Although this protein derives its name from the disease, it is actually a normal protein occurring in the cells of both animals and humans. We all have the gene that produces huntingtin proteins, however, in some people the protein is elongated. This elongated protein aggregates inside nerve cells, producing the protein accumulations characteristic of this disease. The presence of these protein clumps is believed to interfere with normal cellular function. However, there is strong evidence that the protein is formed as a response to stress and is produced as a means of protecting the cell. Whether the aggregation of the protein causes the disease or is a consequence of it is still debated.

In Huntington's disease, huntingtin proteins tend to aggregate in the basal ganglia of the brain, which controls voluntary movement. The basal ganglia is involved in two neurological disorders—Huntington's disease and Parkinson's disease. In Parkinson's disease, neurons in a part of the basal ganglia called the substantia nigra are unable to produce a normal amount of dopamine. In Huntington's disease, cells in another part of the basal ganglia, called the striatum, become hypersensitive to dopamine. Consequently, the symptoms of the two disorders are virtually the opposite. Parkinson's is characterized by gradual loss of the ability to initiate movement, while Huntington's is characterized by an inability to prevent parts of the body from moving unintentionally. While both diseases have cognitive symptoms, especially in their advanced stages, the most prominent symptoms relate to the ability to initiate and control movement. Thus both are classified as movement disorders.

Physical symptoms become manifest first, starting with slight "clumsiness" that progresses to uncontrolled movements such as twitches and muscle spasms; problems with balance and coordination; unsteady walk; head turning to shift eye position; slow, uncontrolled movements; quick, sudden jerking movements of arms, legs, face, and other body parts; and difficulty swallowing. These movements may appear to be very bizarre and include odd body postures. Seizures occur in 30 to 50 percent of individuals with this condition.

Mental and emotional health is also affected resulting in memory loss, lack of concentration, problems in decision making and judgment, changes in speech, disorientation or confusion, irritability, hallucinations, paranoia, depression, and antisocial behavior. All symptoms grow progressively worse over time. The manifestation of symptoms and progression of the disease differs with each person.

Huntington's disease causes progressive disability leading to complete dependence on others. The affected person eventually dies from complications, such as heart failure or aspiration pneumonia. Statistics indicate that people with adult-onset Huntington's disease generally live 15 to 25 years after diagnosis. Those with early-onset Huntington's disease are affected more severely and usually survive only 10 to 15 years after diagnoses.

There is currently no cure or way to stop the progression of the disease. The goal of treatment is to slow down disease progression and help the person function for as long and as comfortably as possible. Treatment consists of drugs to reduce involuntary movements and exercise therapy. Physical fitness is very important. Individuals who exercise and remain active tend to do better than those who do not.

Although Huntington's disease may have a genetic component, environment has a pronounced affect as well. This fact is known from studies with identical twins, each of which carry the same genes. Theoretically, if the genes were in total control, identical twins would develop the disease at the same time. Typically, identical twins who have inherited the huntingtin gene generally develop the disease within a year or so of each other, *if* they live in the same or similar environment. However, if the twins' environment is different, the onset of the disease can vary dramatically.

An example of this is the case of a 71-year-old woman who was diagnosed with Huntington's disease. The onset of the disease began six years prior to diagnoses. Her identical twin sister, however, showed no symptoms of the disease until a year later—seven years after her sister. Why the big difference in time of diagnoses? Investigators determined it was due to the environment.[7] Environmental factors have been shown to influence Huntington's disease in animals.[8]

Both girls grew up in the same house in New Bedford, Massachusetts. Their birth home was across the street from a factory that produced large machines used to manufacture precision cutting tools from the late 1800s to 1987. Numerous chemical spills and leaks had occurred over the years. The air was polluted and in 1993, two years after the factory closed for the second time, the site was designated a federal toxic site requiring cleanup. Both twins had been equally exposed to the factory's toxins until the age of 23 when twin "A" moved out of the original house to a location about 2 miles away. Twin "B," who was first to manifest Huntington's disease, remained in her original house. There was no significant difference in the diet or lifestyle, although twin B used seven prescription drugs and three over-the-counter medications that her twin never took. Both women smoked. Twin A stopped smoking at age 35, while twin B continued to smoke until age 65. Both twins had hypertension, but twin B had the poorer overall health, suffering from rheumatoid arthritis, chronic bronchitis, and type 2 diabetes, as well as being the first to develop Huntington's disease; all of which was presumed to be a consequence of living near the factory and smoking for a longer period of time. The greater exposure to chemical toxins during their lives caused twin B to develop Huntington's disease seven years before her sister. Presumably, if the twins had lived in a cleaner environment and not smoked, the disease may never have manifested itself.

AMYOTROPHIC LATERAL SCLEROSIS (ALS)

In 1939 a rare and little understood disease called Amyotrophic Lateral Sclerosis (ALS) received front page headlines when it was discovered that baseball Hall of Famer Lou Gehrig was diagnosed with the condition. Since that time it has commonly been referred to as Lou Gehrig's disease.

Lou Gehrig was one of the most talented baseball players of all time. He competed with Babe Ruth as baseball's home run king. From 1925 to 1939 he set a record of playing in 2,130 consecutive games. He played well in every game despite broken fingers and toes and recurring back spasms. Late in his career Gehrig's hands were X-rayed, and doctors were able to spot 17 different fractures that had healed while he continued to play. His endurance and strength earned him the nickname "Iron Horse." In 1938, despite his great athletic powers and tolerance to pain, his body began to rapidly waste away and his strength and coordination deteriorated. Teammates noticed that he lacked his former strength and energy and that he began shuffling his feet as he walked. After a dismal and uncharacteristic performance at the start of the 1939 season, he realized he could no longer play baseball and promptly retired. Doctors diagnosed him with ALS. There was nothing they could do for him. He died in 1941, just two weeks before his 38th birthday.

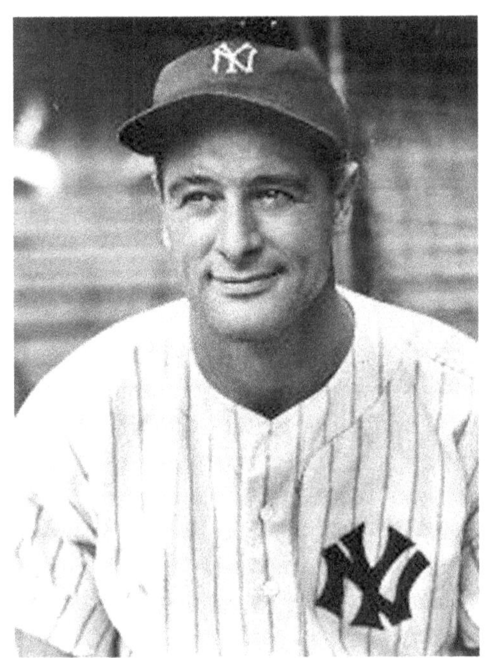
New York Yankees first baseman Lou Gehrig.

Besides Gehrig, other well-known figures who have suffered from this disease include renowned physicist Stephen Hawking, guitarist and composer Jason Becker, actor David Niven, baseball player Jim "Catfish" Hunter, singer Dennis Day, and Chinese revolutionary leader Mao Tse Tung.

ALS was first described in 1869 by French neurologist Jean-Martin Charcot (1825-1893). It is an invariably fatal disorder characterized by progressive muscle weakness eventually resulting in paralysis. The disease attacks the motor neurons in the brain and spinal cord that control voluntary muscles.

Motor neurons are nerve cells that control communication between the nervous system and the voluntary muscles of the body. Messages from motor neurons in the brain are transmitted to motor neurons in the spinal cord and from them to the individual muscles. In ALS, motor neurons in the brain and spinal cord degenerate and die, ceasing to send messages to the muscles. Because the muscles no longer receive messages to function, they weaken from disuse and gradually waste away (atrophy). The ability of the brain to initiate and control voluntary movement is lost. Eventually all muscles under voluntary control are affected and patients lose their strength and ability to move their arms, legs, and body.

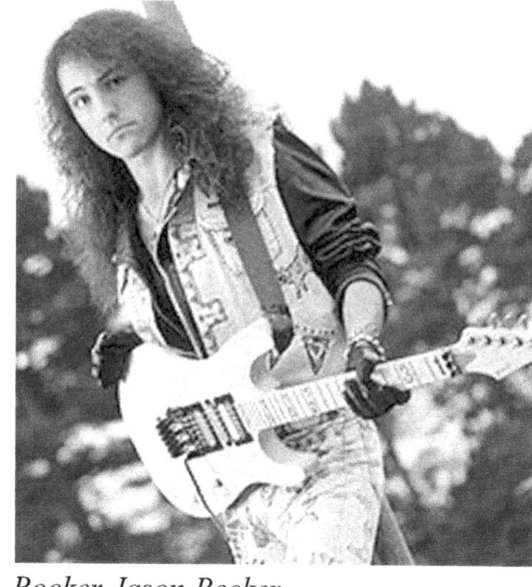

Rocker Jason Becker.

The initial signs of ALS may be so subtle that they are overlooked. The earliest symptoms may include twitching, cramping, stiff muscles, or slurred speech. As muscles deteriorate walking may become awkward accompanied by tripping or stumbling. Hands lose manual dexterity and experience difficulty with mundane tasks such as buttoning a shirt, writing, or turning a key in a lock. Eventually patients will not be able to stand or walk, get in or out of bed on their own, or use their hands and arms. Difficulty swallowing and chewing impair the patients' ability to eat normally and increase the risk of choking. Maintaining weight becomes a problem. While most voluntary muscle control is lost, patients usually maintain control of eye muscles and bladder and bowel functions. When muscles in the diaphragm and chest wall fail, patients lose the ability to breathe on their own and must depend on ventilator support for survival. Most people with ALS die from respiratory failure.

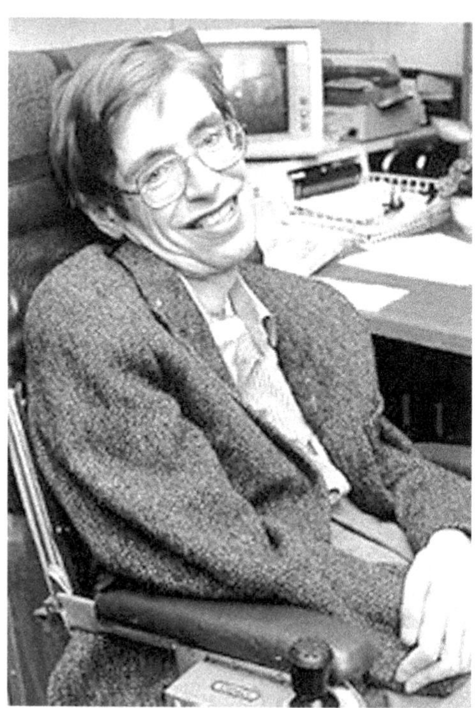

Physicist Stephen Hawking.

ALS predominantly affects just the motor neurons, and in the majority of cases the disease does not impair a patient's mind, personality, intelligence, senses, or memory. American composer Jason Becker is a prime example. Becker was diagnosed with ALS in 1996. He eventually lost the ability to play the guitar, walk, or speak and learned to communicate through eye movements through a system developed by his father. Despite his disability, he remains mentally sharp and continues composing music using a computer.

In a small number of patients frontotemporal dementia may develop, which is characterized by profound personality changes. A slightly larger number of patients experience mild problems with word generation, attention, or decision-making.

ALS occurs worldwide among people of all races and ethnic backgrounds. Men are affected slightly more often than women. Approximately 15 new cases of ALS are diagnosed each day in the United States. Most of those who develop the disease are between 40 and 70 years of age. Approximately 30,000 people in the United States are living with the disease. Worldwide there are about 70,000 people with ALS and one in every 200,000 people develop ALS each year. The average life expectancy after diagnosis for those suffering from ALS is three to five years. Death occurs in half of the people diagnosed within three years and 90 percent within six years. The longest known survivor lived for 39 years after diagnosis.

Scientists have yet to find a definitive cause. The onset of the disease has been linked to several factors including infection, exposure to toxins, DNA defects, immune system abnormalities, occupational factors (military service and elite sports), and enzyme abnormalities. In approximately 5 to 10 percent of cases there appears to be a hereditary factor linked to a mutation in copper/zinc superoxide dismutase, an enzyme responsible for neutralizing free radicals.

Various chemical and natural toxins are highly suspect. A high incidence of the disease occurs among professional football, soccer, and baseball players. An extraordinarily high incidence among Italian soccer players (more than five times higher than normally expected) raised the concern of a possible link between the disease and the use of pesticides on playing fields.

Military veterans are at an increased risk of developing ALS. According to the ALS Association there is nearly a 60 percent greater chance of the disease in veterans than the general population. For Gulf War veterans, the chance is twice that of veterans not deployed to the Persian Gulf, indicating a possible chemical connection.

Several hot spots occur in regions of the western Pacific. The island of Guam in particular has been noted. In these cases the cause seems to be due to prolonged ingestion of a dietary neurotoxin found in the seeds of the cycad, a tropical plant used as food. In the 1950s and early 1960s an epidemic of ALS occurred as a result of eating this toxin.

There currently are no drugs to prevent or cure the disease.

MULTIPLE SCLEROSIS

The tingling began in her right foot. Then, while jogging in New York's Central Park, Terri Garr stumbled. That's odd, she thought. Why am I tripping? Before long, she felt a stabbing pain in her right arm and was overcome by extreme fatigue.

That was 1983, and Garr was 38 years old and at the peak of her acting career. She had won audiences' hearts in such films as *Young Frankenstein* (1974) and *Close Encounters of the Third Kind* (1977). That year she received an Oscar nomination for her portrayal of the scorned girlfriend in *Tootsie* (1982).

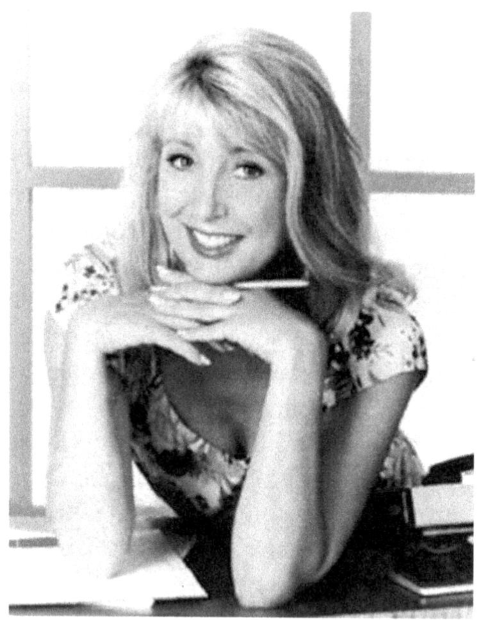
Terri Garr.

Over the next 16 years her symptoms came and went, puzzling the many specialists she consulted. Finally, in 1999 she got a diagnosis: multiple sclerosis (MS)—a chronic, often debilitating disease. In Hollywood a physical disability can spell the end to an otherwise successful career. So Garr kept her diagnosis secret, and tried to hide her symptoms. At home, however, she often tumbled down stairs and dropped dishes. One Christmas, she tripped over a skateboard, crashed into the fireplace and broke her collarbone. Prompted by talk-show host Montel Williams' appearance on "Larry King Live," where he discussed his own struggles with MS, Garr decided to let the world know her secret.

On October 8, 2002, Garr went on "Larry King" and spoke publicly about her illness. King pressed her about the pain and the difficulty of dealing with the disease. But Garr, smiling, upbeat, and cracking jokes, was not about to act like a victim. "I really don't think negatively about any of this stuff," she said. Her message was that people with MS need hope, not discouragement.

Garr now works as a spokesperson for MS LifeLines, an educational and support service funded by the drug companies Serono and Pfizer. She tells listeners about her own symptoms: the sudden, extreme fatigue, the difficulty controlling her right hand, the stumbling. "Another big problem is memory loss," she'll say with a pause. "Now, what was I talking about?"

Besides Garr and Montel Williams, other well-known personalities who have suffered from MS include Annette Funicello, Roman Gabriel, Lena Horne, and Richard Pryor.

MS was first recognized as a distinct disease in 1868 by French neurologist Jean-Martin Charcot. Charcot is also credited with being the first to describe ALS.

Multiple sclerosis is an inflammatory disease characterized by demyelination, or the breakdown of the protective myelin sheath that surrounds the nerve axons in the brain and spinal cord. The loss of myelin affects nerve cell transmission and interferes with the brain's ability to communicate with the rest of the body. The life expectancy for people with multiple sclerosis is about 5 to 10 years less than those without the disease.

A person with MS can suffer almost any neurological symptom including numbness or muscle weakness, muscle spasms, tingling or pain, difficulty moving, problems with coordination and balance, speech problems, visual problems, fatigue, and bladder and bowel difficulties. Also common is cognitive impairment, depression, and mood swings. An electrical shock-like sensation that runs down the back when bending the neck is particularly characteristic of MS, but not specific. People with severe MS may lose the ability to walk or speak. In the early stages of the disease, diagnosis can be difficult because there is no specific test to detect MS and symptoms often come and go.

At least 85 percent of MS sufferers experience unpredictable attacks followed by months or even years of relative quiet with no new signs of disease activity. Between attacks, symptoms may go away completely. Permanent neurological problems often remain and progressively worsen with each succeeding attack. Some 10-15 percent of individuals never have a remission after the initial onset of their symptoms.

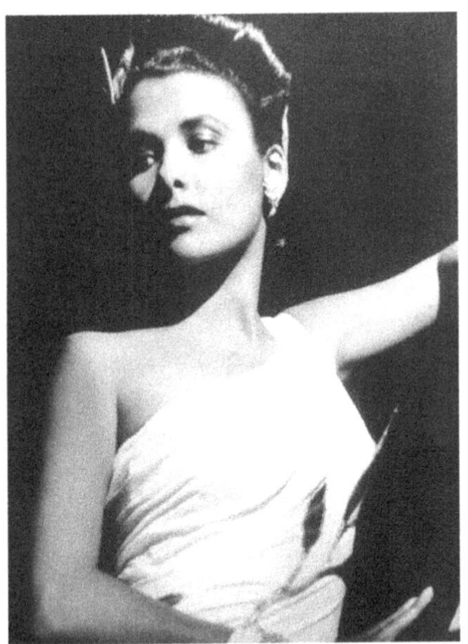

Singer and actress Lena Horne.

More than 2 million people worldwide have MS. About 350,000 Americans are affected, with approximately 200 new cases being diagnosed each week. The disease usually becomes manifest between the ages of 20 and 40, but can occur at any age. Women are more likely to develop MS than are men.

Not much is known about the mechanisms involved in the disease process. It is generally believed to be the result of an autoimmune reaction, in which the body attacks itself. Recent evidence suggests involvement with environmental factors such as chronic infection and nutritional deficiencies.

FRONTOTEMPORAL DEMENTIA

Famed German philosopher and author Friedrich W. Nietzsche (1844-1900) is believed to have suffered from frontotemporal dementia (FTD). In 1886, his friends began to detect changes in his personality. Symptoms gradually grew worse and his behavior became so bizarre that by 1889 he was committed to an insane asylum and later put into the care of his mother until his death. Such was the fate of many of those who suffered from FTD and other forms of dementia that alter one's personality and behavior.

Frontotemporal dementia describes a number of related neurodegenerative conditions that affect the frontal and temporal lobes of the brain—the areas generally associated with personality, behavior, and language. FTD is sometimes referred to as *Pick's disease*, named after Arnold Pick (1851-1924), a professor of psychiatry at the University of Prague, who first described the disease in 1892. However, now the term Pick's disease is reserved for only one subtype of FTD that is characterized by the presence of abnormal protein tangles, called Pick bodies, in degenerating nerve cells.

FTD is characterized by dramatic changes in personality and behavior. Changes in personal and social conduct occur in the early stage of the disease including loss of inhibition leading to socially inappropriate behavior, lack of judgment, impulsiveness, apathy, social withdrawal, decline in personal hygiene, and ritualistic compulsive behaviors. Because of the behavioral changes, FTD is often misdiagnosed as a psychiatric problem, which is why many of those who suffered from this condition ended up being sent to mental institutions.

Some types of FTD are marked by the impairment or loss of speech and the inability to understand written or spoken language. Less frequently, movement disorders occur similar to those associated with Parkinson's disease or ALS, such as, tremor, rigidity, muscle spasms, poor coordination, difficulty swallowing, and muscle weakness.

Unlike Alzheimer's disease patients, who experience severe memory problems, FTD patients may exhibit memory disturbances, but they remain oriented to time and place and recall information about the past and the present.

As many as seven million Americans may be affected with some form of dementia. FTD accounts for about 2 to 5 percent, somewhere from 140,000 to 350,000 cases. The disease progresses steadily and usually rapidly, with survival after diagnosis ranging from less than two years in some individuals to more than 10 years in others. The disease usually occurs after the age of 40 and before age 65, with equal incidence in both men and women. The risk for developing FTD is higher if a parent or sibling has dementia. There are no other known risk factors. While there may be a possible genetic link in some cases, more than half of those who develop FTD have no family history of dementia.

The lesions that develop in the brains of some of those with FTD are of the same type found in those suffering from ALS, suggesting a similar cause. Some forms of FTD and ALS are believed to represent different manifestations of the same disease process; the difference being the location in the brain where the lesions are found. If the motor neurons are affected, ALS occurs; and if the cerebral cortex is affected, FTD occurs. In some cases patients may have lesions in both areas of the brain. Approximately 15 percent of those afflicted with ALS also have FTD.

There is no medical cure for FTD and no effective way to slow down progression of the disease. Treatment relies on managing the symptoms with antidepressants and antipsychotic drugs. For those patients who experience language difficulties, speech therapy may help them learn alternative methods of communication.

A PROGRESSIVE FATAL DISEASE

Neurodegenerative disorders like Alzheimer's and Parkinson's disease are commonly regarded as simply malfunctions of an aging brain. They are often viewed in a similar manner as aging joints or simple memory failure due to advancing years. They are, however, more than just inconveniences or symptoms of advancing age.

Neurodegenerative disease is more accurately described as a progressive fatal disease leading to brain failure. Brain failure is a terminal disease, like cancer, that physically kills patients. When someone experiences heart failure or kidney failure, the end result is death. The brain is no different. The brain is our most vital organ: it controls the heart, the lungs, and all other organs. When it shuts down, so do other vital organs. Dementia is a symptom of a dying brain. People do die from dementia.

The belief that people don't usually die from dementia has skewed death statistics leading to the underreporting of dementia as a cause of death. Dementia, especially Alzheimer's disease, often doesn't get noted on death certificates; other conditions that may be present get the blame. The National Center for Health Statistics ranks Alzheimer's disease as the fifth leading cause of death in the United States of people over the age of 65. This ranking is based on data from death certificates. But according to Melissa Wachterman, MD, MPH of Bringham and Women's Hospital in Boston, death certificates routinely underreport deaths from dementia related illnesses.[9] Wachterman's team checked the death certificates of 165 patients in Boston who had been diagnosed with Alzheimer's disease or other forms of dementia before their deaths. Dementia wasn't mentioned on 37 percent of the death certificates, even as a condition that wasn't the primary cause of death. And of the 114 people who had specifically been diagnosed with Alzheimer's disease before death, Alzheimer's was only mentioned on 27 percent of their death certificates. What this means is that death rates for Alzheimer's and other neurodegenerative diseases may be several times higher than what is reported.

Often patients don't have just Alzheimer's, but they have a combination of neurodegenerative disorders. One study compared clinical and autopsy data on 141 elderly subjects who donated their brains upon death. Annual physical and psychological exams showed that while they were alive, 50 of the 141 had dementia. After death, a neuropathologist, who was unaware of the results of the clinical evaluation, analyzed each person's brain.

Comparison of the clinical and autopsy results showed that only 30 percent of the people with signs of dementia had Alzheimer's disease alone. By contrast, 42 percent of the people with dementia had Alzheimer's disease with vascular dementia and 16 percent had Alzheimer's disease with Parkinson's disease (including two people with all three conditions).

In addition, 33 of the 141 volunteers who died without diagnostic symptoms of dementia had sufficient disease pathology in their brains to fulfill the accepted criteria for Alzheimer's. These diseases don't suddenly happen but occur slowly over many years. When symptoms do become evident, the brain has already sustained extensive damage. This is a good reason to start preventative measures as soon as possible. Beginning in young adulthood is not too early, as conditions at this time can often set in motion the processes that lead to neurodegenerative disease later in life.

After the age of 60, your risk of developing dementia doubles every five years.

4 Premature Aging and Neurodegeneration

THE FREE RADICAL

What do all the following conditions have in common: Alzheimer's disease, Parkinson's disease, Huntington's disease, vascular dementia, ALS, diabetes, multiple sclerosis, and heart disease? You might say that all of these conditions are associated with aging, but some of these conditions can occur at relatively young ages. The thing that ties all these conditions together, as well as most other degenerative disease, is *free radicals*. Free radicals are renegade molecules that attack and destroy other molecules. Any tissue in our body can be damaged by free-radical reactions. It is the accumulation of this damage over many years that results in degeneration of body tissues and loss of function that typifies the symptoms of old age.

Of all the factors that affect human health, the free radical is the most insidious. It doesn't attack suddenly like food poisoning or influenza but is equally as dangerous. A single free radical can do little damage, but the cumulative effect of millions over many years has the power of a stick of dynamite. Like an underwater demolition team, they creep upon us unnoticed, slowly sabotaging our health year after year. Health declines slowly and disease develops so gradually that we take little notice. In the meantime, free radicals are also forming alliances with other health-destroying factors such as viruses and toxins to increase the pain and suffering we endure. In one way or another, free radicals are involved in all major diseases that afflict mankind.

Very simply, a free radical is a molecule with an unpaired electron in its outer orbit. The missing electron makes the molecule highly reactive and unstable. It aggressively seeks to steal an electron from a neighboring molecule. Once an electron is pulled away, the second molecule, now with one less electron, becomes a highly reactive free radical itself and pulls an electron off yet another nearby molecule. This process continues in a destructive chain reaction that may affect thousands of molecules.

Once a molecule becomes a free radical, its physical and chemical properties change in a process called oxidation. The normal function of such molecules is disrupted, affecting the entire cell of which they are a part. A living cell attacked by free radicals degenerates and becomes dysfunctional. Free radicals can attack our cells, literally ripping their protective membranes apart. Sensitive cellular components like DNA, which carries the genetic blueprint of the cell, can be damaged, leading to cellular mutations and death.

Basically, oxidation is a process in which substances combine with oxygen or other nonmetallic elements in such a way as to cause degeneration. In the environment it is seen as rusting in metal, rancidity of oils, and hardening of rubber. One of the classic examples of free-radical deterioration in nature is that of rust. Iron exposed to the elements in the air readily oxidizes. In this process, the corroded iron expands, becomes brittle, and falls apart. The process is one of disintegration or decay. When your body is attacked by free radicals, it essentially "rusts" or disintegrates. The aging process is accelerated.

As cells are bombarded by free radicals, the tissues become progressively impaired. Some researchers believe that free-radical destruction is the actual cause of aging. The older the body gets, the more damage it sustains from a lifetime accumulation of attack from free radicals.

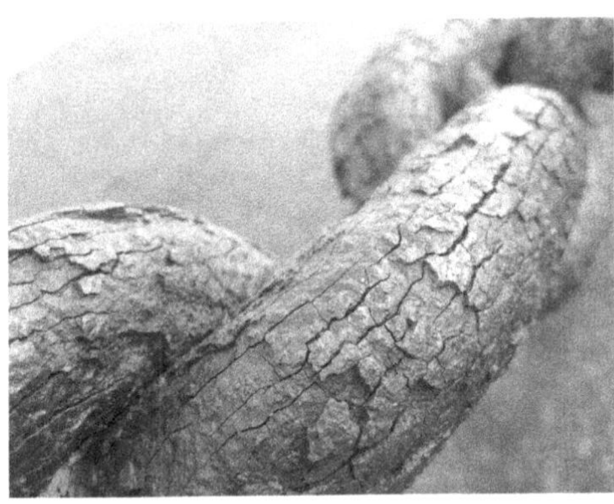

Heavy rust on the links of a chain caused by oxidation. The cells in our bodies break down in a similar manner when attacked by oxidation.

It appears that free radicals are at least partly to blame for the way we look, feel, and function as we get older. Free radicals slowly degenerate body tissues. Aging is a degenerative process. The effects of free-radical degeneration are perhaps most evident in our skin. One of the body tissues damaged most by free radicals is collagen. Collagen acts as the matrix that gives strength and flexibility to our tissues. It is found everywhere in our bodies and holds everything together. It is what keeps our skin smooth, elastic, and youthful. When degraded by free radicals, the skin becomes dry, leathery, and wrinkled—all classic signs of old age.

Free radicals affect the brain in a similar manner. Brain tissues from deceased Alzheimer's, Parkinson's, and other neurodegenerative disease patients are riddled with free radical damage. The brain is uniquely sensitive to oxidative injury because the cell membranes contain a large percentage of highly vulnerable polyunsaturated fatty acids in concentrations among the highest in the body.

It is impossible to prevent all free-radical reactions that occur in the body and in the brain. They are a part of everyday life. Free radicals often form as a natural consequence of normal metabolic processes. The utilization of oxygen and glucose to produce energy also produces free radicals as a side product. Every cell produces free radicals. Our cells, however, are not left defenseless. Antioxidant enzymes are ever-present to quickly squelch these radicals before they can do too much damage. A problem arises when free radical production outpaces the ability of the available antioxidants to neutralize them.

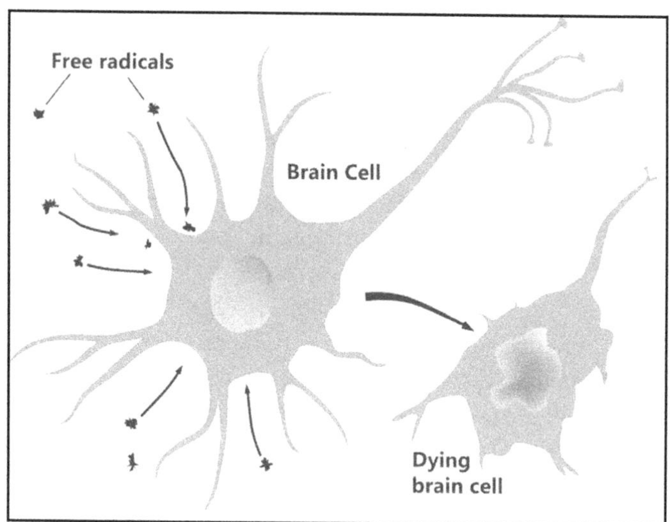

Excessive free-radical exposure cause brain cells to wither and die.

In addition to the normal generation of free radicals inside our bodies, these rogue molecules are also produced by injury, infection, toxins, excessive stress, and various environmental stimuli. Diet is a major source of free radicals. Certain food additives, pesticide residue, chemicals, pollution, and such increase our free radical load. Even the way food is cooked can determine its free radical content. Polyunsaturated vegetable oils are a major source of free radicals in the diet.

The polyunsaturated oils inside natural foods such as vegetables, nuts, and grains are not too much of a problem, so long as they are fresh, because nature always packages them with protective antioxidants to prevent rancidity (oxidation). It's when these oils are extracted and purified into liquid oils that they become troublesome. These oils spontaneously produce free radicals at room temperature. When they are heated, as in cooking, free-radical generation is greatly accelerated. Diets high in polyunsaturated vegetable oils can increase the body's free radical load tremendously. Polyunsaturated oils are so prone to free radical formation that the body's antioxidant reserves are quickly eaten up trying to neutralize them. This can cause not only antioxidant deficiencies but nutritional deficiencies as well, because many of these antioxidants are essential vitamins and minerals important for maintaining good digestive function, hormone balance, a strong immune system, and proper mental function.

THE *AGE*ING BRAIN

Advanced Glycation End Products (AGEs)

Oxidation isn't the only destructive force associated with aging and mental decline. Oxygen is a very reactive molecule and readily causes oxidation and free-radical generation. Likewise, glucose can react in a similar manner to cause *glycation*. The process of glycation is essentially the same as oxidation but with glucose taking the place of the oxygen. To glycate something is to combine it with glucose. Like oxidation, glycation of proteins and polyunsaturated fats produce free radicals and other highly reactive and destructive molecular entities.

Glucose is a very sticky substance and combines easily with other molecules. It can stick to fats but is especially attracted to proteins. The glycation of proteins forms what are called advanced glycation end products (AGEs).

The effects of advanced glycation end products are aptly expressed in the acronym "AGE" because that's what they do—they age the body. Aging is the accumulation of damaged cells. The more AGEs you have in your body, the "older" you become functionally, regardless of how many years you've lived. AGEs adversely affect other molecules, generating free radicals, oxidizing LDL cholesterol (thus creating the type of cholesterol that collects in arteries and promotes atherosclerosis, heart attacks, and strokes), degrading collagen (the major supporting structure in our organs and skin), damaging nerve tissue (including the brain), and wrecking havoc on just about every organ in the body. AGEs are known to play an important role in the chronic complications of diabetes and in the development of Alzheimer's, Parkinson's, ALS, and other neurodegenerative diseases.[1-3]

The AGEing hypothesis of aging was prompted by multiple observations that aged tissues are characterized by the accumulation of a variety of AGE products. AGEs are involved in a vicious cycle of inflammation, generation of free radicals, amplified production of AGEs, more inflammation, and so on.

We all experience the effects of AGEs to some extent. It is just a part of living. As we grow older, we accumulate more AGEs and our bodies respond with the loss of elasticity and tone to skin and other tissues, decreased functional efficiency of organs, failing memory and motor skills, reduced ability to fight off infections, and all the other symptoms associated with aging. Some people are exposed to more AGEs than others. Diabetics are particularly troubled by these rogue molecules. The major complications associated with diabetes—failing eyesight, nerve damage, kidney failure, and heart disease—are all directly linked to AGEs.

Why are diabetics so vulnerable to these troublemakers? The answer is glucose, or more specifically, blood glucose. Chronically elevated blood glucose levels expose our cells and tissues to high concentrations of glucose for extended periods of time. The longer glucose is in contact with proteins, the greater the opportunity they have of forming advanced glycation end products. High blood sugar causes accelerated AGEing.

We are not totally defenseless against AGEs. They are so harmful that the body has a means of getting rid of them. Our white blood cells have receptors specifically designed for them. They latch onto the damaged proteins and remove them.

However, some glycated proteins, like those in collagen or nerve tissues, aren't easily removed. They tend to stick to each other and to other proteins, accumulating and causing damage to surrounding tissues. This plaque-like material becomes a more or less permanent fixture and a continual source of irritation. When a white blood cell encounters a glycated protein, it sets off an inflammatory reaction. The receptors for AGEs are known by the acronym RAGE, which is fitting since the reaction of white blood cells with AGEs can lead to chronic inflammation.

Chronic inflammation is a characteristic of many degenerative conditions including Alzheimer's disease, heart disease, and diabetes.

The formation of AGEs in our body is a normal process. While they can't be completely avoided, we can keep them to a minimum by reducing our sugar and refined carbohydrate consumption. Your brain will thank you, as will the rest of your body.

Dietary Advanced Glycation End Products

Advanced glycation end products form not only inside our bodies but outside as well. When you roast a chicken in the oven, you are creating glycated proteins. The browning of the chicken skin is caused by AGEs.

When proteins and sugars are cooked together at high temperatures in the absence of water, AGEs are formed. You don't need to combine high-protein foods, such as meats, with carbohydrates (sugars) in cooking to develop AGEs. Most foods contain both protein and sugar naturally. All grains, vegetables, fruits, and nuts contain enough protein and sugar to form AGEs under the right conditions.

You can tell when AGEs form by the color of the cooked food. It turns brown. This browning effect imparts a tasty flavor we enjoy in many of our foods. The "golden brown" color that tells you a baked item is fully cooked is the result of AGEs. The brown coloration on cookies, bread crust, roasted and barbequed meats, and even roasted coffee beans are the result of AGEs formed during the cooking process. The making of caramel candy from sugar and milk involves the formation of glycated proteins. In fact, in the food industry they use another word for glycation; the word they use is caramelization. AGEs caramelize the brain. Candies containing caramel are loaded with AGEs. Unlike a loaf of bread where only the outside crust is affected by browning, in caramel the destructive chemical reaction involves every single molecule in the entire product. Not good.

Not all methods of cooking cause AGEs. Cooking with water prevents sugars from binding to proteins and forming these toxic molecules. While frying, baking, and grilling can create AGEs, boiling and steaming with water do not, or at least not to the same extent.

Fortunately, most of the glycated protein products you ingest pass through the body without too much harm. However, approximately 10 percent is absorbed, and about two-thirds of that is deposited in your tissues—your arteries, kidneys, eyes, and brain.[4] Obviously, the more foods you eat that contain these products, the more effect they will have on your health.

Will the small amount of glycated protein that is absorbed into your tissues be of any concern? It definitely can. Dietary-derived AGEs are major contributors to the body's total pool of glycated proteins. Diets high in AGEs accelerate the consequences of natural aging and initiate or contribute to the development of degenerative disease.

In one study, 20 patients were given a low-AGE meal and later a high-AGE meal. The meals contained the same ingredients but different amounts of AGEs, which were obtained by varying the cooking time and temperature. After the high-AGE meal, blood flow-mediated dilation (an indicator of blood vessel function) decreased by 36.2 percent, compared to 20.9 percent after eating the low-AGE meal.[5] In other words, blood flow was restricted more after the high-AGE meal. Reducing blood flow tends to increase blood pressure and restrict flow of nutrients and oxygen into the brain and other vital organs. So this is an important finding.

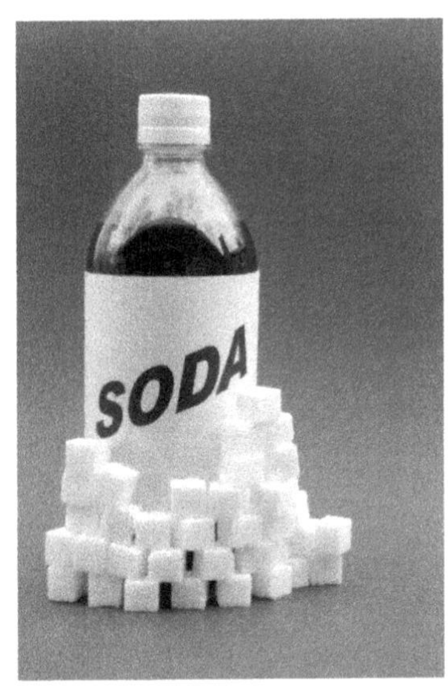

A 32-ounce bottle of soda contains over 30 teaspoons of sugar, usually in the form of high-fructose corn syrup.

Reducing the amount of AGEs in the diet can have a positive affect on health. In another study researchers reported that putting mice on a low-AGE-containing diet not only reduced AGE accumulation but also ameliorated insulin resistance and kidney dysfunction with age. Animals on the low-AGE diet (50 percent lower than the controls) also had a significant increase in lifespan compared to the controls.[6]

As we age we tend to accumulate greater amounts of AGEs. Research suggests that diets high in AGEs accelerate the consequences of natural aging and associated degenerative diseases such as diabetes and Alzheimer's.[7] One study reported that in a comparison of 172 young subjects (under 45 years of age) and older subjects (over 60 years), circulating AGEs increased with age. This was to be expected, but the researchers also found that indicators of inflammation, oxidative stress, and insulin resistance increased with AGEs regardless of the subject's chronological age.[8] So AGE levels were more important at determining physical or functional age than was chronological age. It's not how old you are but how much accumulated damage you have sustained that really determines your level of health.

Environmental factors can contribute to AGEs as well. It may not come as a big surprise to learn that tobacco smoke is another major source of AGEs. Smokers have significantly higher risk than nonsmokers for developing coronary heart disease and stroke, both consequences of AGEs. Blood levels of AGEs in smokers are higher than in nonsmokers.[9] Second-hand smoke is just as harmful.

Most of the AGEs in our bodies come from eating sugar and refined carbohydrates. Sugar and refined carbohydrates (i.e. white flour) raise blood sugar, which in turn increases the rate at which AGEs are formed. While we most often think of glucose when we talk about glycation, two other sugars, fructose and galactose, undergo glycation at about 10 times the rate of glucose.

Milk sugar or lactose is made from a combination of 50 percent glucose and 50 percent galactose. When milk is cooked at high temperatures the galactose glycates with milk proteins, forming AGEs.[10]

A more disturbing problem is fructose. In recent years fructose, in the form of high-fructose corn syrup, has overtaken sucrose (table sugar) as the primary sweetener in commercially prepared products. The reason for this is that fructose is nearly twice as sweet as sucrose, therefore, less of it can be used to impart the

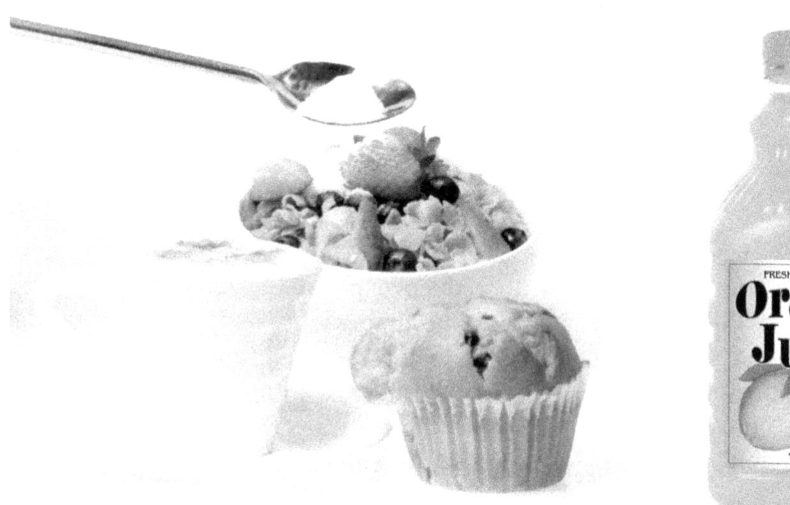

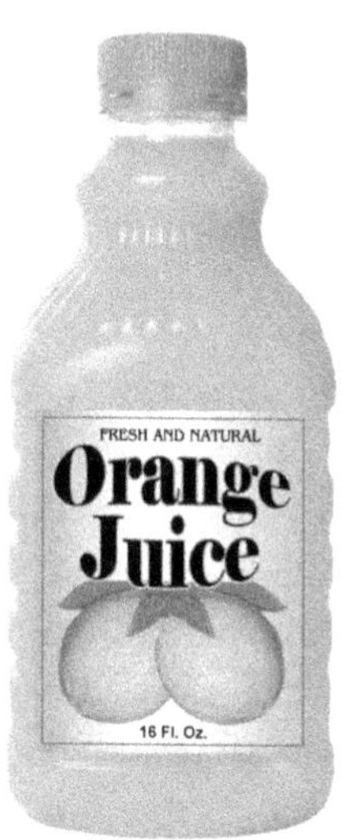

Candy, soda, and desserts aren't the only sources of sugar. Many everyday foods such as breakfast cereal, coffee, muffins, fruit juice, pancakes, and waffles are loaded with sugar in one form or another.

same amount of sweetness. In other words, it's cheaper and reduces manufacturing costs. High-fructose corn syrup is used in the majority of packaged foods in place of sucrose or other sugars. Look at the ingredient labels of ice cream, candy, cookies, breads, and other prepared foods. If sugar is added, it most likely is in the form of high-fructose corn syrup.

Fructose is recommended to diabetics and those with insulin resistance because it has less of an effect on raising blood sugar than table sugar. Ironically, however, while fructose does not affect blood sugar as dramatically as sucrose, it has a much greater overall damaging effect because it increases AGE generation and intensifies insulin resistance, making conditions worse.

All sources of fructose have the same affect on the body. It does not matter if the fructose is from high-fructose corn syrup or a natural source such as agave syrup (a popular sweetener used in the health food industry). The effects are all the same.

An interesting study was conducted in Europe. Researchers took two groups of non-diabetic subjects; one group was vegetarian and the other ate a mixed diet. Diet histories were recorded and blood tests measured AGE levels. The results were surprising. You would expect that the vegetarians, who ate no meat (grilled, fried, or otherwise), consumed less milk, ate more fruits and vegetables, and generally used lower temperatures in cooking, would have lower AGE levels. But this was not the case. The mixed diet subjects had significantly lower AGEs compared to the vegetarians. The vegetarians ate two to three times as much fresh fruit as the mixed diet subjects, three times as much dried fruit, four times as much honey, and about the same amount of commercial sugar. The vegetarian's sugar intake was significantly higher, particularly in fructose. The researchers attributed the higher AGE levels in the vegetarians to their high fructose consumption.[11]

It is interesting that despite eating foods that were lower in AGEs than the mixed diet subjects, the sugar content of the vegetarians' diet had a much greater impact on AGE formation in their bodies. This illustrates that the types of foods eaten have a greater impact on AGE levels in the body than does the way the foods are prepared. Foods high in sugar, especially fructose, have a dynamic affect on AGE formation. This is not to say that cooking methods are not important. They are, but sugar consumption is a far greater concern.

While it may be impossible to totally avoid glycated proteins and fats, or so-called glycotoxins, it is possible to reduce exposure by changing the way you prepare your food and by using cooking methods with a low potential for stirring up these troublemakers. Limit frying, broiling, and grilling at high temperatures and prepare more meals by steaming, boiling, lightly stir-frying, or using a slow cooker. When frying, add a little water and let the hot steam do most of the cooking. Cook meats at lower temperatures and eat them rare or medium-rare. Eat more raw foods and avoid cooking altogether. You need to be particularly careful about prepared, packaged foods such as ready-to-eat breakfast cereals, crackers, chips, cookies, donuts, and other pre-cooked, high-carbohydrate foods. Food manufacturers intentionally cook foods to increase caramelization and browning to enhance flavor. These are major sources of AGEs. If possible, choose raw milk over pasteurized. Eat more fresh vegetables, both raw and cooked. Vegetables are rich sources of antioxidants that can help protect against AGE formation. Antioxidants and foods high in antioxidants help to reduce glycation and AGE formation.[12-13]

ABNORMAL PROTEINS: PLAQUES, TANGLES, AND AGGREGATES

Amyloid Beta and Neurofibrillary Tangles

The brain of an Alzheimer's patient is characterized by the progressive accumulation of amyloid plaques and neurofibrillary tangles. Amyloid plaques and tangles are structures that are believed by some researchers to be the prime suspects in damaging and killing brain cells in Alzheimer's disease.

Amyloid plaques build up between the nerve cells. They contain deposits of a protein fragment called amyloid beta. Amyloid is an insoluble protein deposit that cannot be broken down and interferes with or alters the normal function of tissues on which it forms.

Neurofibrillary tangles are insoluble twisted fibers that form inside the dying brain cells. These tangles consist primarily of a protein called tau, which forms part of a structure called a microtubule. The microtubule helps transport nutrients and other important substances from one part of the nerve cell to another. In Alzheimer's however, the tau protein becomes abnormal and the microtubule structures collapse.

We all develop some plaques and tangles as we age. Those with Alzheimer's, however, tend to accumulate five to ten times more than normal. The plaques and tangles begin to form in areas important in learning and memory and eventually spread to other regions in the brain.

In Alzheimer's disease, plaques first develop in the hippocampus, a structure deep in the brain that helps to encode memories, and in areas of the cerebral cortex that are essential in thinking and making decisions.

Plaque formation starts with a normal blood protein called *amyloid precursor protein* (APP). Although not fully understood, APP is believed to be involved in protecting nerve cells and appears to be important in helping neurons grow and survive. They help damaged neurons repair themselves and help parts of neurons regrow after injury.

Free radicals and AGEs accelerate the formation and aggregation of amyloid proteins and induce inflammatory responses. As the disease progresses, protein accumulation increases, neurons die and shrivel away, and the brain shrinks. Ventricles—hollow spaces within the brain that contain cerebrospinal fluid—become enlarged. Brain mass is lost.

Plaques and tangles are found not only in Alzheimer's disease, but also in the brains of patients with other neurodegenerative disorders, including Parkinson's disease, Huntington's disease, and amyotrophic lateral sclerosis (ALS).

Lewy Bodies

Lewy bodies are abnormal aggregates of protein found inside degenerating dopamine-producing nerve cells. Lewy bodies are commonly found in the brains of people who have Parkinson's disease and Lewy body dementia. In Parkinson's disease, Lewy bodies are found in large numbers in the substantia nigra of the brain stem, which controls voluntary movement. These protein deposits deplete the neurotransmitter dopamine, causing the physical symptoms characteristic to Parkinson's disease. In Lewy body dementia, they are dispersed throughout the brain, including regions in the cerebral cortex which are involved in thinking and memory.

The primary structural component of the Lewy body is a protein called alpha-synuclein. Alpha-synuclein proteins are normally involved in regulating the transport activities of dopamine in the synapses between nerve cells. Under excessive oxidative stress, these proteins tend to aggregate into Lewy bodies. Their presence in the cells alters normal cellular functioning and processes. This has led researchers to assume that they cause the cells to degenerate and die, and much research has pursued this line of reasoning. Some evidence, however, indicates that Lewy bodies are not haphazard formations, but produced as a defensive response to protect the cell. They are found in damaged cells, not because they caused the damage, but because the cell was damaged by free radicals or other factors and initiated Lewy body formation as a coping response. Their presence may interfere with cellular function, but in the process extend the life of the cell. Whether Lewy bodies cause the cell to degenerate or are formed as a means of self preservation is still under investigation.

Huntingtin Proteins

The distinguishing feature of Huntington's disease is the presence of aggregates of a protein within brain cells called huntingtin protein. Huntingtin protein is a normal protein that occurs in all of our cells. The exact function of this protein is not known, but it is believed to play an important role in nerve cell function. Within cells, huntingtin protein appears to be involved in signaling, transporting materials, binding other proteins, and regulating lifespan of the cell.

The length of this protein is variable depending on the number of glutamine (an amino acid) molecules it contains. Huntingtin normally contains 3,144 amino acids (the building blocks of proteins) with a string of from 6 to 35 glutamine molecules attached to one end.

In Huntington's disease, the huntingtin protein is elongated with additional glutamines. The longer the huntingtin protein is (i.e., the more glutamine molecules attached to the end), the more severe the disease. No cases of Huntington's disease have been diagnosed when the huntingtin protein contains a sequence of less than 36 glutamines, which is the normal number. People with 36 to 40 glutamine segments may or may not develop the disease; while people with more than 40 will develop the disorder if they live long enough. When there are more than 60 glutamine segments on the protein, the disease is severe and the person likely develops early-onset Huntington's disease.

According to the most popular theory, Huntington's disease is believed to be caused by mutated genes that produce the elongated huntingtin proteins. Being hereditary, the gene would be passed to offspring. However, unlike other genes, this gene apparently can change from generation to generation, which stirs doubt about it being strictly a genetic defect. As the gene is passed from one generation to the next, the size of the huntingtin protein apparently can change, either increasing or decreasing. Parents who don't have the disease can pass it on to their offspring and parents that do have the gene can have children without the disease.

What causes the gene to change from one generation to the next is still a mystery. Since the length of the huntingtin protein can change, apparently there are some environmental influences that must be in play. One of these influences may be the amount of stress one experiences.[14] Other influences may include such things as diet, lifestyle, toxic exposure, and infections. Disease conditions such as insulin resistance or diabetes may also be a factor. If this is so, then there are things that those people with this disease can do to improve their condition and decrease the risk of passing the defective genes to their children.

The presence of the elongated huntingtin protein itself does not seem to be harmful. Enzymes in the cell often cut this elongated protein into fragments. These protein segments tend to clump together, forming protein aggregates inside brain cells. The areas of the brain most affected are the striatum (a part of the brain that coordinates movement) and the frontal cortex (which controls thinking and emotions). These huntingtin protein aggregates influence cellular functions, which have generally been interpreted as being harmful to the cell and capable of promoting premature cell death.

At one time it was thought that the presence of these protein clumps played the primary role in the development of Huntington's disease and that they were the consequence of a defective gene. Further research, however, has undermined this belief. Researchers have discovered that aggregated proteins such as huntingtin aggregates in Huntington's disease, like the amyloid plaques in Alzheimer's disease, do not cause neurodegeneration as was once thought. Brain cell death can occur in the absence of any detectable aggregates. Aggregates can exist in the absence of disease pathology or symptoms.[15] Furthermore, these protein aggregates appear to be formed as a protective response to injury or stress. Studies now show that the presence of huntingtin aggregates actually *extends* the life of neurons and acts to reduce damage to neighboring neurons.[16] Elongated huntingtin proteins, therefore, may not be genetic flaws but normal and natural products designed to protect the cells from injury or stress. The length of the protein being an indication of the degree of stress in the system and not the random consequence of a mutated gene.

The evidence suggests that huntingtin aggregates only occur when the brain is under some type of stress. This is why they are found in abundance in those with Huntington's disease. Neurodegenerative disease, including Huntington's disease, is a process that occurs gradually over many decades. Therefore, elongated huntingtin aggregates can be present in brain tissues long before symptoms ever develop. The amyloid plaque in Alzheimer's disease and Lewy bodies in Parkinson's disease and Lewy body dementia may be defensive responses to stress within the central nervous system.

The belief that Huntington's disease has a genetic component is based to a large extent on the observation that children of Huntington's disease parents often end up developing the disease as well. This, however, does not mean the disease is strictly genetic. Parents who suffer from health problems due to poor nutrition, infection, toxic exposure, and such can pass onto their children a variety of health problems such as spina bifida and heart defects or predispose them to develop certain health problems such as allergies, insulin resistance (type 2 diabetes), cognitive impairment, heart disease, frequent infections, and others.[17-25]

Having a genetic predisposition to develop a health problem does not guarantee the problem will occur. It means it has a higher chance of occurring given the right circumstances. Huntington's disease appears to be like this. Those who are predisposed to Huntington's disease will develop the disease sooner and more severely than those who are not, but anyone who is exposed to the stresses that lead to this disorder can develop it. This is why some have early-onset neurodegenerative disease while others don't get it until later in life, or not at all.

TDP-43

Amyotrophic lateral sclerosis (ALS) and some forms of frontotemporal dementia (FTD) are characterized by the accumulation of a protein called TDP-43. Little is known about this protein, which is found throughout the body. In ALS and FTD it is believed to have been "tagged" by the body's natural defensive forces to be destroyed and eliminated. When the removal process fails, the tagged protein can build up into aggregates. In the case of ALS, this occurs in the motor neurons, and in the case of frontotemporal dementia, it occurs in the frontal and temporal lobes of the cortex.

TDP-43 is a normal protein found in the nucleus of the nerve cells. The nucleus is where the cell stores the information (DNA) required to make proteins needed for normal cell function. In ALS and frontotemporal dementia, variants of this protein accumulate in the cytoplasm outside the nucleus. Scientists speculate that the accumulation of TDP-43 in the cytoplasm causes cellular degeneration. However, like other abnormal proteins, it may be that the protein is there in response to toxins or oxidative stress and is a consequence of this stress rather than the cause.

Recent studies have shown that TDP-43 protein can be detected in blood samples and that levels of this protein are elevated in FTD and ALS as well as in some Alzheimer's patients.[26]

Pick Bodies

Another protein that accumulates in some forms of FTD are Pick bodies. In this case the disease is called Pick's disease. Like other forms of FTD, these proteins accumulate in the frontal and temporal lobes of the brain that control personality, behavior, and language.

Pick bodies are spherical aggregations of tau protein found inside dying neurons. They are composed of numerous tau fibrils arranged in a disorderly array. While Tau protein is the major component of Pick bodies, they may also contain alpha-synuclein, the same protein that is involved in the formation of Lewy bodies.

Amyloid beta, tangles, Lewy bodies, huntingtin proteins, TDP-43, Pick bodies, and other proteins accumulate at different rates as the brain ages. When any one or more of these proteins accumulate in unusually large amounts, brain function can be seriously affected. Any one or more of these proteins can be found in the various forms of neurodegeneration. Amyloid beta proteins, for example, are not restricted to only those who suffer from Alzheimer's disease but can affect those with no outward symptoms as well as those with Parkinson's disease or any other neurodegenerative disease. The same is true with Lewy bodies or TDP-43, although there is a tendency for one to predominate in any given disease.[27]

As neurodegenerative disease progresses and more protein deposits accumulate in the brain, it becomes increasingly difficult to distinguish between one disease and another.

CHRONIC INFLAMMATION

While each of the neurodegenerative diseases can be identified by their respective symptoms and the accumulation of specific protein aggregates, one unifying feature that is common to all the neurodegenerative conditions is chronic inflammation.[28]

Chronic inflammation in the brain begins early in the development of neurodegeneration and strongly correlates with disease progression.[29-30] Therefore, inflammation is believed to play a very significant role in the origin and progression of the disease. In Huntington's disease, for example, chronic inflammation has been detected in the brain as early as 16 years before the onset of symptoms with the level of inflammation increasing as the disease progresses.[31]

Inflammation is a normal and natural response to injury and stress. It stimulates the influx of blood and oxygen into the injured area to facilitate healing. The blood brings in platelets to stop bleeding, if necessary, along with other proteins to rebuild damaged tissues. Ordinarily, inflammation is of brief duration. Once repair is well underway, inflammation abates and everything goes back to normal. However, if irritation and injury remain, so does inflammation. Chronic irritation leads to chronic inflammation. Chronic inflammation itself can cause additional irritation creating a vicious cycle of more inflammation and more irritation.

Inflammation always appears to be present and, if chronic may even contribute to the problem, but it is not the cause of neurodegeneration. What causes inflammation? Postmortem analysis of human brain tissue, studies on animals, and clinical trials point to excessive oxidative stress (membrane lipid peroxidation in particular), AGE accumulation, and impaired neuronal glucose uptake and utilization. When this stimulation becomes chronic, so does the inflammation. These conditions establish the underlying cause to all the major neurodegenerative diseases.[32]

What causes oxidative stress, AGE accumulation, and disrupts glucose metabolism? While genetics may play a role in some cases, by far the major influences involve a combination of diet, trauma, drugs, stress, toxins, and infection.[33] Each of these will be discussed in the following chapters.

5 Insulin Resistance and Neurodegeneration

NEURODEGENERATION: THE NEW DIABETES

When you hear a doctor give a diagnosis of Alzheimer's disease, you should automatically think of diabetes or, more specifically, insulin resistance—the underlying cause for both of these conditions. Those with diabetes are at higher risk of developing Alzheimer's and other neurodegenerative diseases than the general population. Diabetes often progresses into Alzheimer's disease. The relationship between these two conditions is so close that Alzheimer's disease is now recognized as another form of diabetes.[1]

Diabetes is a major cause of disability leading to blindness, lower-limb amputation, kidney disease, and nerve damage. Currently 23.6 million people (7.8 percent of the population) in the United States have diabetes. Nearly 6 million more are living with diabetes but are totally unaware of it. More than 23 percent of all adults age 60 and older have diabetes: that's one out of every five older adults! But it's not just an old-age disease; nearly 200,000 people under the age of 20 have been diagnosed with the disease as well. In all age groups, over 1.6 million new cases are diagnosed each year. Most of these people are at risk of developing Alzheimer's disease at some point in their lives. The younger the age at the time of diagnosis of diabetes, the greater the risk. Diabetes is the 6th leading cause of death, just ahead of Alzheimer's.

Diabetes occurs as a result of the body's inability to properly regulate blood sugar. When we eat a meal, much of the food is converted into glucose, or blood sugar, and sent into the bloodstream. When blood sugar levels rise too high (or fall too low), the body can be thrown into a panic, metabolically speaking. Insulin, a hormone secreted by the pancreas into the bloodstream, brings blood sugar levels back to normal. However, if for some reason blood sugar is not normalized in a reasonable amount of time, cells and tissues become damaged. This is what happens in people with diabetes.

There are different types of diabetes. Type 1 diabetes occurs when the pancreas stops producing insulin or produces too little to properly regulate and control blood glucose. Type 1 diabetes is typically diagnosed in early childhood. It used to be known as juvenile-onset diabetes or insulin-dependent diabetes mellitus. Type 1 diabetics require a lifetime of regular injections of insulin to keep blood sugar in balance. This form of diabetes can develop in older individuals due to dysfunction of the pancreas by alcohol abuse or disease. It comprises about 10 percent of all cases of diabetes in the United States.

In type 2 diabetes, the pancreas may be capable of producing a normal amount of insulin, but the cells of the body have become unresponsive or resistant to its action. A larger amount of insulin is needed in order to accomplish its task. This condition is referred to as insulin resistance. This is by far the most common form of diabetes. About 90 percent of diabetics are of this type. Type 2 diabetes typically occurs in adulthood, usually after the age of 45. It used to be called adult-onset diabetes mellitus, or non-insulin-dependent diabetes mellitus. These names are no longer used because type 2 diabetes does occur in younger people, and some people with type 2 diabetes need to use insulin. Early in the course of the disease the pancreas is usually capable of producing the large amounts of insulin needed to overcome the insulin resistance of the cells. But over time the high demand for insulin takes its toll on the pancreas and insulin production begins to decline. More than half of all those with type 2 diabetes eventually require insulin to control their blood sugar levels as they get older. Type 2 diabetes is usually controlled with diet, weight management, exercise, and medication.

Gestational diabetes is temporary form of type 2 diabetes that occurs in women during the second half of pregnancy. Gestational diabetes typically goes away after delivery of the baby. Women who have gestational diabetes are pre-diabetic and are more likely than other women to develop type 2 diabetes later in life.

A third form of diabetes called type 3 has recently been recognized. This new form of diabetes links insulin resistance with neurodegeneration and most specifically with Alzheimer's disease. Type 3 diabetes combines characteristics of both type 1 and type 2 diabetes. The brain has an insulin deficiency like in type 1 diabetes and is insulin resistant like in type 2 diabetes. Insulin resistance is the primary distinguishing feature. In this book, when I speak of "diabetes" I am generally referring to type 2 diabetes. If a distinction needs to be made between types 1, 2 or 3, I will be more specific.

The fact that Alzheimer's is recognized as a form of diabetes is not as strange as it might sound. Diabetes has long been known to adversely affect nerve tissue throughout the body, including the brain. Studies show that diabetics have substantially smaller brain volumes in comparison to non-diabetic subjects. The decrease in size is due to the death of brain cells. The brains of people with diabetes age prematurely. Sudha Seshadri, MD, a neurologist at Boston University, says that the brains of diabetics are about "10 years older" than the brains of same-age people without diabetes. "Even if it were not a direct cause, diabetes may hasten the onset of clinical manifestations of Alzheimer's disease because the brain goes downhill faster," she says.

Insulin does a lot more than regulate blood sugar. Insulin plays a role in normal cognitive function. Dysregulation of insulin increases risk for cognitive impairment, Alzheimer's and other neurodegenerative diseases. Recent studies confirm that diabetes leads to a significant cognitive decline and increases the risks of dementia and Alzheimer's disease by up to 150 percent.[2]

While research at this time has linked neurodegeneration in general and Alzheimer's specifically to disturbances in insulin metabolism, other disorders such as vascular dementia, Parkinson's disease, Huntington's disease, and ALS also exhibit features suggesting insulin resistance as either an important underlying factor or as a contributor to the initiation and progression of the disease.[3-4]

All of the major neurodegenerative diseases display a marked decline in energy metabolism leading to cell death and loss of brain volume. Any disturbance in normal insulin function can dramatically affect energy metabolism and consequently brain function. In that sense, they might all be viewed as various manifestations of type 3 diabetes.

With further research the connection between other neurodegenerative conditions and insulin resistance will likely become more evident. Research is just now beginning to uncover the relationships between Parkinson's and insulin resistance.[5] Abnormal glucose tolerance has been reported in up to 80 percent of Parkinson's disease patients. Dysfunction of insulin metabolism in the brain is known to precede the death of the dopamine-producing neurons in the development of Parkinson's disease.[6] Insulin resistance also exacerbates the severity of the symptoms and reduces the therapeutic efficacy of levodopa and other dopaminergic agents.[7]

Evidence shows that those who have diabetes are at greater risk of developing Parkinson's. In one of the largest studies of this kind to date, researchers followed a group of more than 50,000 men and women over a period of 18 years. The researchers found that those people who had type 2 diabetes at the start of the study were 83 percent more likely to be diagnosed with Parkinson's disease later on in life than non-diabetics.[8] If the study had extended longer, no doubt there would have been an even greater correlation since risk of Parkinson's increases with age.

Even Huntington's disease, which is considered primarily an inherited condition, appears to be influenced by insulin resistance. Studies show that those with Huntington's disease are more likely to have diabetes than those without the disease.[9-10]

The changes that take place in the body that lead to diabetes and eventually to neurodegeneration occur long before either of these diseases becomes apparent. Glucose metabolism becomes abnormal one to two decades before type 2 diabetes is diagnosed.[11] Neurodegenerative disease may surface another couple of decades after that.

Diabetes is on the rise. According to the Mayo Clinic, diabetes has doubled in the United States over the past 15 years. Worldwide diabetes has increased from 30 million to 230 million cases over the past 20 years. This is a huge increase. Scientists have expressed concern that today's mushrooming diabetes epidemic may become tomorrow's Alzheimer's epidemic or Parkinson's epidemic. The epidemic may have already begun—as witnessed by the increasing rates of Alzheimer's, Parkinson's, and other neurodegenerative diseases.

GLUCOSE POWERS OUR CELLS

The neurons, or brain cells, as well as every other cell in the body, require energy to perform their various functions. We derive energy from the three major nutrients in our foods—carbohydrate, protein, and fat. While protein and fat can be used to produce energy, their primary function is to provide the basic building blocks for tissues, hormones, enzymes, and other structures that make up the human body. The primary purpose of carbohydrate, on the other hand, is to produce energy. It is the body's preferred choice for fuel. Typically, 55-60 percent of our energy needs are supplied by carbohydrate with the remainder coming from protein and fat.

Carbohydrates are found in virtually all plant foods. Milk is the only animal derived food that contains carbohydrate. Plants are made predominantly of carbohydrates. Carbohydrates are constructed out of sugar. Sugar molecules provide the basic building blocks for all plants. The grass in your front yard, the flowers on your porch, the apples and oranges on your kitchen countertop, and the vegetables in your refrigerator are composed almost entirely of sugar and water.

There are three basic types of sugar molecules that are important in our diet—glucose, fructose, and galactose. All the carbohydrates in our diet consist of some combination of these three. *Simple carbohydrates* consist of only one or two units of sugar. For example, table sugar, or sucrose, consists of one molecule of glucose and one of fructose. Milk sugar, or lactose, consists of one molecule of glucose and one of galactose. *Complex carbohydrates* are composed of many sugar molecules linked together by chemical bonds. Starch, for example, consists of long chains of glucose. Glucose is by far the most abundant sugar molecule in plant foods.

When you eat a slice of bread, you are eating mostly glucose in the form of starch. Along with the starch, you get some water, fiber (which is also a type of carbohydrate), vitamins, and minerals. The same thing is true when you eat an apple, a carrot, corn, potatoes or any other plant derived food.

When food containing carbohydrate is consumed, digestive enzymes break the bonds between the sugar molecules, releasing the individual glucose, fructose, and galactose molecules. These sugars are then transported to the bloodstream. Here glucose, also referred to as blood sugar, is delivered throughout the body to supply the fuel needed by the cells. Fructose and galactose in their current form cannot be used by the cells to produce energy. They are taken up by the liver, converted into glucose, and then released back into the bloodstream. Foods high in glucose produce a rapid rise in blood sugar concentration. Fructose and galactose increase blood sugar as well, but not as rapidly because they must pass through the liver first.

Dietary fiber is also a carbohydrate, but the human body does not produce the enzymes necessary to break the chemical bonds holding these sugars together. Therefore, fiber passes through the digestive tract and out of the body mostly intact. Since fiber releases little or no sugar, it does not raise blood sugar levels.

Most cells cannot store glucose. They take up and use what is necessary for their immediate needs. The liver and muscle cells are exceptions; they have the ability to store a small amout of glucose for later use.

If food is not consumed for a period of time and the stored glucose becomes depleted, the body begins to metabolize fat and protein to meet its energy needs. Fat serves as the primary alternative source of energy when blood glucose levels decline. To a limited extent, protein can be converted into glucose, fat however, cannot. It is released as individual fat molecules known as fatty acids. Some of these fatty acids are converted into molecular units called ketone bodies or ketones. Fatty acids and ketones can be used by the cells in place of glucose to supply energy needs.

THE ROLE OF INSULIN

As glucose circulates throughout the body, it is picked up by the cells and transformed into energy. The cells, however, cannot absorb glucose by themselves. They need the help of the hormone insulin. Insulin unlocks the door on the cell membrane which makes it possible for glucose to enter. Without insulin, glucose cannot enter the cells. Your blood could be saturated with glucose, but if insulin was not present, glucose could not pass though the cell membrane, and the cells would "starve" and die.

Every cell in your body needs a continuous supply of glucose to function normally. Just like us, if we don't get enough food at regular intervals, our health fails and we die. Likewise, if the cells don't get enough glucose on a continual basis, they degenerate and die.

But an overabundance of glucose is not good either. Too much glucose is toxic. In order to avoid the dire consequences of too little or too much glucose, the body has built in feedback mechanisms that maintain a narrow range of glucose levels in the blood.

Every time we eat, blood sugar levels rise. As sugar levels increase, special cells in the pancreas are triggered to release insulin into the bloodstream. As insulin shuttles glucose into the cells, blood sugar levels drop. At some point, another signal triggers the pancreas to stop insulin secretion. If blood sugar levels fall too low, the pancreas is prodded to release another hormone called glucagon. Glucagon induces the release of glucose stored in the liver, thus increasing blood sugar levels. In this way, blood sugar is continually maintained within a narrow boundary.

Blood sugar levels naturally fluctuate slightly throughout the day. Whenever we eat, blood sugar levels increase. Between meals or during times of heavy physical activity, as the body's demand for energy increases, blood sugar levels decline. As long as the body is capable of compensating for both upward and downward spikes in blood sugar, balance is quickly reestablished and maintained.

What we eat profoundly affects the workings of this system. High carbohydrate meals, especially if they contain a significant amount of simple carbohydrates and a lack of fiber, fat, and protein, can cause blood glucose levels to rise very rapidly. Refined starches such as white flour have been stripped of most of their fiber and bran and tend to act like sugar, spiking blood glucose levels as well.

Fiber, protein, and especially fat slow down the digestion and absorption of carbohydrate so glucose trickles gradually into the bloodstream, providing a steady, ongoing supply. The larger the quantity of simple and refined carbohydrate in meals, the greater the spike in blood sugar and the greater the strain placed on the body and especially the pancreas, which produces both opposing hormones—insulin and glucagon.

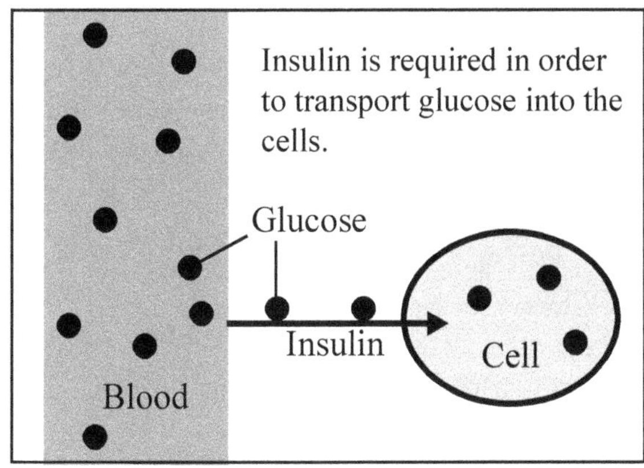
Insulin is required in order to transport glucose into the cells.
Glucose
Insulin
Cell
Blood

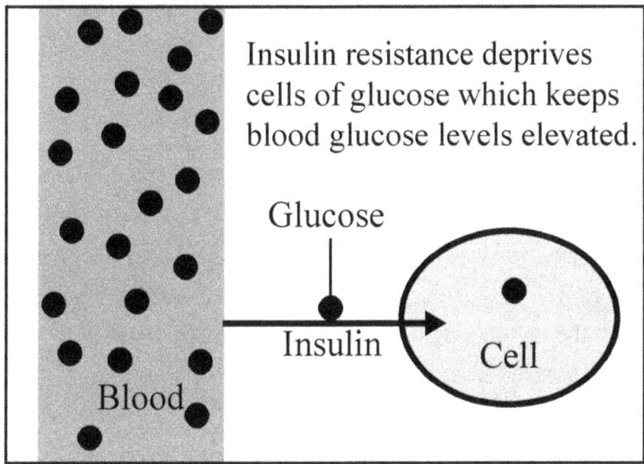
Insulin resistance deprives cells of glucose which keeps blood glucose levels elevated.
Glucose
Insulin
Cell
Blood

If a high carbohydrate meal is eaten every four or five hours, along with one or two high carbohydrate snacks such as a candy bar, soda, donut, or coffee with sugar between meals, insulin levels are going to be raised continually for a substantial part of the day. When cells are continually exposed to high insulin levels, they begin to lose their sensitivity to the hormone. It is like walking into a room with a bad odor. When you first enter the room the smell can be overpowering, but if you have to stay in the room for any length of time, the smell receptors in your nose become desensitized and you will not notice the odor any longer. The smell is still there, but your ability to detect the smell has declined. If you left the room for a while and your sense of smell became resensitized, as soon as you walked back into the room you would again notice the odor. Our bodies react in somewhat the same way with insulin. Chronic exposure to high insulin levels desensitizes the cells, and they become unresponsive or resistant to the action of insulin. This is referred to as *insulin resistance*. In order to move glucose into the cells, a higher than normal concentration of insulin is needed, which puts more stress on the pancreas to produce more of the hormone. Insulin resistance is the first step toward developing diabetes. It is also the first step toward Alzheimer's disease. Diet, therefore, has a direct affect on the development of insulin resistance and consequently, diabetes and neurological dysfunction.

INSULIN RESISTANCE

If you are an average, non-diabetic individual, when you wake up in the morning, your blood contains between 65 and 100 mg/dl (3.6-5.5 mmol/l) of glucose. This is known as the fasting blood glucose concentration. Fasting blood sugar measurements are taken after a person has not eaten for at least eight hours. The ideal fasting blood sugar range is between 75-90 mg/dl (4.2-5.0 mmol/l).

When you don't eat and as your cells continue to draw glucose out of the blood, your glucose level gradually falls. Most people experience a feeling of hunger at about 65 mg/dl (3.6 mmol/l), the low end of the normal range. The normal response to this sensation is to eat; which raises blood sugar. Normally, your blood sugar should not rise to more than 139 mg/dl (7.7 mmol/l) after eating a meal. This is called postprandial glucose level. Elevated fasting and postprandial glucose levels indicate insulin resistance.

Diabetes is diagnosed when fasting blood sugar is 126 mg/dl (7.0 mmol/l) or higher. People with fasting blood sugar levels between 101 and 125 mg/dl (5.6-6.9 mmol/l) are considered to be in the early stages of diabetes, often referred to as "pre-diabetes." Fasting blood sugar levels over 90 mg/dl (5.0 mmol/l) indicate the presence of insulin resistance. As insulin resistance increases, so do blood sugar levels. The higher the blood sugar, the greater the insulin resistance.

The level at which a person is considered to have full-blown diabetes is more or less arbitrary. For many years a fasting blood sugar reading of 140 mg/dl (7.8 mmol/l) was considered the point which defined diabetes. In 1997 The American Diabetes Association lowered the definition to 126 mg/dl (7.0 mmol.l). Does that mean if you have fasting blood sugar of 125 mg/dl (6.9 mmol/l) you are not diabetic? Not hardly. The 126 mg/dl (7.0 mmol/l) is just as arbitrary as 140 mg/dl (7.8 mmol/l). Insulin resistance is usually present in anyone who has a fasting blood sugar level over 90 mg/dl (5.0 mmol/l). Although levels up to 100 mg/dl (5.5 mmol/l) are generally considered to be normal, they are viewed this way only because so many people fit into this category. They are not really "normal" for a healthy individual. Having insulin resistance is not a state of health, even if the condition is relatively mild.

While about 24 million Americans have been diagnosed with diabetes, another 41 million are insulin resistant enough to be considered pre-diabetic. All are at increased risk for Alzheimer's. You don't need to be diagnosed as a diabetic in order to develop Alzheimer's disease—even pre-diabetes significantly increases the risk.

A study conducted by researchers from Stockholm's Karolinska Institute demonstrated this. The researchers followed the participants of the study for nine years and kept track of how many patients developed Alzheimer's. People who had pre-diabetes at the start of the study were found to have a 70 percent increased risk of developing Alzheimer's. This percentage likely would have increased if the study continued longer, allowing more of the participants to develop the disease.

Over the past several decades a tenfold increase in the incidence of type 2 diabetes has occurred. This has been documented in the Japanese, Israelis, Africans, Native Americans, Eskimos, Polynesians, Micronesians, and others.[12] This is believed to be caused by the increased consumption of refined carbohydrates. Animal studies have shown that diets very high in sugar cause insulin resistance and diabetes. It is reasonable to conjecture that the change in dietary habits in humans is at the core of our current diabetes epidemic.

Some people are more susceptible to developing diabetes or insulin resistance than others. This susceptibility comes from their parents. Children of diabetic parents are at higher risk of developing insulin resistance and becoming diabetic themselves.[11]

If just one parent is insulin resistant, even if it is not severe enough to be diagnosed as full-fledged diabetes, the children can be at greater risk of developing insulin resistance. Mothers who develop gestational diabetes predispose their children to develop insulin resistance later in life. This is why diabetes sometimes seems to run in families. Susceptibility does not come from poor genes but from nutritional deficiencies. In other words, it is passed on to future generations as a consequence of a poor diet. To make matters worse, poor eating habits are taught to children, who pass it down to their children. Consequently, people are developing diabetes at increasingly earlier ages.

In 1997, the United States government recommended that all adults be tested for diabetes by the time they reach age 45, before diabetic complications can progress and become difficult to treat. Testing people at 45 may be too late.

The average age at which diabetes is diagnosed is now 37. Researchers from the Centers for Disease Control and Prevention (CDC) are recommending that people should be tested for type 2 diabetes at age 25.

Inheriting a susceptibility for insulin resistance or diabetes doesn't guarantee these conditions will become manifest. They will only develop under the right conditions. In this case, the right conditions are consuming high amounts of carbohydrate, especially refined carbohydrates and sweets. A susceptible person can live a long and healthy life without the slightest trouble with insulin resistance as long as he or she eats a healthy diet.

BRAIN DIABETES

Type 3 Diabetes

Insulin resistance can have an adverse effect on virtually every organ and system in the body. Nerves are highly sensitive to elevated blood sugar and insulin levels. Chronic insulin resistance causes nerve damage, a condition known as diabetic neuropathy. Diabetic neuropathy is the most common serious complication of diabetes. About 60 to 70 percent of people with diabetes have some form of neuropathy. Symptoms include pain, tingling, or numbness in the hands, arms, feet, and legs. The legs and feet are most commonly affected, but nerve damage can develop throughout the body, including the brain.

Population-based studies have shown that those with type 2 diabetes have an increased risk of cognitive impairment, dementia, and neurodegeneration.[13] The damage done to the nerves by insulin resistance increases the risk of developing Alzheimer's disease as well as other neurodegenerative diseases. Diabetics have almost twice the risk of getting Alzheimer's disease as the general population.[14] The younger a person is when he or she develops insulin resistance, the greater the risk. If diabetes occurs before the age of 65, it is associated with a 125 percent increased risk of eventually developing Alzheimer's disease.[15] Even pre-diabetics are in danger of developing Alzheimer's. The common denominator between pre-diabetes, diabetes, and Alzheimer's disease is insulin resistance.

The underlying cause of type 2 diabetes—insulin resistance—appears to be essential for the development of Alzheimer's disease. Every cell in your body depends on glucose to supply its energy needs. Your brain cells are no different. Your brain cells are continually active, even while you are sleeping, so they are continually drawing on the supply of glucose in the fluid surrounding them. To maintain the supply, a steady stream of blood moves past these cells, replenishing the glucose as the cells use it up. A disruption in the availability of glucose can be catastrophic. Without glucose to keep them functioning, neurons weaken and die.

In Alzheimer's disease, the brain has a lower than normal level of insulin, thus reducing its ability to take up and utilize glucose.[16] Reduced glucose utilization and deficient energy metabolism occurs early in the course of the disease, suggesting a causative role in the disease process and thus giving rise to the discovery that Alzheimer's disease is actually a third form of diabetes similar yet distinct from either type 1 or type 2 diabetes.

Medical researchers at Brown Medical School first reported on this novel third form of "brain diabetes" in 2005, after discovering that insulin and its related proteins are reduced in the brain of Alzheimer's disease patients.[1] The term "type 3 diabetes" was coined by Dr. Suzanne de la Monte, a neuropathologist and lead researcher of the group.

This was the first study to provide direct evidence of the suspected link between diabetes and Alzheimer's. New evidence continues to emerge, adding to the concept that Alzheimer's disease is a type of brain diabetes.

Alzheimer's disease isn't the only neurodegenerative condition associated with insulin resistance. Studies of Parkinson's disease patients have also provided evidence for altered glucose metabolism in this disorder.[17] The alterations are, in general, similar to those in Alzheimer's and include abnormal glucose tolerance and increased insulin resistance. These findings are particularly interesting because studies in rodents indicate that chronic high blood sugar can cause dysfunction of dopaminergic transmission.

Since the 1950s glucose intolerance has been reported in a significant percentage of patients with ALS.[18-19] Researchers in Paris found that in 21 non-diabetic ALS patients compared to 21 age- and sex-matched normal subjects, the ALS patients showed abnormal glucose tolerance and higher risk of insulin resistance.[20]

Insulin Resistance and the Brain

Brain insulin resistance and Alzheimer's disease appear to be strongly influenced by whole body insulin resistance. The details have yet to be worked out, but in a nutshell, here is the general theory. As a person develops insulin resistance, insulin levels in the blood rise. Since insulin in the brain comes primarily from the pancreas and is delivered to the brain by way of the bloodstream, you might expect brain insulin levels to rise as well. This is not the case. When insulin in the bloodstream rises, insulin levels in the brain actually fall, dipping *below normal*. High blood insulin leads to low brain insulin. The primary reason for this is that insulin resistance causes the blood-brain barrier to become resistant to insulin. Insulin passage through the blood-brain barrier is restricted. With less insulin getting to the brain, less glucose is able to enter the neurons and power brain cell functions. Neurons deprived of nourishment begin to starve, degenerate, and die.

The shortage of brain insulin isn't the only problem. Insulin-resistant individuals also have elevated blood glucose levels. Unlike insulin, glucose is not barred from passing through the blood-brain barrier. Consequently, brain levels of glucose increase. With low insulin levels in the brain, glucose levels remain elevated. If glucose does not go into the cells, it lingers in the blood, where it tends to spontaneously bond to blood proteins and fats forming harmful substances that promote inflammation, glycation, and oxidation, contributing to the formation of amyloid beta peptides and amyloid plaque—a prime feature associated with neurodegenerative disease.

Brain levels of insulin and the insulin receptors in the nerve cells fall sharply during the early stages of Alzheimer's, indicating a primary role of insulin deficiency in the neurodegenerative process. Insulin levels continue to drop progressively as the disease becomes more severe.

It is apparent that insulin plays a central role in the development of Alzheimer's disease. Keeping insulin levels in balance is essential for good mental health. In diabetics, if the pancreas is not producing enough insulin, this hormone is delivered by injection into the bloodstream. A similar process has been suggested for treating brain diabetes.

Injecting insulin into the general bloodstream, however, will not benefit a brain that suffers from insulin resistance. In fact, it may make the situation worse by increasing blood insulin levels, thus making the blood-brain barrier more insulin resistant and reducing insulin passage further.

To avoid raising blood insulin levels or causing hypoglycemia (low blood sugar), the insulin must be injected directly into the brain. A novel way to accomplish this is to deliver the insulin through the nasal passage using a spray. The insulin is absorbed from the nasal passage into the brain without affecting the general circulation. When insulin is delivered daily in this manner, brain insulin levels increase and cognitive function temporarily improves. Only the brain is affected; blood glucose and insulin levels in the rest of the body are unchanged. In early Alzheimer's disease intranasal delivery of insulin has shown to improve memory and increase attention span. It also appears to reduce the levels of sticky amyloid beta.[21]

Researchers have also had success using standard diabetic drugs, such as Avandia, that improve insulin sensitivity—at least in brain tissue cultures in the laboratory. Avandia is a common oral drug taken by those with type 2 diabetes as a treatment for insulin resistance. As with any drug, there are risks of unwanted side effects. The side effects that have been reported with Avandia include blurry vision, breathing problems, chest pain, stomach pain, increased appetite or thirst, skin rashes, swelling in legs and feet, and less commonly confusion and/or disorientation, paralysis, heart attack, and stroke.

Are drugs and nasal sprays the answer? Drugs must be taken daily for life. They are only temporary fixes and don't solve the underlying problem causing the disease. There is a better solution that involves making better dietary choices.

With a dietary approach, you have no costly drugs to buy, don't have to worry about harmful side effects, and best of all, the root cause of the disease, insulin resistance, is corrected naturally. Drugs don't cure the underlying problem; they only mask the symptoms. With Alzheimer's the underlying problem is insulin resistance. Insulin resistance can be successfully treated with diet and lifestyle modifications.

Most neurodegenerative disorders involve the disruption of normal glucose metabolism in the brain. Systemic insulin resistance or type 2 diabetes is a strong risk factor for Alzheimer's and other neurodegenerative disorders. Yet, not all diabetics progress to Alzheimer's, even when insulin resistance is severe. Insulin resistance alone is not enough. There is more involved in neurodegeneration then just a disruption in glucose metabolism. Other factors commonly associated with neurodegeneration include excessive oxidative stress and free-radical destruction, chronic inflammation, and AGE accumulation. There are a number of things that can trigger these conditions, including poor diet, physical trauma, toxins, and infection. It is the combination of insulin resistance with other insults on the brain that ultimately lead to neurodegeneration. In the following chapters you will see how each of these can have a detrimental effect on brain function.

6 Trauma

BLUNT TRAUMA

Blunt trauma is any injury caused by physical force, such as a blow to the head. There is no doubt that blunt trauma can cause brain and spinal cord injuries that affect brain function. This is no more evident than in the sport of boxing where the goal is to slug the opponent so hard as to cause a concussion—a brain injury.

Boxers have one of the highest rates of brain injury of any profession and, consequently, experience a high rate of neurodegeneration. Doctors have a special name for the type of brain damage caused by repeated physical trauma to the head: dementia pugilistica. The symptoms may include memory loss, tremors, lack of coordination, inappropriate behavior, unsteady gait, and speech problems which can mimic the appearance of being drunk. For this reason, it is often called *punch-drunk syndrome*. The loss of neurons, scarring, and build-up of protein aggregates in the brains of boxers who suffer from dementia pugilistica is very similar to those found in other neurodegenerative diseases.

Trauma to the head and neck has long been known to affect cognitive ability and motor skills. The effects are not always immediately noticeable, especially if the trauma is relatively minor. Injuries, even minor ones, cause the release of free radicals, stimulate inflammation, and promote the creation of abnormal proteins such as amyloid beta that are associated with neurodegen-erative diseases.[1] When injuries, regardless of their intensity, are repeated over the course of many years, as typical in numerous sports, inflammation becomes chronic. Over time, brain cells degenerate and abnormal pro-teins build up, forming the characteristics seen in neuro-

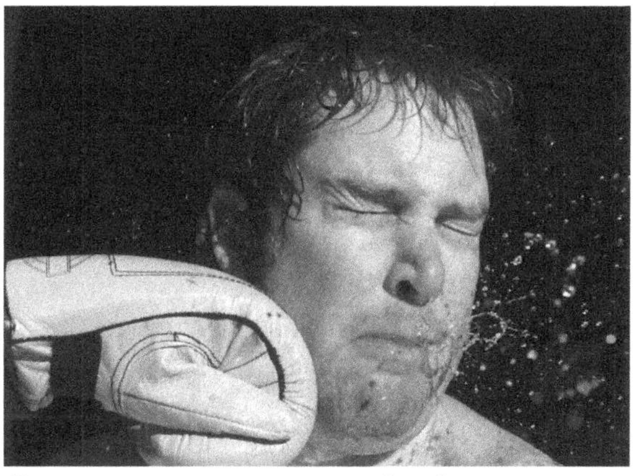

Boxers experience extensive head trauma.

degenerative diseases. For this reason, it is common for retired boxers to develop neurodegenerative disorders later in their lives.[2] Among the many boxers who have fallen prey to neurodegenerative disease are Muhammad Ali (Parkinson's), Joe Louis (dementia), Floyd Patterson (Alzheimer's), Jack Demsey (Parkinson's), Jerry Quarry (dementia), Sugar Ray Robinson (Alzheimer's), Ezzard Charles (ALS), and Leon Spinks (dementia), to mention just a few.

Brain trauma isn't limited to just boxers but can occur in those who participate in any number of sports or recreational activities. It is also seen in many non-athletic situations such as car accidents and falls.

Amyotrophic lateral sclerosis (ALS) is frequently associated with athletes and head trauma. It's the disease that took the life of baseball legend Lou Gehrig. An unusually large number of boxers, football players, baseball players, soccer players, jockeys, and other professional athletes develop ALS. Although the disease normally surfaces after retirement, in some cases it occurs while the players are still actively involved in sports, as was the case with Lou Gehrig, World Heavyweight boxing champion Ezzard Charles, and Houston Oilers football player Glenn Montgomery.

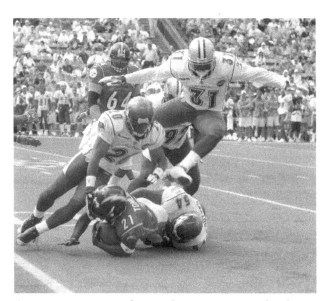

Some sports provide ample opportunity for brain injury.

While some notable athletes had come down with ALS over the years, the connection to head trauma wasn't fully recognized until it was discovered that an unusually large number of European soccer players were developing the disease. It is believed that the repetitive jarring that occurs when players are controlling and advancing the ball with their heads may cause brain injury which can eventually lead to ALS. Studies have since confirmed the connection between head, neck, and back injuries to increased risk of ALS.[3] Even mild repetitive injury as you would receive by bouncing a soccer ball on the head can increase the risk of ALS.[4]

Multiple minor injuries have an accumulative effect, but a single injury of more severity can be just as risky. In one study, questionnaires were sent to patients with ALS who had developed the disease before the age of 45. Out of 135 patients who responded, 78 (58 percent) of them reported having sustained injuries severe enough to have required medical attention prior to the onset of the illness. The findings of this investigation showed that suffering a single severe head or neck injury is a high risk factor in ALS.[5]

The more head injuries sustained, the greater the risk. Another study showed that for those who had multiple head injuries with the latest occurring in the past 10 years, risk was elevated to more than 11 times the risk of those who had suffered only one head injury. Injury to other parts of the body like the arms, legs, and trunk were not related to ALS risk.[6]

Studies with Alzheimer's patients have shown similar results.[7] There appears to be a strong link between head injury and future risk of neurodegenerative disease. Those people who sustain head and neck injuries are two to three times more likely to develop ALS, FTD, Alzheimer's and other neurodegenerative disease later in life.[8-10]

Injuries don't have to come as a result of professional sports. Many everyday head injuries can promote neurodegenerative disease. A 38-year-old man struck his forehead against the windshield in a near head-on motor vehicle accident. He immediately began experiencing neck pain radiating down the left arm and weakness in his left hand. Five months after the accident he was diagnosed with ALS.

Symptoms may surface within months of an accident or may not appear until years later. In some cases, brain injury associated with neurodegeneration has been traced back to childhood. A serious childhood accident may set the stage for problems in the future.

HYPOXIA

Another form of trauma is hypoxia. Hypoxia occurs when the brain is starved of oxygen. Brain cells can survive only a few minutes without oxygen. This may occur during birth: a baby's brain cannot tolerate a lack of oxygen for more than about five minutes. At any age, hypoxia may occur as a result of cardiac arrest (stoppage of the heart), cerebrovascular accident (stroke), respiratory arrest (cessation of breathing), poisoning, drowning, electric shock, or status epilepticus (prolonged convulsions).

Interfering with the normal blood flow and delivery of oxygen to the brain is one of the most prominent causes of brain dysfunction. Hypoxia resulting from asphyxiation during birth is one cause of cerebral palsy. Later in life, cerebral hypoxia can result from accidents such as choking or from arrest of breathing and heart beat following electrocution or drowning. From middle age onward the most common cause of hypoxia of the brain is stroke.

When a major artery, such as the carotid artery that feeds the brain, suddenly becomes clogged or ruptures, a stroke accompanied by severe and life-threatening symptoms occurs. Symptoms may include the sudden onset of numbness or weakness in the face, arms, or legs on one side of the body, confusion, trouble speaking or understanding, visual difficulties, trouble walking, dizziness, loss of balance, and severe headache. If a person survives a stroke, he or she is often left with some permanent brain damage that may affect motor or cognitive skills.

A less severe stroke that affects smaller arteries, called a transient ischemic attack, is a temporary interruption of blood flow to a part of the brain. The signs and symptoms are the same as for a stroke but last for a much shorter period (several minutes to 24 hours) and then disappear without leaving noticeable permanent effects. These attacks can and often do recur. They may be so subtle that they go unrecognized, being attributed to fatigue, aging, or some other cause. Although the effects may seem to go away, these mini-strokes cause damage that can build over time, leading to dementia, Alzheimer's, and other forms of neurodegenerative disease.

Although the precise cause is still unknown, the major risk factors for stroke include high blood pressure, overweight, diabetes, atherosclerosis (hardening of the arteries), and smoking. Risk factors associated specifically with stroke-induced dementia include all the above in addition to living in a rural area, occupational exposure to pesticides or fertilizers, depression, living in an institution, and taking aspirin.[11] Recently, bacterial and viral infections have been added to this list,[12] along with consuming foods containing trans fatty acids.

Trans fatty acids are toxic fat molecules found in hydrogenated and partially hydrogenated vegetable oils. Margarine and shortening are hydrogenated vegetable oils. Liquid vegetable oils are hydrogenated to make them solid at room temperature and to give them an extended shelf life. Liquid vegetable oils oxidize very quickly and easily, imparting a rancid flavor to foods. By hydrogenating the oil, foods oxidize or go rancid more slowly and maintain their flavor longer. Hydrogenated vegetable oil is found in a wide variety of processed foods including chips, crackers, cookies, candy, bread, frozen waffles, toaster pastries, soups, frozen dinners, pizza, pot pies, ice cream, salad dressings, tacos, burritos, beans—the list goes on and on. Almost all deep fried foods, whether they come from a grocery store or a restaurant, are cooked in hydrogenated vegetable oils—French fries, onion rings, donuts, chicken nuggets, battered fish, hushpuppies, okra, etc. Hydrogenated oil is popular for deep frying because it can be used far longer than liquid vegetable oils before going rancid. Saturated fats like beef tallow or coconut oil would be far healthier to use in frying because they do not break down like liquid vegetable oils do under normal cooking temperatures, and they contain no trans fatty acids.

Recently, researchers at the University of North Carolina, Chapel Hill announced that diets high in trans fatty acids significantly raise the risk of stroke. The study involved over 87,000 participants as part of the Women's Health Initiative. Of those who had high intakes of trans fat—approximately 7 grams a day—there was an associated 30 percent increased risk of stroke.

Trans fatty acids have been linked to a number of health problems, including diabetes, autoimmune disease, obesity, and heart disease, as well as stroke. Researchers at the Institute of Medicine of the United States spent three years reviewing and evaluating all the published studies on hydrogenated oils and trans fatty acids. At the end of their review they made a public announcement. They warned that no level of trans fatty acids was safe in the diet. What surprised everyone was the Institute of Medicine didn't give a recommendation as to what percentage of trans fats were safe to consume, as is often done with food additives, but flatly stated that *no* level of trans fats is safe to eat. Because of this announcement, the FDA enacted a new regulation requiring all food manufacturers to state the amount of trans fats contained in their products. This statement is found in the nutritional side panel on all packaged foods sold in the United States. Canada and some other countries have similar requirements.

Factors that seem to protect against stroke include eating shellfish, getting regular exercise, and, believe it or not, eating saturated fat. Numerous studies have consistently shown that saturated fat intake in animals and humans reduces incidence of stroke.[13-16] One of the most notable of these studies was conducted by researchers from Harvard Medical School. The aim of the study was to examine the association of stroke incidence with intake and type of fat during 20 years of follow-up among middle-aged men participating in the Framingham Heart Study. The study involved 832 men between the ages of 45 and 65 who were initially free of cardiovascular disease. In conformity with previous studies, intakes of saturated fat were associated with reduced risk of ischemic stroke. The study also showed that the highest incidence of stroke was associated with the highest polyunsaturated fat consumption.

The fact that saturated fat protects against stroke is a surprise for most people. The prevailing opinion for many years has viewed saturated fat as detrimental to the cardiovascular system. This belief is beginning to change as new research emerges. This topic will be discussed in more detail in a later chapter.

7 Drugs

One of the most memorable anti-drug public service commercials ever aired on television showed a man who held up an egg and said, "This is your brain." He then shows a hot frying pan and adds, "This is drugs." He proceeds to crack open the egg and drop the contents into the sizzling hot pan. As the egg crackles and fries in the hot grease, he says, "This is your brain on drugs." Finally he looks up at the camera and asks, "Any questions?" Although this public service announcement was meant to discourage the use of street drugs, it is applicable to many prescription and over-the-counter drugs as well.

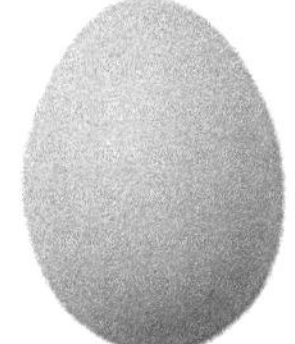

This is your brain.

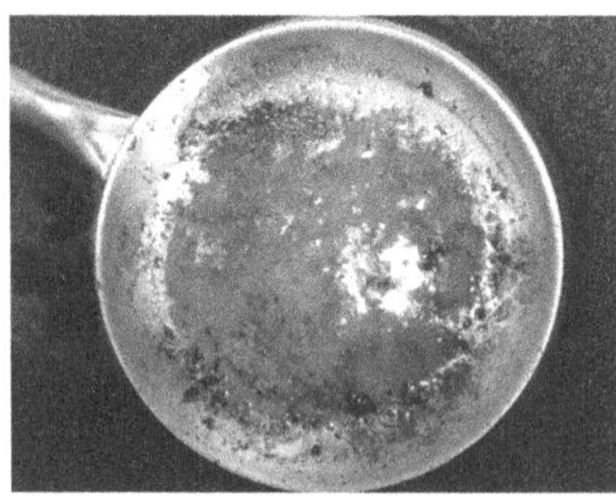

This is drugs.

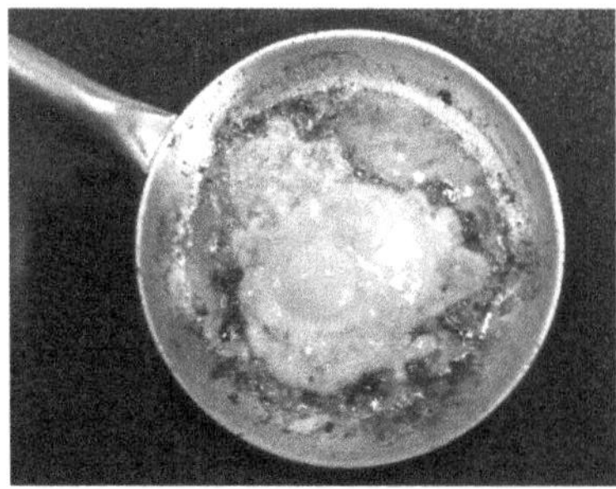

This is your brain on drugs. Any questions?

There are many drugs that disrupt normal brain chemistry and function, some of which people use nearly every day. They include Valium, Xanax, Klonopin, Ativan, Prozac, Ritalin, Zoloft, and Haldol, which are prescribed for patients with psychiatric disorders; Lunesta, Ambien, Rozerem, Halcion, Sominex, and Sonata for insomnia; Reglan, Octamide, and Metozolv for stomach disorders; Zantac, Pepcid, and Tagamet used to treat excess stomach acid; Tylenol PM, Anacin PM, Excedrin PM, Advil, Motrin, and Aleve for pain relief; Dristan, Dimetapp, Sinutab, Contac, NyQuil, and Benadryl for colds and allergies; and Harmonyl and Cardura for high blood pressure, among others. Chronic use of any of them can lead to a variety of mental problems. Reglan, for instance, which is given to patients who suffer from digestive disorders such as GERD, interferes with neurons that process dopamine, and can cause irreversible and incurable involuntary repetitive movements like those of Parkinson's disease. Frequent users of Zantac and other antacids have a 2.5 times increased risk of developing dementia.[1] The cholesterol-lowering statin drugs, which are commonly prescribed for the middle-aged and elderly, are among the most frequently prescribed drugs associated with memory loss, mental confusion, depression, and suicide.

In this chapter we cannot cover all the drugs that may have adverse effects on the central nervous system. What is provided is a sample of some of the more common or interesting drugs that can affect mental health, especially those that promote neurodegenerative disease.

ANESTHETICS AND PAINKILLERS

"My dad (age 71) was outside taking the seats out of his van, to clean," says Danette. "He ended up falling over the seat, onto his back, on the concrete driveway. He ruptured several disks and cracked his vertebrae. His only option was to have back surgery...*My dad had no previous signs of Alzheimer's*...Then immediately following his surgery 'boom'...almost like he had just had Alzheimer's inserted into his brain during surgery or something. From that point, it was on, full blast. His memory quickly deteriorated and five years later, he lies in a hospital bed in my mother's home, in diapers and plastic sheets, never to even walk again."

An estimated 200 million patients worldwide undergo surgery each year. Some of the side effects of the general anesthetics used in surgery include cognitive impairment, delirium, and confusion. This problem is particularly pronounced in the elderly and especially in those who already display some cognitive difficulties. Postoperative neurologic impairment can affect as many as 61 percent of elderly patients undergoing surgery.[2] In most cases the mental disturbance is only temporary, but in some cases it can be permanent. If the patient already has symptoms of neurodegeneration, such as the early stages of Alzheimer's, it can worsen and accelerate the condition. Several studies have shown that general anesthetics can lead to Alzheimer's disease and Parkinson's disease, even when neither of these conditions existed prior to surgery.[3-4]

Unfortunately, many people go into surgery unaware of the potential danger. Incidences such as the one described above are all too common. "My father was just diagnosed with a progressive form of Alzheimer's disease," says Sherrie. "A year ago he underwent an operation. After this operation he quickly began to lose his math skills, being an estimator for a paving company he lost his job. He went downhill fast, emotionally. Six months later he was getting lost in the house. Frantically, I tried to get my mom to get him tested so we could see what was wrong. She begged me to wait until after he underwent yet another oral surgery to have four titanium implants put into his lower jaw. He again, in less than a year, went under anesthesia. His condition worsened at an alarming rate! He started having delusions, confusion, conversations that one word didn't go with the next! I *know* for a fact that anesthesia does exacerbate Alzheimer's, if it's there, but it also *accelerates* it! *Why are we not being told?* The doctor mentioned that 85 percent of his Alzheimer's patients are there because of anesthesia! My dad may have had Alzheimer's disease before, but it would have progressed more slowly! My dad is only 67."

"My dad is only 63," says Amy. "He was just diagnosed with early Alzheimer's in the last 3 years. On October 1 (a week before his 63rd birthday), he had to have a kidney stone crushed. They used anesthesia. He hasn't been the same since! He's in the hospital now. I'm going crazy! All of his tests have come back negative (as far as infections, heart problems, diabetes, etc.). He's hallucinating, talking gibberish, can't remember his birthday. It's like his Alzheimer's went off a cliff and progressed 30 years in a week!"

Although mental disturbances are frequently seen in the elderly after surgery, it has often been viewed as a temporary and minor side effect. But recent studies are showing it isn't necessarily temporary or minor. Permanent damage often occurs.

A number of studies have shown that applying anesthetics to cultured brain cells can lead to the formation of amyloid beta proteins—the hallmark feature of senile plaques seen in the brains of Alzheimer's patients—and to the cell-death process known as apoptosis. "Our studies have shown that isoflurane (a common anesthetic gas) may induce a vicious cycle of apoptosis, amyloid beta generation, and further rounds of apoptosis leading to cell death," says Zhongcong Xie, MD, PhD, of the MassGeneral Institute for Neurodegenerative Disease.[5]

When isoflurane is given to laboratory animals in doses comparable to what is given to human patients during surgery, they develop the same degenerative features found in treated cell cultures. Insults to the brain from anesthetics "may lead to long-term brain damage," says Dr. Xie and "may promote Alzheimer's disease."[6]

Brenda Plassman, PhD, and colleagues at Duke University Medical Center agree. "Short-term postoperative cognitive dysfunction is common among the elderly," she says. Her team of investigators examined the long term effects (over 6 months) of anesthesia in human patients after surgery. They evaluated 856 surgical patients aged 70 years or older. "Our findings suggest an increased risk of dementia after surgery with general anesthesia among older adults," says Plassman. "This increased risk for dementia may be an important factor to consider when making decisions about surgery, especially those that are elective, in later life."[7]

Anesthetic gases such as isoflurane and halothane seem to cause more trouble than intravenous anesthetics. But most general anesthetics are risky. If surgery is needed, it may be best to opt for intravenous anesthetics as opposed to anesthetic gas. Better yet, if possible, choose local anesthesia, which does not carry the same risk as general anesthesia.

Anesthetics are used in a hospital setting to deaden pain or render a patient unconscious. Other milder forms of painkillers can be prescribed by doctors or purchased over the counter. These too, can have detrimental effects on brain health.

Research suggests that older people who want to avoid Alzheimer's disease or other forms of dementia might want to avoid taking anti-inflammatory painkillers such as ibuprofen (Advil, Motrin), naproxen (Aleve), and celecoxib (Celebrex).

Since chronic brain inflammation is a well-known feature of Alzheimer's disease as well as other neurodegenerative diseases, scientists have speculated that reducing inflammation through the use of nonsteroidal anti-inflammatory drugs (NSAIDs)

Hospitals Could Be Detrimental to Your Mental Health

If you want to maintain your mental health, stay out of the hospital. That is the conclusion that may be made based on a study that appeared recently in the *Journal of the American Medical Association*.[22]

The study reported that older people are likely to suffer a significant decline in cognitive abilities and have an increased risk of developing dementia after being hospitalized. It has long been observed that older patients develop long-term cognitive impairment after a hospital stay. This study set out to determine the risk of cognitive decline and dementia in older individuals who are hospitalized as compared to those who are not.

The study followed almost 3,000 people 65 and older for more than a decade. None of the participants had dementia at the start of the study. Those who were hospitalized for any reason, on average, experienced a statistically significant drop in performance on cognitive tests when compared to age-matched people who had not been hospitalized. Those who had been hospitalized for relatively minor, noncritical illnesses faced a 40 percent increase in dementia after the hospitalization, and those who experienced critical conditions, like a severe infection or cardiac arrest, were more than twice as likely to develop dementia afterwards.

While some of the cognitive impairment could stem from the illness itself, the researchers said side effects of treatment, including medications administered in the hospital, were likely the primary cause for the cognitive decline.

might prevent or improve the symptoms of Alzheimer's disease. Some studies using aspirin seem to support this hypothesis.

To test this hypothesis further, researchers evaluated the effects of two common anti-inflammatory pain killers (Vioxx and Aleve) on Alzheimer's patients and compared them with patients taking dummy pills (placebos). They found that the anti-inflammatory painkillers had no benefit in slowing the decline of Alzheimer's disease. In fact, those taking the drugs displayed greater mental decline than the subjects taking placebos. In addition, the treatment group also experienced a higher percentage of adverse effects such as fatigue, dizziness, and hypertension. Vioxx was later taken off the market because it was found to increase the risk of heart attacks and strokes.[8]

A few years later a larger study was conducted using more than 2,000 people aged 70 and older with a family history of Alzheimer's but no cognitive problems themselves. The anti-inflammatory painkillers Aleve and Celebrex (a drug similar to Vioxx) were compared to a placebo. The study was to continue for several years, but was halted early when heart risk turned up in those taking Celebrex. Researchers also noticed more heart attacks and strokes in the people taking Aleve. Despite the study's early end, the data showed that both the Celebrex and Aleve users had lower cognitive scores than those who had been given placebos.[9]

The following year another study was published that involved 2,700 subjects age 65 and older. In this study, investigators checked the subject's usage of Advil and Aleve. They found that people who used these drugs frequently were 66 percent more likely to develop dementia than those who used them less often.[10] Each of the above studies showed that the use of the painkillers tested accelerated mental decline. Other NSAIDs such as indomethacin (Indocin), oxaprozin (Daypro), and piroxicam (Feldene) caused various neurological disturbances ranging from mental confusion and vertigo to Parkinson's and epilepsy.

Although aspirin and Tylenol also carry risks of side effects, they don't appear to be as harmful to the central nervous system as many other painkillers. But when these painkillers are combined with other drugs and marketed as treatments for conditions other than just relieving pain, problems may arise. Case in point: Tylenol PM, which is marketed as a sleep aid and treatment for allergies.

Public attention was first brought to Tylenol PM by neurologist Amarish Dave, MD. He tells of a 57-year-old patient who experienced memory loss, confusion, and difficulty concentrating for over a year. Initially the symptoms suggested early-onset dementia. Dr. Dave reviewed all the medications she was on and found that Tylenol PM was being taken as a sleep aid. Knowing one of the active ingredients can aggravate mental decline, he eliminated the medication from the patient's regimen. Improvement was almost immediate. The patient described herself as "coming out of a fog" after stopping the Tylenol PM.

Tylenol PM contains two ingredients known to affect the brain, the pain numbing drug acetaminophen and the antihistamine diphenhydramine (the active ingredient used in the allergy/cold medication Benadryl). Diphenhydramine is a member of a class of drugs known as anticholinergics. This drug exerts a number of adverse effects on the central nervous system. Other Tylenol products to watch out for include Tylenol Cold Relief, Tylenol Sore Throat Nighttime, Extra Strength Tylenol Aches and Strains, Extra Strength Tylenol Allergy, and even medications for children such as Children's Tylenol Cold and Children's Tylenol Allergy. Anacin PM and Excedrin PM contain the same two chemically active ingredients as Tylenol PM.

"I find that many of these patients are on medications that have anticholinergic properties that can cause memory problems, and by eliminating them, the memory problems can sometimes lessen or improve, and sometimes improve dramatically," says Dr. Dave. "Typically anticholinergic side effects are thought of as mainly a concern for elderly patients, however, in this case, my patient was in her 50's. If you think about how many patients in midlife are on medications like Tylenol PM that have anticholinergic side effects, it's astounding, and that has major implications for evaluation of memory loss in this age group."

Anticholinergics include not only antihistamines but also a wide variety of medications often given to middle-aged and elderly patients, all of which can have adverse side effects on mental ability and motor skills.

ANTICHOLINERGICS

Anticholinergics are a class of medications that inhibit the function of cholinergic neurons (neurons in the parasympathetic nervous system and motor neurons supplying skeletal muscles) by blocking the action of the neurotransmitter acetylcholine. Blocking this neurotransmitter prevents nerve transmissions that control involuntary movements of the smooth muscles present in the gastrointestinal tract, urinary tract, lungs, and blood vessels.

Anticholinergic drugs are used to treat a variety of disorders such as stomach ulcers, gastritis, acid reflux (GERD), heartburn, diverticulitis, ulcerative colitis, cystitis, urethritis, prostatitis, urinary incontinence, asthma, chronic bronchitis, motion sickness, muscular spasms, high blood pressure, Parkinson's disease, poisoning with certain toxic compounds, and as an aid in anesthesia. Most antihistamines used for allergies and colds are anticholinergics. These drugs are also used to induce sleep.

As you might expect, any drug that alters brain chemistry and affects so many body systems is bound to have some adverse reactions. Below are some of the common side effects associated with anticholinergic drugs.

General Side Effects:
Apnea (failure in breathing)
Burning pain in the throat
Loss of coordination
Decreased mucus production in the nose and throat
Dry mouth
Drowsiness
Cessation of perspiration
Headache
Hypotension (low blood pressure)
Increased body temperature
Muscle pain
Muscle weakness
Nausea
Pupil dilation and sensitivity to bright light
Blurred or double vision
Rapid heart rate (tachycardia)
Constipation
Restlessness
Shaking
Urinary retention

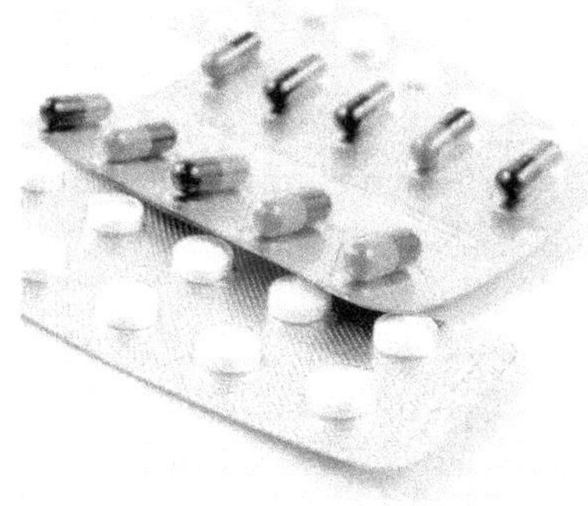

Central Nervous System Side Effects:
Anxiety
Delirium
Confusion
Disorientation

Dizziness
Agitation
Memory loss
Hallucinations
Inability to concentrate
Inability to sustain a train of thought
Incoherent speech
Involuntary muscle twitching and jerking
Unusual sensitivity to sudden sounds
Illogical thinking
Seizures
Coma

It is of interest to note that anticholinergics were some of the first drugs prescribed for the treatment of Parkinson's disease and are still currently being used. If you look at the list of side effects you will notice many of the classic symptoms of Parkinson's disease such as muscle weakness, involuntary muscle twitching and jerking, shaking, and speech problems are included! In fact, some anticholinergics can produce parkinsonism. So why would doctors give a drug to someone who is already suffering from these symptoms?

Since all drugs carry risks, doctors must weigh the risks of the drugs they prescribe with the benefits. Many doctors feel the benefits, at least initially, outweigh the risks.

In a normal healthy brain there is a balance between the neurotransmitters dopamine and acetylcholine. In Parkinson's disease dopamine-producing neurons are lost, decreasing the amount of dopamine in the brain. However, acetylcholine levels remain fairly normal. This imbalance is believed to contribute to some of the symptoms associated with Parkinson's disease. Anticholinergic drugs suppress the action of acetylcholine, bringing back a balance between dopamine and acetylcholine. However, this also means instead of having only one deficient neurotransmitter, there are now two. This might help with some symptoms but create others.

The anticholinergic drugs used for Parkinson's disease include benztropine, biperiden, diphenhydramine, ethopropazine, orphenadrine, procyclidine and trihexyphenidyl. Perhaps these drugs help temporarily, but in the long run they will accelerate the progression of the disease.

It has been known for some time that people with dementia should not be given anticholinergic drugs because their symptoms worsen. Even those with normal cognitive skills can be adversely affected.

This discovery started with a simple observation from Jack Tsao, MD, a neurologist at the Uniformed Medical Services University in Bethesda, Maryland. Dr. Tsao was examining a 74-year-old woman who had suddenly started having hallucinations and memory problems. Surprised at the sudden onset of symptoms, before conducting extensive tests to see whether she had Alzheimer's, he looked for any medicines she was taking that could be responsible. She had recently begun taking 2 milligrams of Detrol, a medication for overactive bladder. The symptoms seemed to coincide with the medication. She stopped taking the medication and within weeks her symptoms disappeared.

This experience prompted Dr. Tsao to conduct a study to see to what extent anticholinergics have on those with normal cognitive abilities. He compared 191 people who had never taken medication with anticholinergic properties with 679 who had. The average age of the participants was 75 years. Over an eight year period the rate of cognitive decline among the group taking the medications was 1.5 times as fast as those not taking the drugs. Evidentially, anyone taking anticholinergic drugs experiences some cognitive decline.

In some people the loss of mental ability is transient and will reverse itself once the drugs are discontinued, while in others it can be permanent. Studies are now showing that the frequent use of anticholinergic drugs may not only produce short-term cognitive effects but also increase the risk for irreversible brain damage leading to dementia and parkinsonism.[11]

Some classes of drugs should always be avoided for the elderly because the risks outweigh the benefits. Yet these drugs are still routinely prescribed, when there are often better and safer alternatives. Thirty percent of the hospital admissions of elderly patients are linked to adverse effects from drugs.[12] One nursing home study showed that 66 percent of the residents had adverse drug reactions over a four-year period, with 1 in 7 requiring hospitalization.[13]

In 1997 Mark H. Beers, MD, and an expert panel of doctors identified a number of medications which they deemed inappropriate for persons older than 65 years of age, regardless of the patient's level of health or severity of illness.[14] The panel agreed that the potential risks associated with these drugs outweighed the potential benefits and should not be used by this age group. The list of drugs is known as the "Beers Criteria for Potentially Inappropriate Medication Use in Older Adults." The list was updated in 2003.[15] Among the classes of drugs listed are the anticholinergic drugs. The reasons for this is evident when you look at the long list of side effects accompanying these drugs, not the least of which are the effects on brain health.

Many of the conditions for which anticholinergic drugs are used are common in middle-aged and elderly people. Consequently, many older adults frequently use these drugs. However, anticholinergics are expressly singled out as not appropriate for seniors. Yet doctors still prescribe them to older adults and many are available over the counter and marketed to this age group.

Anticholinergics include some of the most recognized drugs on the market. Among them are Dristan, Benadryl, Contac, Sominex, Vicks Formula 44m, Zantac, and all the many forms of Tylenol (i.e., Tylenol Cold Relief, Tylenol PM, etc.) although not Tylenol itself. For an extensive list of anticholinergics and other medications that adversely affect the central nervous system, see Appendix C: Drugs Seniors Should Avoid.

Seniors take, on average, between two and six prescription drugs and one to three over-the-counter drugs regularly. It is unfortunate that many elderly people live for years and die with dementia, parkinsonism, or other neurological disorders that were drug-induced. In many cases simply removing the drug would have brought substantial relief.

Ironically, some of the drugs used to treat neurodegeneration accelerate the progression of the disease or cause troubling side effects that are as bad as the condition they are meant to treat.

Since blocking the neurotransmitter acetylcholine with anticholinergic drugs often causes degenerative processes that promote dementia, doing the opposite might improve brain function. Using this logic, drugs (cholinesterase inhibitors) that inhibit the enzyme which breaks down acetylcholine would allow more of this neurotransmitter to be used by the brain. The popular Alzheimer's drugs Aricept (donepezil), Exelon (rivastigmine), and Reminyl (galantamine) work in this way. But like all drugs, these have adverse side effects, including death. In a recent study involving 648 patients taking Aricept and 326 taking a placebo, the treatment group had 11 deaths after just 24 weeks of use. The placebo group had none.[16]

The study showed these drugs have "questionable" value, yet sales for these three drugs accounted for over $861 million in 2004. These drugs are not temporary medications; they are meant to be taken for life, even though that life may be cut short.

These drugs sell well not because they are effective but because of the marketing skills of the drug industry. The successful strategy to sell Alzheimer's drugs is based on hope, fear, and guilt: hope that one of these drugs might "work," fear that if one of these drugs is not started quickly all will be lost, and guilt if family members do not make the decision to "fight" the disease with these expensive, minimally effective drugs.

Any drug that messes with brain chemistry can have serious consequences. Ironically, doctors often prescribe Aricept along with anticholinergic drugs. The effects of each cancel the other out, destroying any therapeutic value of either, while both continue to mess with the brain and produce undesirable side effects as a result.

STATINS

The statins are the most profitable prescription drugs of all time, generating billions of dollars a year in profits for drug manufacturers. While they are touted as safe, they have a long list of troublesome side effects including digestive problems, muscle degeneration and pain, liver failure, kidney failure, mental deterioration, and brain damage leading to memory loss, mood swings, and behavioral changes. Next to muscle pain, the most frequently reported side effect to statin therapy is cognitive problems.[17]

The most popular statins are Lipitor, Crestor, Pravachol, Zocor, and Mevacor, with Lipitor being by far the most commonly prescribed. Another statin, Baycol, was pulled off the market in 2001 because of an alarming number of users suffered from severe muscle wasting, kidney failure, and death.

Beatrice A. Golomb, MD, PhD, heads the Statin Study Group at the University of California at San Diego. Her group is actively researching the side effects of statin medications. She has collected thousands of case reports from patients about statin side effects. She says common complaints from patients taking statins include being unable to remember the name of a grandchild, walking into a room and forgetting why you are there, or starting a sentence and being unable to finish. Some complain of personality changes or irritability.

One typical example is 69-year-old Jane Brunzie. Brunzie was so forgetful that her daughter was investigating Alzheimer's care for her and refused to let her babysit her 9-year-old granddaughter. Then Brunzie stopped taking the statins. "Literally, within eight days, I was back to normal—it was that dramatic," says Brunzie. Doctors put her on different statins three more times. "They'd say, 'Here, try these samples.' Doctors don't want to give up on it," she says. "Within a few days of starting another one, I'd start losing my words again," says Brunzie. With a clear mind she has gone back to volunteering at the local elementary school she loves. "I feel very blessed—I got about 99 percent of my memory back," she adds. "But I worry about people like me who are starting to lose their words who may think they have just normal aging and it may not be."

While all the statins carry the risk of neurological problems, the most popular statin, Lipitor, appears to be the most troublesome in this regard. Memory problems can occur within five days after taking a statin drug but may not surface until after several years of statin therapy. Memory loss can occur suddenly, causing complete amnesia accompanied by confusion and disorientation. After discontinuing the drug, memory may return. However, in some cases cognitive problems may continue indefinitely.

STEROIDAL HORMONES

During his five years as a backup quarterback for the San Francisco 49ers in the 1960s, Bob Waters suffered his share of bumps, bruises, and broken bones. At the age of 44 he began to experience some shakiness in his right arm but simply chalked it up to an old playing injury that had been repaired with a metal plate. His doctor suggested it might have something to do with the metal. Waters went on with his life as the football coach at Western Carolina University in Cullowhee, NC. During the next four years the muscle spasms and weakness gradually spread to both arms. Waters became alarmed. There was something more going on than a reaction to the metal plate. In 1985 further evaluation by doctors confirmed his worst fear—he was suffering from ALS.

Waters' random stroke of misfortune soon began to play out like a scene from a medical mystery. Shortly after his diagnosis, Waters learned that former 49ers teammate Gary Lewis, a fullback, was also stricken with ALS. Lewis, died from the disease in December of 1986 at the age of 44. The following month, Waters heard that another teammate from the 1964 squad, 53-year-old Matt Hazeltine, a linebacker, had just died from ALS. All three played for the same team during the 1964 football season. Waters' physical condition continued to deteriorate as he dropped 20 pounds and lost the use of both arms. Within three years he too was dead, at the age of 50.

The only known link between Waters, Lewis, and Hazeltine is that they played for the same team during the 1964 football season. Is it just a coincidence that they each died from the same rare disease? ALS typically strikes about 1 in 50,000

Americans a year, yet it hit three teammates on a 55-man squad. While it could possibly be due to chance, three out of 55 is way out of proportion.

This trio of cases is just one of many clusters of ALS. In Ohio three teachers who taught in the same high school classroom developed the disease. So did six people living on the same hillside behind the Berkeley campus of the University of California. Approximately 85 people who once worked or lived at Kelly Air Force Base in San Antonio, Texas contracted the disease, and at least 17 of them worked in the same building. These clusters of cases suggest that there was something toxic in the diet or environment common to all the victims. Many culprits have been suggested including infection with poliovirus, exposure to heavy metals or pesticides, eating toxic substances, employment in the plastics industry, and a history of traumatic injuries. In the case of the 49ers, the suspect was a fertilizer used on the team's practice field, although this was never proven. Another suspect was provided by Waters himself. He admitted using steroids during his time with the 49ers. Perhaps steroid use combined with repeated head trauma from playing football for so many years contributed to the problem. Or perhaps a combination of head trauma, steroids, and some environmental factor such as contaminated fertilizer or pesticides used on the playing field or some other unrecognized factors collectively contributed to the problem.

Steroid use is a strong possible contributing factor. Anabolic steroids are artificial male sex hormones that are taken as pills or injections to build muscle quickly. Anabolic steroids build bulging muscles but shrink the brain. Research shows they cause a dramatic loss of brain cells. In animals they have been shown to impair learning and memory. Long-term users often suffer from mood swings, hallucinations and paranoia, depression, irritability, and aggressive and suicidal behavior, as well increased risk of stroke, including multiple mini-strokes detrimental to the brain. Steroid-induced aggression is well known in the bodybuilding world, where it is referred to as *roid rage*.

Steroids can cause healthy cells to become "suicidal," causing neuron death and brain shrinkage, which has been implicated in some cases of Alzheimer's, Huntington's, and other neurodegenerative diseases.

Although steroids are banned by the National Football League, many players still use them. Why then, aren't there more cases of neurological disorders? Maybe there are. Players may not always develop ALS, but rather Parkinson's, Alzheimer's and other forms of dementia.

In 2005, neurologist and forensic pathologist Dr. Bennet Omalu made a shocking discovery. Arriving at the Allegheny County coroner's office in Pittsburgh awaiting him for autopsy was the body of Terry Long, a professional football player. Terry Long was a starting offensive lineman for the Pittsburgh Steelers from 1984 to 1991. He had died from drinking antifreeze. In 1991 he was suspended from the team for steroid use. He later rejoined the team but was released at the end of the season. Terry Long had a clinical history of depression, memory loss, and crazy behavior which led him in and out of psych wards. He was bankrupt, living destitute and alone. He attempted suicide using rat poison and other cocktails, but failed until he tried antifreeze.

Dr. Omalu wondered, how did this big athletic man end up so crazy in the head? He was thinking dementia pugilistica (or punch-drunk syndrome, as it is known in boxers). Omalu figured if chronic bashing of the head could destroy a boxer's brain, it could also destroy a football player's brain. When he examined Terry Long's brain, however, it appeared to be normal. There was none of the obvious contusions often seen in dementia pugilistica. There had to be an answer. People don't go crazy for no reason.

Omalu took Terry Long's brain, sliced it, and examined it under the microscope. He was shocked. The brain was riddled with tau proteins. "This stuff should not be in the brain of a 45-year-old man." He said. "This looks more like a 90-year-old brain with advanced Alzheimer's."

Terry Long's brain looked surprisingly like a brain autopsy Omalu performed three years earlier, on former Steelers center Mike Webster, who had died at age 50.

Mike Webster was a nine-time Pro Bowler and Hall of Famer. "Iron Mike" was a legendary Steelers center for 15 seasons. He too exhibited erratic behavior before his death, such as urinating in his own oven and squirting Super Glue on his rotting teeth. Mike Webster bought himself a Taser gun and used it on himself to treat his back pain. He would shock himself into unconsciousness just to get some sleep. Despite his success in his career, when he died he was penniless. How did he lose it? He forgot. Mike Webster forgot how to eat, too. In the end, he was homeless and living in a truck.

Over the next several years Omalu and associates examined the brains of 11 more former football players who suffered from dementia and erratic behavior. All displayed similar brain wasting. Since many of these players had used steroids, it has been suggested that the wasting was most likely a result of a combination of repeated trauma and steroid use—a one-two punch that destroyed their brains.

Another group of steroids that are associated with brain cell death are glucocorticoids.[18] Glucocorticoids are produced in our bodies by the adrenal glands. They are called stress hormones because they are secreted in higher levels during times of stress. Glucocorticoids stimulate the release of glucose into the bloodstream, raise blood pressure, inhibit immune function, and reduce inflammation. Glucocorticoids oppose the action of insulin, inducing a state of insulin resistance. These changes help us cope with stressful situations for brief periods of time. Once the stress has passed, glucocorticoid levels decline and body functions return to normal.

Chronic stress, however, causes excessive amounts of glucocorticoids to be pumped into the bloodstream for extended periods of time. This can bring about many detrimental effects, among which are the death of brain cells and memory loss. Studies show that elevated glucocorticoid levels are especially damaging to the hippocampus, the area of the brain associated with memory.[19] The extent of exposure to glucocorticoids influences the rate of neuron loss to such an extent that chronic stress can accelerate hippocampal degeneration. Chronic stress has been observed in many Alzheimer's patients and is believed to contribute to the development and progression of this disease.[20] Consequently, people who live stressful lifestyles are at greater risk for developing Alzheimer's disease or other forms of dementia later in life.[21]

Cortisol is the most important human glucocorticoid. Cortisol medications are used to treat a wide variety of inflammatory conditions such as arthritis, colitis, asthma, psoriasis, eczema, and allergies. There are numerous preparations of cortisol steroids including tablets, capsules, liquids, topical creams and gels, inhalers, eye drops, and injectable and intravenous solutions. Many can be purchased without a prescription. Excessive use of these products can contribute to insulin resistance, hamper cellular energy production, and kill neurons.

THE CASE OF THE FROZEN ADDICTS

Drugs derived from opium such as heroin, methadone, and morphine can destroy brain cells. These drugs produce low-grade inflammation in the brain along with protein build-up. In autopsies of young drug abusers the damage seen is comparable to what is normally seen in much older people in the early stages of Alzheimer's disease. Synthetic or "designer" opiates can be even more detrimental.

There was an interesting breakthrough in Parkinson's disease that has since become known as "The Case of the Frozen Addicts." A book with that same name was published in 1996 describing the details of seven heroin addicts who mysteriously developed Parkinson's disease. The story begins in 1982 when 42-year-old George Carillo shuffled into the Santa Clara Valley Medical Center in San Jose. He seemed more like a mannequin than a living person. The heroin addict was bent over and twisted, drooling, and unable to speak; nearly every muscle in this body seemed to be stiffened as if frozen. Carillo's symptoms suggested that he had been suffering for at least a decade from Parkinson's disease. Yet, only days earlier he was completely normal. What had happened in those few days to transform an otherwise healthy individual into an advanced case of Parkinson's? The doctors were stymied.

Unable to speak, Carillo managed with his stiffened fingers to scrawl answers to the doctors' questions. The symptoms had appeared suddenly after he tried a synthetic form of heroin that had recently hit the streets. He used the drug for three days and two days later was transformed into a living statue.

In time, clinics in the Santa Clara area reported six more cases of heroin addicts with the same advanced form of Parkinson's disease. All of them had used the synthetic heroin just before the onset of symptoms. A toxicologist at the county crime laboratory recalled a case in 1976 of a Maryland chemistry graduate student who had developed Parkinson's symptoms after injecting himself with a homemade synthetic heroin. The student had been trying to produce a substance similar to the pain-killer Demerol, but had accidently created a related chemical called MPTP. Investigators obtained samples of the drug used by Carillo and tested it. Sure enough, it contained MPTP.

Once MPTP enters the bloodstream, it is converted into another similar but highly toxic chemical (called MPP+) that attacks the substantia nigra, the area of the brain that produces the majority of dopamine, causing the damage found in all Parkinson's patients.

This incident led to some important developments in Parkinson's research. For years research on Parkinson's disease had been limited by the lack of an animal model on which to test new drugs and treatments. MPTP is now being used in animal research to help scientists understand and develop treatments for the disease. In addition, this incident led scientists to suspect that most Parkinson's disease is caused by exposure to toxic substances similar to MPTP. If exposure is heavy, symptoms can occur quickly, as in the case of the seven addicts, but if exposure is light and continued for an extended period of time, Parkinson's symptoms can develop gradually.

USE CAUTION WHEN TAKING DRUGS

In this chapter we have seen that drugs can induce severe neurodegeneration, sometimes quickly as with MPTP and sometimes slowly with chronic use of milder drugs. Drugs that adversely affect the central nervous system may not always lead to permanent injury, but they do contribute to inflammation and free-radical destruction, thus fanning the flames of neurodegeneration and accelerating the onset of dementia, parkinsonism, or ALS.

Most drugs have adverse side effects of one sort or another; often they affect the nervous system, including the brain. Caution should be used whenever you consider taking drugs, regardless whether they are prescription or over-the-counter. You should research the known and suspected side effects of all drugs before taking them. Even seemingly innocent drugs such as antacids and painkillers could have devastating effects on the health of your brain. Doctors often are unaware of many of the side effects to the drugs they prescribe, so you have to research this yourself. The standard reference book for drug side effects is the *Physicians' Desk Reference*. This book is available at most good libraries. You can also search for side effects on any drug in question on the Internet.

Sometimes drugs may be necessary for certain conditions. Avoid those drugs listed in Appendix C and choose safer medications. If possible, it may be better to use a "natural" solution to pharmaceutical drugs—natural being interpreted as herbs, vitamins, homeopathics, diet, exercise, and the like. Two good resources for natural solutions to drugs are *Natural Alternatives to Over-The-Counter and Prescription Drugs* by Michael Murray and *Drugs That Don't Work and Natural Therapies That Do!* By David Brownstein.

8 Environmental Toxins

PESTICIDES

Jackie Christensen was 32 and had just returned to work after the birth of her second child when she noticed something was wrong. When she tried to type, two fingers on her left hand refused to cooperate. "They wouldn't go where I would want them to on the keyboard," says Christensen. "I also had what they frequently call frozen shoulder, with a very low range of motion in my left arm."

She went a few times to doctors but they didn't have any answers for her. Over the next few years her symptoms progressively got worse. She finally consulted with a neurologist. The diagnosis shocked her. She had Parkinson's disease. "I can't have Parkinson's, I'm not old," Christensen exclaimed. But the diagnosis was confirmed when her symptoms immediately improved after taking the Parkinson's drug L-dopa. She was just shy of her 35th birthday.

Why did a disease that usually strikes people after their fifth decade of life and affects men more often than women suddenly attack her? Christensen believes it was caused by her exposure to pesticides as a teenager. Growing up in rural Minnesota, she spent summers working on local farms. She and other teens would engage in a practice known as "walking beans." A pickup truck would drop her and other workers off at the end of the field and they would walk the rows of soybeans, weeding as they went. Later, they would ride a "bean buggy"—a rig attached to the front of a tractor from which they would spray Roundup. The herbicide was often dyed purple so they could see where it was landing, carefully aiming for the weeds and trying to avoid the beans. She frequently dressed in nothing more than a bathing suit and a baseball cap. "I had a great tan those summers." She said. "I had no idea nor gave any thought whatsoever to what I might be exposing myself to, or what the effects might be. After the first day or two of spraying, I could no longer smell the odor of the herbicide. I do remember that when I would come home, my mother would immediately tell me to take a shower because I smelled like chemicals."

Although there is no direct proof that Christensen's exposure to herbicides as a youth caused her disease, research does support her belief. Parkinson's disease has been reported to occur at high rates among farmers and in rural populations, contributing to the hypothesis that agricultural pesticides may be partially responsible. Studies have shown that animals exposed to certain pesticides—specifically maneb, a fungicide, and paraquat, an herbicide—cause Parkinson's symptoms in animals. Researchers at UCLA have provided evidence that the same process may occur in humans as well.

Pesticides applied from the air or ground often drift from their intended treatment sites with measurable concentrations subsequently detected in the air, in plants, and in animals up to several hundred meters from the application sites. The UCLA researchers studied residents from California's Central Valley who lived within 500 meters of fields sprayed with maneb or paraqual. Residents exposed to either chemical had a 75 percent increased risk of Parkinson's disease. The researchers also found that patients who developed early-onset Parkinson's (prior to age 60), such as Christensen, experienced twice the risk if exposed to either chemical alone, and four to six times the risk if exposed to both chemicals.[1]

The researchers concluded that the study uncovered strong evidence that pesticides can cause Parkinson's disease in humans. It shows that exposure to multiple chemicals increases the toxic effects of each. This is important, since we are often exposed to more than one pesticide in the environment.

Exposure to toxins may occur years before the onset of symptoms. This indicates that toxins can set in motion degenerative changes in the brain that, if not stopped, may continue in a downward spiral of neurodegeneration. This is very important because it means that many people who have been exposed but currently do not have any symptoms, may be gradually developing Parkinson's disease or some other neurodegenerative condition without knowing it. Exposure may come not just from pesticides, but from an assortment of chemicals, drugs, and even certain foods. Preventative measures, which we will discuss in coming chapters, can dramatically reduce the risk.

Several studies have shown a relationship between dairy consumption and Parkinson's disease. For instance, in one study, dairy consumption was associated with modest but significant increased risk of developing Parkinson's disease.[2] The more dairy consumed, the greater the risk. The association was stronger in men and was mostly explained by milk consumption. The results could not be attributed to any specific nutrient in the dairy such as calcium, vitamin D, or fat. Since milk and dairy frequently contain trace amounts of pesticides associated with Parkinson's disease, the researchers reasoned that this was the reason for the increased risk.

Feed given to dairy cows is often heavily sprayed, and residual pesticides accumulate in the milk. Not all dairy is contaminated with chemicals. Cows raised under organic conditions are given pesticide-free feed, so the milk is free from industrial chemicals, including growth hormones and antibiotics often added to livestock feed.

NATURAL NEUROTOXINS

Some plants used as food contain natural neurotoxins that can promote neurodegeneration and have been associated with Parkinson's, ALS, and Alzheimer's disease. For years scientists were perplexed by an epidemic of Parkinson's disease in the French West Indies in the Caribbean, particularly on the island of Guadeloupe.

An epidemic of Parkinson's disease gripped the island's population. Investigators discovered that the culprit was one of the popular foods on the island—a heart-shaped, yellow-green fruit known as *soursop* or *pawpaw* (*Annona muricata*).[3] A similar epidemic on the island of New Caledonia in the South Pacific was attributed to the same fruit—which was transplanted from the French West Indies and commercially cultivated.

Various species of pawpaw are native to the Caribbean as well as North and South America. It has been cultivated in many tropical countries around the world. In Spanish-speaking countries it is called *guanabana* and in Portuguese-speaking Brazil it is called *graviola.*

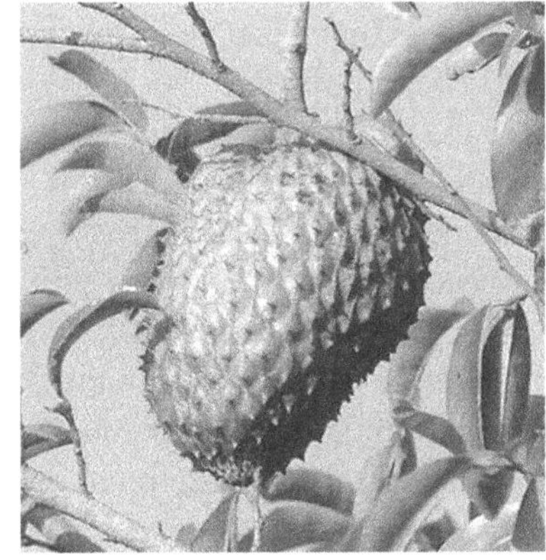

Pawpaw (Annona muricata) *commonly found in the Caribbean and South America.*

The fruit is sold in local markets. Tea is sometimes made from the leaves, and the slightly sour-tasting fruit pulp is made into drinks and sherbets. Historically, the native people used all parts of the tree in herbal medicines for a variety of remedies. The fruit was used to expel worms and parasites. The bark, leaves, and roots were used as sedatives.

Pawpaw is a member of the annonaceae family of plants. These plants contain a chemical toxin called annonacin. Annonacin has been investigated for a number of years as a possible treatment for cancer because it is highly toxic to cancer cells. Unfortunately, it also kills brain cells. It is particularly toxic to neurons in the substantia nigra—the brain cells that produce dopamine. Annonacin is 1,000 times more toxic to neurons than MPP+, the toxic chemical associated with synthetic heroin.[4] Fortunately, the fruit contains much smaller doses than typically used in recreational drugs.

An average fruit is estimated to contain about 15 mg of annonacin. A can of commercial nectar contains 36 mg. As an indication of its potential toxicity, an adult who consumes one fruit or can of nectar a day is estimated to ingest over a period of one year the amount of annonacin shown to induce brain damage in lab animals.[5]

While pawpaw is infrequently consumed in the United States, some varieties of the fruit are native to North America, ranging from Florida to the Midwest as far as Nebraska. The most popular is the species *Asimina triloba,* which produces a sweet fruit similar in texture to a banana. It is sometimes called the Indiana banana. The state of Ohio recently declared the pawpaw its "official native fruit." It isn't seen in stores much because it doesn't ship or store well. However, there is a movement to make the fruit more commercially available. It is enticing to growers because most insects and animals avoid the tree, reducing the need for pesticides. Annonacin, which is most concentrated in the leaves and bark, is marketed and sold as a "natural" insecticide and animal repellent. The pulp of the fruit is often combined with other fruit juices and sold commercially. Its historical medicinal properties are often touted as a "healthy" reason to eat the fruit. Several companies sell it in the form of a dietary supplement and market it as a natural aid to cancer treatment. It is often promoted in various forms on websites under the Brazilian name graviola. While most Americans are still generally unfamiliar with pawpaw, it appears that it will become better known in the future as marketing efforts increase.

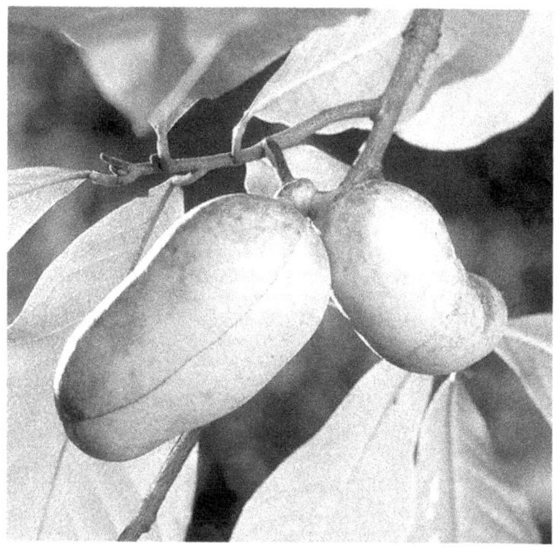

Pawpaw (Asimina triloba) *species native to North America has a banana-like texture with large seeds.*

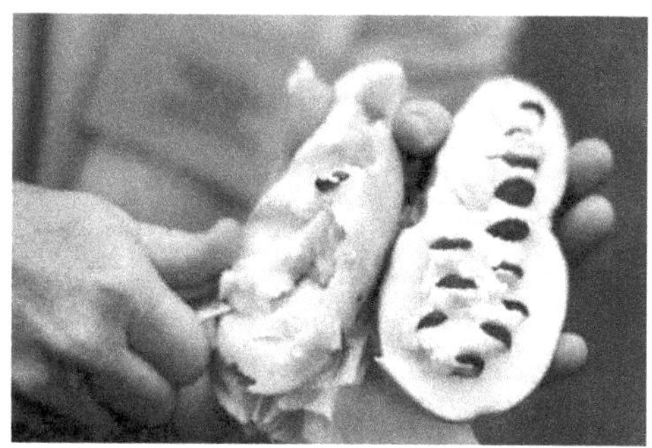

Pawpaw isn't the only plant used for food that contains neurotoxins. The grass pea (*Lathyrus sativus*), a legume that grows in Asia, Africa, and the Middle East contains a neurotoxin called beta-N-oxalylamino-L-alanine (BOAA). This toxin causes a neurodegenerative disease in animals and humans called *lathyrism,* which is very similar to ALS. While not a normal food item, the grass pea is eaten in times of poverty or famine. The disease is prevalent in some areas of Bangladesh, Ethiopia, India, and Nepal.

The toxic effect of the cycad plant that grows in many tropical and subtropical areas of the world is well known. It is believed to be the cause of a severe form of neurodegenerative disease that progresses to Parkinson's, ALS, and Alzheimer's disease. Epidemics of the disease have appeared on the islands of Guam and Rota, on the Japanese peninsula of Kii, and among the coastal people of West Papua (New Guinea).

The cycad contains various toxins, some that provoke liver disease and some that attack the brain. The seeds of the cycad contain a high concentration of a neurotoxin known as BMAA, a compound that resembles BOAA found in grass peas. Animal studies have shown that large doses of BMAA cause ALS-like symptoms and somewhat lower doses cause Parkinson's disease-like symptoms. Both can progress to Alzheimer's-like dementia.

The cycad is a common source of food in the South Pacific. The seeds are often ground into flour and made into mush or flatbread. Ordinarily, the toxins are washed away during processing, reducing the amount to very low levels.

A particularly severe epidemic of this ALS/parkinsonism dementia complex (ALS/PDC) occurred on the American governed island of Guam. Cases of ALS were up to 100 times higher on the island than in the rest of the world. Between 1940 and 1965 ALS/PDC became the leading cause of death among the adult

Chamorro—the native inhabitants of the island. During this time period one out of every five deaths was attributed to this disease.

Prior to 1900 the disease was completely unknown on the island. In 1902 the American vice-governor William Safford reported that the Chamorro were "remarkably free from disease and physical defects, and lived to a great age." However in 1904 three death certificates mentioned a form of paralysis that apparently was due to ALS. The number of cases grew until it reached a peak in the 1950s, and then slowly died off. Although older people continued to die from the disease through the 1960s, no one born since 1961 has been affected by it.

The Chamorro had been eating flour made from cycad seeds for generations without apparent problems. Investigators were puzzled as to why the disease suddenly appeared and just as suddenly disappeared. Some pointed out that the amount of BMAA consumed by the Chamorro from cycad flour wasn't enough to cause the numerous ALS and Parkinson's cases on the island. There had to be another explanation. It was apparent that it had something to do with the Chamorros' native diet because non-natives who lived on the island were not affected. Genetic causes were ruled out.

The solution to the mystery was found to be due to biomagnification.[6] Although eating flour made from cycad seed could have contributed to the problem, eating fruit bats was a more likely suspect. Flying foxes—the fruit bats that inhabited the island—were frequently hunted for food. The bats were boiled in coconut milk and eaten whole—muscle, skin, organs, and all. These bats fed on the cycad seeds, building up toxins in their tissues. BMAA binds with proteins in the body, allowing it to accumulate. The concentration of BMAA in the bats was 400 times greater than in the cycad seeds.

The traditional method of catching the fruit bats was to sneak up to them as they slept in breadfruit trees and snare them with nets. The bats have sensitive hearing so accomplishing this feat was difficult and resulted in only an occasional catch. However, with the modernization of the island in the early 1900s, the Chamorro began to acquire guns, making it much easier to kill the bats. A newly acquired cash economy allowed the hunters to sell the bats in the markets. Fruit bats were a prized delicacy and consumption greatly increased. Along with it came an increase in ALS/PDC. The Chamorros' love for bat meat caused the flying fox population to dwindle rapidly. One species on the island became extinct and the other seriously endangered. With the bat population falling, the Chamorro turned to other sources of meat and ALS/PDC cases declined.

ALS/PDC was thought to be unique to Guam and the nearby island of Rota, but in 1962 a disease that resembled it was found among the coastal people of West Papua and a third focus on the Kii peninsula of Japan. In both places cycads are used as food and medicine, but the people don't consume cycad-eating bats. How these populations get the disease is still unknown, but it may be due to some form of bioaccumulation from other foods in their diets.

While these outbreaks may seem remote, what scientists discovered in their investigations could have a direct connection to many cases of ALS, Parkinson's, and Alzheimer's in other parts of the world, including places where cycads do not grow, such as the United States and Europe.

CYANOBACTERIA

In 2002 researchers discovered that BMAA is not manufactured in the cycad itself. It is produced by cyanobacteria that live within the cycad's roots.[7] These microorganisms provide nitrogen, an important nutrient, for the cycad. Along with nitrogen, they produce BMAA, which is absorbed by the cycad and concentrated in the seeds. This is the source of the toxins in the cycad.

Cyanobacteria is common in moist soil and surface waters. Although it is a form of bacteria, it was once believed to be an algae—a simple rootless aquatic plant. It forms large blooms in lakes and slow-moving pools of water, where it is commonly referred to as blue-green algae or simply "pond scum." There are many species of cyanobacteria, some toxic and some not. Spirulina, a popular dietary supplement, is made from a non-toxic form of cyanobacteria. It is grown and harvested in controlled conditions to maintain its purity. Blue-green algae harvested from open water carries the risk of contamination from toxic forms of cyanobacteria and caution should be taken when using dietary supplements from these sources.

When the weather is warm, blue-green "algae" flourishes. Lakes, ponds, and slow-moving water can be covered in floating mats of green bacteria. Fish and crustaceans that feed on or near the bacteria can build up a concentration of toxins in their tissues. Even the water itself can become toxic because the poisons are released into the water when the bacterial cells rupture or die. Drinking the water or eating fish from the water can be dangerous. Boiling the water may kill the bacteria, but it does not neutralize the toxins or make the water safe to drink.

Clusters of Parkinson's, Alzheimer's, and ALS cases have been found near lakes that are often covered in cyanobacteria blooms. Researchers from Dartmouth-Hitchcock Medical Center have been investigating clusters of these diseases in lakeside communities in New Hampshire, Vermont, and Maine where algae blooms frequently form. The Dartmouth investigators indicate that ALS cases are nearly triple for people living near waterways with cyanobacteria blooms. In one hot spot, Mascoma Lake in New Hampshire, nine people living near the lake have been diagnosed with ALS. This is at least 10 times greater than what is normal nationally.

Brain samples from deceased ALS and Alzheimer's patients show traces of BMAA, strengthening the evidence for the cyanobacteria connection.[8] Investigators from the University of Miami examined brain tissues from 13 ALS patients and 12 Alzheimer's patients and compared them with 12 age-matched controls who were free from any neurological disease. BMAA was found in the ALS and Alzheimer's samples, but not in the controls.[9] Researchers from the Institute for Ethnomedicine in Hawaii discovered BMAA in the brain tissues of nine Canadian Alzheimer's patients. The toxin was not detected in 14 Canadians who died of causes unrelated to neurodegeneration.[10]

The presence of blue-green algae does not always mean the water is contaminated. Samples taken from various parts of the world indicate that 50 to 70 percent of cyanobacterial blooms are potentially harmful because they contain at least one toxic species. But the toxin is only produced during certain periods of the bacteria's life cycle, so it may be harmless most of the time. Since there is no obvious way to tell if a particular bloom is toxic, it is safest not to eat fish from, swim in, or use such water.

FOOD ADDITIVES

Excitotoxins

Many of the foods in your local grocery store contain neurotoxins. That hot dog you ate for lunch or the diet soda you drank to wash it down could damage your health and destroy precious brain cells. "Carol Hamm was a close friend," says James Bowen, MD. "We played cards together a couple of times per week and she constantly had diet drinks in her hands while she played. She, over a short period of a few weeks use, visibly deteriorated physically right in front of my eyes, and mentally. Her card playing deteriorated as well! She would defiantly look me right in the eye as she drank diet drinks to let me know that she didn't care that I had warned her of what I knew about aspartame. She was going to satisfy her addiction by damn! Come what may! What came was that, one night she didn't show for cards, and her daughter Debby called the police. When we arrived at her house she was lying dead in bed with bloody fluid running out of her mouth."

Carol was a victim of what has come to be known as *aspartame disease*—poisoning caused by consuming foods containing the artificial sweetener aspartame (AminoSweet, NutraSweet, Equal, Spoonful, and Equal-Measure). Aspartame accounts for over 75 percent of the adverse reactions to food additives reported to the FDA each year. There are over 90 different adverse effects that have been reported with aspartame consumption; among them are headaches, memory loss, slurred speech, tremors, irritability, anxiety, depression, seizures, and even death. An entire weight-loss industry has been built around aspartame. It is added to thousands of diet and low-calorie desserts, snack foods, sugar-free chewing gum, and beverages.

Aspartame is made up of three chemicals: phenylalanine (50 percent), aspartate (40 percent), and methanol (10 percent). Methanol, also known as wood alcohol, is toxic. Methanol breaks down into formic acid and formaldehyde in the body. Both are poisonous. Formaldehyde is a potent neurotoxin. The Environmental Protection Agency (EPA) recommends a limit of consumption of 7.8 mg/day. A single 1 liter sized beverage sweetened with aspartame contains about 56 mg of methanol—seven times the EPA limit. Heavy users of aspartame-containing products consume two or three times this amount, as much as 168 mg of methanol daily, which is 22 times the EPA limit.

Phenylalanine is an amino acid found naturally in some foods. Persons with the genetic disorder phenylketonuria (PKU) cannot metabolize phenylalanine. This leads to dangerously high (even fatal) levels of phenylalanine in the brain. It has been shown that ingesting aspartame, especially along with carbohydrate, can lead to excess levels of phenylalanine in the brain even in persons who do not have PKU. Excessive levels of phenylalanine in the brain can cause the levels of serotonin, a neurotransmitter, in the brain to decrease, leading to emotional disorders.

The name "aspartame" is a derivative of the third ingredient—aspartate. Aspartate is an amino acid. It is similar to another amino acid—glutamate. Both aspartate and glutamate are found in various levels in foods. Our cells can convert aspartate into glutamate and vice versa. Aspartate and glutamate are important neurotransmitters. In fact, they are the most abundant neurotransmitters in the brain. Aspartate and glutamate in the diet can become potent *excitotoxins*—substances that cause overstimulation leading to cellular death.

Glutamate and aspartate are excitatory neurotransmitters. Too many of them can overstimulate the neurons, exciting them into a feverish frenzy of electrical activity, exhausting the neuron's energy reserves, causing them to die. In the process, a large number of destructive free radicals are generated that promote inflammation and cellular damage, compounding the problem.

The body is capable of handling a certain amount of excess neurotransmitters. Receptors and enzymes keep them under control. But if the influx of neurotransmitters is greater than the body's ability to control them, brain cells can be stimulated to death. A few dead brain cells won't be noticed at first. But if the situation is repeated over and over again, then more and more brain cells will be killed. In time, the accumulative loss of brain cells will manifest itself as various neurological abnormalities.

A growing number of studies are linking glutamate excitotoxicity to neurodegenerative diseases including Alzheimer's, Parkinson's, ALS, Huntington's, dementia, and stroke.[11-22] Even the typical memory loss, mild intellectual deterioration, and loss of coordination that frequently occurs in late middle age may be related to excessive consumption of excitotoxins.

The most frequent source of aspartate is from the artificial sweetener aspartame. The biggest source of glutamate comes from monosodium glutamate (MSG)—a flavor enhancer. MSG is added to a large assortment of commercially packaged foods—soups, frozen dinners, pizza, gravies, sauces, chips, croutons, lunch meats, bouillon, canned tuna, and salad dressings. It is frequently found in restaurant foods. You can even buy MSG by itself as a flavor enhancer in the spice section of the grocery store. It is sold under the brand name Accent.

The negative effects of glutamate were first observed in 1954 by a Japanese scientist who noted that direct application of glutamate to the central nervous system caused seizure activity. This report, unfortunately, went unnoticed for several years. The toxicity of glutamate was then observed in 1957 by two ophthalmologists, D.R. Lucas and J.P. Newhouse, when the feeding of monosodium glutamate to newborn mice destroyed the neurons in the inner layers of the retina. Later, in 1969, neuropathologist John Olney repeated Lucas and Newhouse's experiment and discovered the phenomenon was not restricted to the retina, but occurred throughout the brain. He coined the term "excitotoxicity" to describe the neural damage that glutamate, aspartate, phenylalanine, cysteine, homocysteine, and other excitotoxins can cause.

In 1994 Russell L. Blaylock, MD, who at the time was a clinical assistant professor of neurosurgery at the University of Mississippi Medical Center, published a book titled *Excitotoxins: The Taste That Kills*. Both of his parents were afflicted with Parkinson's disease, which compelled him to research the disease in depth, seeking for the cause and an effective treatment. His research led him to an understanding of the devastating effects of excitotoxic food additives and their influence on various forms of neurodegeneration. His book summarizes the research linking excitotoxins to neurodegenerative disease and provides details on the types of foods to avoid.

If only a few foods contained glutamate or aspartate, it wouldn't be much of a problem. Small amounts in the diet can be handled without too much worry. The problem is that the vast majority of processed, packaged and restaurant foods contain excitotoxins. It is very difficult to find a canned, frozen, packaged, or prepared food in the grocery store that does not contain excitotoxic additives in some form.

Aspartame and MSG are the most common and the most recognizable. Because of the public's growing awareness of the dangers of MSG, food manufacturers often disguise this ingredient by putting it in a different form. Additives that contain MSG include hydrolyzed vegetable protein, sodium caseinate, calcium caseinate, yeast extract, autolyzed yeast, soy protein isolate, and textured protein. Of these, hydrolyzed vegetable protein is probably the worst because it also contains two other excitotoxins—aspartate and cysteine. Some food manufacturers have attempted to sell the idea that this additive is "all natural" or "safe" because it is made from vegetables, but it is not. Dr. Russell Blaylock says, "Experimentally, one can produce the same brain lesions using hydrolyzed vegetable protein as by using MSG or aspartate." One very ambiguous but common ingredient is "natural flavorings." Despite the word "natural," this is a general term that often includes MSG. You should get into the habit of reading the ingredient labels on everything you buy and avoiding all foods containing these additives or any additives that have similar sounding names.

Amino acids have become popular as dietary supplements. You can find individual purified excitotoxins being peddled as dietary supplements labeled as L-glutamine, L-cysteine, and L-phenylalanine. You may also see them in combination with other amino acids. Despite health claims, they are nothing more than brain-destroying drugs, and it is best to avoid them all.

Some people are more sensitive to excitotoxins than others and display allergy-like reactions. This has been called Chinese Restaurant Syndrome because MSG is commonly used in Asian cooking. Symptoms may include headaches, nausea, diarrhea, heart palpitations, dizziness, difficulty concentrating, mood swings, heartburn, skin rashes, and others. Those who are allergic to MSG are lucky. They know to avoid eating foods with this additive. But the rest of us can be completely oblivious to the damage that is being done.

Those people who defend the use of MSG state that glutamate is a natural substance commonly found in many foods; if glutamate-containing foods are not harmful, then MSG is not harmful either. Our bodies can handle natural dietary sources of glutamate that are found in meats, cheeses, vegetables, and such. This is clearly seen in those who are allergic to MSG. They can eat mushrooms, tomato sauce, red meat, and other foods high in natural glutamate without problem, but when they eat foods with MSG added they experience immediate adverse reactions. Obviously there is something very different between the glutamate that is found naturally in foods and the glutamate in food additives.

Protein is built out of amino acids. Glutamate is one of some 22 amino acids that make up the proteins in the human diet. Many of the plant and animal proteins in our foods contain glutamate. Glutamate in foods is always attached to other amino acids. The process of breaking proteins down into individual amino acids takes time, so the amino acids are released slowly. Blood levels of glutamate are kept within reasonable bounds that the body is capable of handling. Also, glutamate bound to other amino acids or proteins cannot pass through the blood-brain barrier, so it doesn't pose a problem. The glutamate in MSG, on the other hand, is in its free form and does not have to be broken off a protein, so you absorb a higher dose more quickly. MSG in this more purified form acts like a drug, passing through the blood-brain barrier with an immediate effect.

Excess glutamate in the brain is so detrimental that it is carefully regulated by a special cleanup and recycling system. When glutamate is released by nerve cells in the normal action of relaying messages across the synapse, some of it tends to drift away into the extracellular space. Special glutamate transport proteins are waiting, ready to bind to this extracellular glutamate. These transport proteins shuttle this excess glutamate to cells where it is stored for future use. Certain conditions, such as an influx of glutamate from the bloodstream, exposure to toxins, infection, and the release of free radicals formed by peroxidation of polyunsaturated fats can interfere with the action of the glutamate transporters.[23-25]

High blood levels of free glutamate in the diet tend to open up the blood-brain barrier, allowing more glutamate as well as other neurotoxins, to enter the brain.[26] This extracellular glutamate, along with other neurotoxins, interferes with glutamate transporters, triggers inflammation, and stimulates free-radical production. This excitotoxicity causes the release of intracellular glutamate stored in the brain cells (primarily the astrocytes). The brain is flooded with glutamate, causing more inflammation and producing more free radicals, which in turn releases more glutamate. A vicious cycle continues, leading to neuron destruction.[27]

Even small concentrations of excitotoxins entering the brain can trigger this destructive cycle. Anyone who wants to avoid developing neurodegenerative diseases as they grow older and anyone who is already experiencing the effects of these disorders should stop eating foods with excitotoxic additives immediately. That means most processed, packaged convenience foods sold at the grocery store. Replace them with fresh, natural foods and make more meals from scratch rather than using packaged ingredients. When you go out to eat at a restaurant it is difficult to avoid all possible sources of MSG, but you can reduce a lot if you tell them that you do not want MSG in your food. Often they can accommodate you, but sometimes the packaged foods they use already have the ingredient in it.

Nitrates, Nitrites, and Nitrosamines

Which of the following two meals supports good brain health and which can contribute to poor mental health?

1) Scrambled eggs cooked in butter, topped with cheese and sour cream

2) Tossed salad with croutons and diced lean turkey topped with low-fat Thousand Island dressing

Number 1 is the better choice. Eggs are very nutritious and actually support good brain health. However, as nutritious as the salad may sound, it can be a cause of many problems. While the vegetables are good, the toppings may not be. The croutons, turkey, and salad dressing may contain a number of additives that harm the brain, including MSG, aspartame, and, in the turkey, nitrite. Nitrite in itself is not so bad, but when eaten it can transform into one of many nitrosamine compounds, and that can spell big trouble.

Nitrosamines are potent cancer-causing chemicals formed in the stomach by a reaction between nitrite added to foods and amines (found in proteins normally present in the body). They are carcinogenic in large doses and cause liver damage, insulin resistance, and neurodegeneration at smaller doses.

Nitrite is added to many processed foods, especially processed meats such as bacon, sausage, ham, bologna, salami, pepperoni, pastrami, olive loaf, hot dogs, polish sausage, bratwurst, jerky, beef sticks, corned beef, smoked meats, preserved fish, and fish byproducts. It can be found in some processed vegetables, nonfat dry milk, and cheeses.

Nitrosamines are present in substantial amounts in beer and tobacco. The nitrosamine levels in smokers have been found to be up to eight times that of nonsmokers. Tobacco use also increases the body's burden of destructive free radicals and promotes atherosclerosis, which reduces blood flow to the brain. Some studies show an increased risk of dementia with tobacco use.[28]

People often use the words nitrite and nitrate interchangeably. Although chemically similar, they are two distinct substances. We are exposed to nitrite primarily from processed foods. Nitrate, to a lesser extent, is also added to foods, however, it is a greater problem in contaminated drinking water. Nitrate from fertilizers and human and animal waste may be carried by rain, irrigation, and other surface water through the soil into ground water, ultimately contaminating drinking supplies. Well water is the most susceptible. Nitrate is converted into nitrite in the digestive tract, which in turn can be converted into nitrosamine. Nitrite is ten times more toxic than nitrate.

Nitrates are also found naturally in some leafy green and root vegetables, but these sources are of little concern because they are always combined with antioxidant nutrients such as vitamins C and E, beta-carotene, and flavonoids that prevent their conversion into nitrosamines. The meat industry often tries to dispel fears about the nitrites added to their products by pointing out that nitrates (not nitrites) are found naturally in some vegetables. They fail to mention that nitrates are 10 times less dangerous than nitrites—the type most commonly used in the meat industry. Nor do they mention that nitrate toxicity is rendered impotent by other substances in the vegetables that are not found in processed meat products.

You will usually see nitrite listed on food labels as *sodium nitrite* or *potassium nitrite*. It is added to foods as a preservative. It prevents toxin production by the bacterium *Clostridium botulinum*, which is responsible for causing botulism. Because of nitrite's high carcinogenic potential, this has been an important issue within the food industry. Regulatory agencies would like to ban the chemical completely from all foods, but that would increase the risk of botulism poisoning. To limit risk of cancer, yet still provide safety against botulism, the United States government limits the addition of sodium or potassium nitrite to 120 parts per million. This is the lowest level found to be effective in controlling growth and toxin production by the bacterium.

Awareness of the danger of nitrosamines was first sounded in the early 1970s, after an epidemic of liver cancer occurred in Norwegian farm animals. The problem was traced to herring meal that was fed to the animals. The herring meal had been preserved using sodium nitrite. The sodium nitrite had reacted with the amine dimethylamine in the fish and produced the nitrosamine dimethylnitrosamine. Since then, the carcinogenic nature of nitrosamines has been well established.

Nitrite and nitrosamine intake is linked with an increased risk of cancer of the lungs, stomach, esophagus, pancreas, bladder, colon, and liver in humans.[29-32] More recently, it has been discovered that nitrosamines not only can cause cancer but also diabetes, fatty liver disease (steatohepatitis), and Alzheimer's disease. Nitrosamines cause DNA damage, oxidative stress, lipid peroxidation, and inflammation, which lead to increased cellular degeneration and death, thus promoting neurodegeneration.[33]

Drs. Ming Tong and Susan de la Monte at the Department of Pathology, Warren Alpet Medical School at Brown University, Providence, Rhode Island, claim that the epidemic of type 2 diabetes and Alzheimer's disease we are experiencing right now is directly related to the overconsumption of nitrite-containing processed foods.[34-35] Their studies have shown that nitrites cause degenerative changes in the brains of lab animals and promote insulin resistance, a known factor in Alzheimer's disease. They contend that high levels of nitrites in the diet cause cancer, while lower subcarcinogenic levels lead to insulin resistance and Alzheimer's disease.

Their studies are supported by many others that show nitrosamine-like compounds cause cancer in high doses and diabetes and Alzheimer's type neurodegeneration at lower doses.[36-38]

Does this mean you should never eat bacon, sausage, or ham? Yes...and no. It would be wise to avoid all processed foods containing sodium and potassium nitrite. This includes most cold cuts and cured meats and products that contain them, such as pizza and canned soup. These foods also often contain MSG and sometimes aspartame as well. Read ingredient labels. Fortunately, supermarkets are increasingly offering brands of processed meats that are nitrite-free. You have to search for them at regular food stores, but they are readily available in most health food stores. Fresh meats are almost always free of added nitrites.

9 Toxic Metals

Metals meddle with the mind. In human tissues, some metals actively promote oxidation and act as catalysts, accelerating the aging process. Exposure to iron, manganese, copper, zinc, aluminum, nickel, cobalt, cadmium, chromium, mercury, and lead can cause antioxidant depletion and free-radical generation. They may also promote inflammation and interfere with normal enzyme action and energy metabolism. In medicine, these elements are loosely referred to as the "heavy metals" and more specifically as "toxic metals." Some are more toxic than others. A few, such as iron, manganese, copper, zinc, and chromium, are required by the body in minute quantities, acting as nutrients in small amounts but toxins in larger amounts. The others have no known purpose in the body and are toxic at any level. Many of these metals are dangerous pollutants in our environment. Exposure to heavy metals can come from industrial, environmental, dietary, or medical sources.

Studies have shown that Alzheimer's, Parkinson's and ALS patients often have higher concentrations of heavy metals in brain tissues, indicating excessive exposure at some point in their lives.[1-3]

Manganese is an essential nutrient yet can be the direct cause of serious neurodegeneration. Parkinson's disease is known to be caused by manganese poisoning. Manganism, as it is called, is prevalent in such occupations as mining, welding, and steel manufacturing. Exposure comes primarily from inhaling manganese particles in the air. Parkinson's from manganese exposure continues to progress clinically even years later, when traces of manganese can no longer be detected in the body. Manganese isn't the only heavy metal that is associated with Parkinson's disease: iron, copper, mercury, and other heavy metals have all been linked to Parkinson's.[4-5]

Researchers from Case Western University Medical School in Ohio presented findings at the American Academy of Neurology in 2000 indicating that workers exposed to lead, such as in lead smelters and the manufacture of lead-containing batteries, pottery, pipes, and ammunition, had more than double the risk of developing Alzheimer's. It has long been known that children exposed to lead can develop brain damage. Low-level exposure to lead in children is characterized by low IQs, lessened school success, increased school drop-out rates, reduced attention spans, and antisocial behaviors. Higher levels can lead to seizures, coma, and death. But lead poisoning is not just a childhood problem. Adults who have been exposed to lead as children are at a higher risk of developing Alzheimer's later in life.[6] Lead exposure is also associated with ALS and Parkinson's disease.[7-8]

Working in the metal or mining industry or living near a factory that produces toxic waste increases the risk of neurodegeneration of all types. While exposure to toxic metals can occur through industrial sources, dietary sources are perhaps of greater concern because they affect many more people and do so without warning. If you live or work around toxic metals, you know there is a risk of exposure. But people consuming foods or medicines may have no idea that they are exposing themselves to potential harm. The three toxic metals we are probably exposed to the most from dietary and medical sources are aluminum, iron, and mercury. These are also the metals that are most commonly found to accumulate in elevated amounts in neurodegenerative disease.[9-10]

ALUMINUM

Of all the toxic metals, aluminum is the most commonly associated with Alzheimer's disease. Aluminum has long been known to be toxic to living tissues. The connection to Alzheimer's was made in the 1960s when aluminum was added to neurons in tissue cultures. This caused changes in the nerve tissue similar to those seen in the brains of humans with Alzheimer's disease. In addition, when aluminum was added to the diets of lab animals, the animals developed neurological damage. The connection was strengthened when it was reported that several dialysis patients developed dementia related to elevated aluminum levels in the dialysis liquid.[11] Once the dialysis liquid was cleared of aluminum, the dementia disappeared. Further evidence came when researchers discovered aluminum in senile plaques and neurofibrillary tangles in brain tissues from deceased Alzheimer's patients.[12] This discovery was hailed by the popular press as the long-sought cause of Alzheimer's and gained a lot of publicity. Numerous studies have been published on this subject, some even show a possible link between aluminum and ALS and Parkinson's disease as well.[13] The overall evidence, however, has been mixed. Some studies showed no evidence of elevated aluminum in Alzheimer's patients in general. This caused many to doubt the Alzheimer's aluminum connection. Later studies, however, using more sensitive methods of measurement, confirmed the presence of elevated aluminum in affected areas of the brains of many Alzheimer's patients.[14] While aluminum may not be the only factor involved in Alzheimer's disease, it definitely is toxic to brain tissue and can be a contributing factor.

Aluminum is a common element in the environment. Public water supplies contain trace amounts of minerals, including aluminum. Some areas have higher concentrations than others. Therefore, there is a possibility for low-dose chronic exposure in some areas. The presence of aluminum, as well as copper, in drinking water has been shown to adversely affect the progression of Alzheimer's disease.[15] Nine out of 13 published epidemiological studies of aluminum in drinking water and Alzheimer's disease have shown a statistically significant positive relationship.[16] Elderly people who drank water high in aluminum had 4.4 times higher incidence of

Alzheimer's than those who drank water with lower levels.[17] This evidence argues for the use of water filters. Fortunately, silica, a common mineral that is also found in trace amounts in water, binds with aluminum, reducing its absorption in the digestive tract. So in areas where the silica content is high, the risk of aluminum toxicity may be reduced.[18]

Water typically contributes 1-2 percent of our daily aluminum intake, while food and medicine supply over 95 percent.[19] Therefore, food and medical sources of aluminum are of greatest concern.

We are exposed to varying amounts of aluminum from products we use every day. Aluminum is found in processed cheese, baking powder, table salt, antacids (Di-Gel, Maalox, Gelusil, Mylanta, and Rolaids), buffered aspirin (Bufferin), antidiarrheal preparations (Donnagel, Kaopectate and Rheaban), antiperspirants, deodorants, and in foods cooked in aluminum pots and coffee made in aluminum percolators. Aluminum cans may also transfer significant amounts of aluminum to beverages. Foods wrapped in aluminum foil may absorb the mineral, especially if the food is acidic. Aluminum may also be found as an added ingredient in some canned fish and shellfish, liquid or frozen whole eggs and egg whites, dried eggs, beer, and pickles.

Medicines can supply large doses of aluminum. A person can consume thousands of times more aluminum from antacids than from drinking water.[20] Vaccines often contain aluminum, as well as mercury. The amount of these metals in vaccines is high enough to cause chronic inflammatory reactions in some individuals after immunization.[21-22]

You can avoid the dietary sources of aluminum by choosing your foods carefully and reading ingredient labels. Avoid all foods that list any ingredient containing the word "aluminum," such as aluminum ammonium sulfate, calcium aluminum silicate, sodium aluminosilicate, and sodium aluminum phosphate. Baking powder commonly includes sodium aluminum phosphate. Most baked goods containing baking powder will have this ingredient. This includes almost all donuts, muffins, cakes, and similar goods purchased at grocery stores and restaurants, as well as pancake, muffin, and cake mixes. You can purchase aluminum-free baking powder, but most commercial

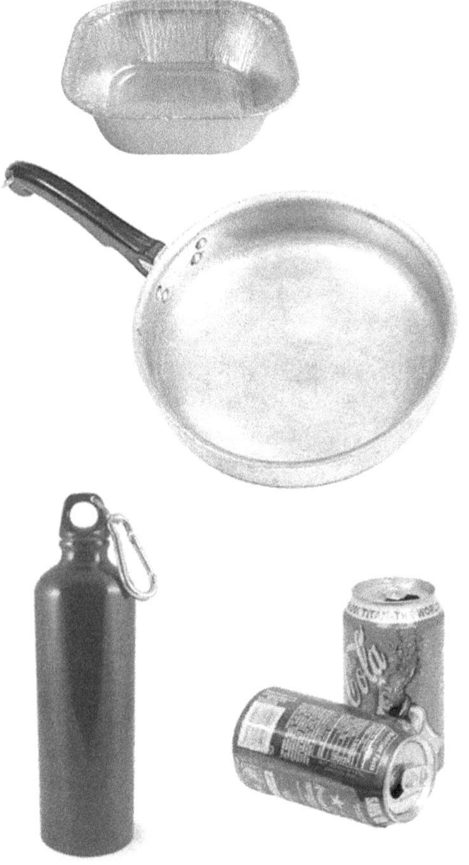

Aluminum cookware, soda cans, and water bottle.

baked goods that list baking powder use the aluminum-containing variety. Table salt typically contains aluminum as an anticaking agent, but you can buy salt without it. Natural sea salt is a good choice. Some processed (soft) cheese contains aluminum, but real cheese does not. You can tell processed cheese from real cheese because it is labeled as "pasteurized prepared cheese" or some similar term.

IRON

Every living cell contains iron. Without iron, cells could not generate energy to fuel metabolic processes. New cells could not be made and neither could hormones and enzymes.

Iron plays an essential role in the distribution of oxygen. Our red blood cells pick up oxygen in the lungs and distribute it throughout the body. Each red blood cell carries about 300 million molecules of hemoglobin, the iron-containing substance that grabs the oxygen.

We need some iron in our diet, but too much can spell trouble, and lots of it. Just like most other nutrients, if consumed in excess, it can be hazardous. But how can we get too much? Isn't iron deficiency one of our major health concerns? This may be a concern in some cases, but iron excess is a bigger problem that affects a much greater number of people. Too much iron can lead to heart disease, liver damage, diabetes, cancer, and neurodegenerative disease.[23-24]

Our bodies are the ultimate recycling machines. Proteins, fats, minerals, and other substances are continually being broken down and recycled to make new compounds. Iron, too, is recycled. It is extracted from old red blood cells and stored in special proteins called ferritin. Ferritin is a huge spherical protein molecule. Inside there is room for up to 4,500 iron atoms. We have millions of ferritin molecules roaming around in our blood and organs. This iron is used to make new red blood cells, enzymes, and other compounds.

Iron is so vital to life that it is stockpiled as a precaution against iron deficiency. Such a situation was common to our ancestors during times of winter or famine when food was scarce.

The body goes to great lengths to recycle iron. Once it is absorbed into the bloodstream, the body doesn't want to give it up. In fact, the body has no mechanism for getting rid of iron. Almost all the iron we consume is stored away in the body.

Because of the efficiency of the recycling of iron, our daily requirement for iron from food is really very small. We do lose about 1 mg of iron per day in sweat and urine as well as in cells that naturally slough off from the intestinal wall, hair, skin, and nails. The biggest loss of iron occurs with the loss of blood. Iron-filled red blood cells and ferritin molecules are lost and the body pulls out iron from its storage sites to replenish what was lost.

Premenopausal women lose iron on a regular basis, which is why women are considered more at risk of low iron levels than men. The Recommended Dietary Allowance (RDA) of iron for premenopausal women is 15 mg; for men and postmenopausal women it is 10 mg. The body absorbs approximately 10 percent of the iron in our foods, so consumption of 10-15 mg of dietary iron would supply 1 to 1.5 mg to body stores. This gain equals about the same that is lost every day. Consuming more than 10-15 mg of iron means that all of the excess will go into storage.

If the diet becomes iron deficient, a signal is sent to the digestive tract and more iron is absorbed from the food in the intestines. It is an efficient system to make sure the body gets all the iron it needs when dietary intake decreases. Most menstruating women are not iron deficient because this absorption mechanism performs effectively. In addition, if more iron is needed, the body can pull more out of its ferritin reserves.

The average diet supplies more than enough iron for all our needs. Most of us eat far more than the RDA. All excess iron is packed neatly away in our tissues. Because we normally take in more iron than we lose, iron reserves increase with age, even in most premenopausal women.

So what's so terrible about having a little extra iron stored away in our body? It might come in handy if we ever need it. And if iron is such an important nutrient that the body makes special efforts to stockpile it, how can it be bad?

When iron is bound to hemoglobin or ferritin, it causes no harm. However, some of the iron that is stored in ferritin leaks out and roams around the body as free iron. The larger our iron reservoirs, the more free iron we have wandering about inside our bodies.

The trouble with free iron is that it is a powerful oxidizer and unleashes a horde of destructive free radicals. Polyunsaturated fatty acids and other compounds quickly fall prey to these molecular renegades. This damage caused by an iron-catalyzed reaction is extensive and can affect all cells and tissues. The brain, being mostly fat with a relatively high amount of polyunsaturated fatty acids, is particularly vulnerable.[25]

Randall Lauffer, PhD, professor of biochemistry at Harvard Medical School, describes iron this way: "Free iron can unleash a destructive chain reaction that makes use of iron's special property of combining with different forms of oxygen. When bound to hemoglobin, iron is a little chemical angel, carefully escorting oxygen in the blood and benevolently delivering it to the neediest tissues. But free—alone and bare—iron is a little devil, a neighborhood brat playing with a dangerous chemistry set and a tank of oxygen. The interaction between iron and oxygen then becomes destructive, and our tissues are the victims."[26]

Iron is recognized as a carcinogen. Some researchers believe increased iron reserves are directly involved in the development of cancer, diabetes, heart disease, stroke, Parkinson's disease, and Alzheimer's disease.[26]

It has been known for a long time that sufferers of Parkinson's disease have abnormally high levels of iron in their brains. A healthy adult brain might contain 50 mg of iron per gram of tissue. However, in Parkinson's suffers, this figure can rise to 250 mg per gram of tissue. Iron is stored throughout the brain, accumulating rapidly during adolescence and early adulthood.

Studies at the University of Washington have shown that diets high in iron increase the risk of Parkinson's disease. Researchers showed that people in the top 25 percent of iron consumption are 1.7 times more likely to develop Parkinson's disease than those in the lowest 25 percent. People who have diets high in iron and take multivitamins that contain iron are 2.1 times more likely to develop Parkinson's disease. Adding excess manganese increases the risk, and the risk of both minerals together are greater than for either one alone.[27]

Excess iron intake increases Alzheimer's risk as well. Iron accumulates in the brain with age, and evidence shows that iron stimulates the production of destructive free radicals that contribute to the amyloid beta deposition and neurofibrillary tangles that characterize this disease.

Iron-induced free-radical reactions have also been shown to damage arteries, promoting atherosclerosis, heart attacks, and strokes. The risk of multiple mini-strokes that lead to vascular dementia and are often associated with Alzheimer's is increased with high iron intake.

According to Randall Lauffer, PhD, the reason why more middle-aged men experience a greater number of heart attacks than middle-aged women is because men have higher stores of iron in their bodies. Once women reach menopause and are no longer losing iron through menstruation, their iron stores increase rapidly—and so does their rate of heart disease.

Another mechanism whereby iron can cause oxidative damage is injury. Mechanical or chemical injury to tissues can cause cells to rupture and release their contents into the surrounding area. These contents include metal ions such as iron which accelerate free-radical reactions in extracellular fluids. These radicals can accelerate fat peroxidation because fats are the most vulnerable segments of our tissues.

It has been proposed that injury to the brain by head trauma or by oxygen deprivation (stroke) can result in release of iron ions into the surrounding area. Iron ions could facilitate further damage to these surrounding areas by accelerating free-radical reactions.

Because disease causes tissue injury and the release of iron, almost any disease is likely to be accompanied by increased formation of free radicals. Much of the damage caused during illness is the result of free-radical reactions.

Since the iron content of human tissues increases as we age, injuries to older tissues result in the release of a greater amount of iron. Free radical damage, therefore, also increases as we age.

Most of our foods contain iron. It is found naturally in all produce, grains, nuts, seeds, eggs, and meats. Dairy, however, is comparatively low in iron unless it has been fortified. Oils and fat also lack iron.

One of the highest dietary sources of iron is white flour. When whole wheat flour is processed, iron along with several other nutrients are removed. In a society where wheat constitutes the main source of food, taking out vital nutrients has had a drastic effect on health. For many people, bread or flour is the basis of their diet. When the processing of white flour became common over a century ago, the lack of nutrients resulted in people developing deficiency diseases. The government mandated that white flour be "enriched" with certain nutrients to prevent these diseases. One of these nutrients was iron. Although some 20 nutrients are removed in the process, only four or five are added back. To make the bread even "healthier," food processors add more iron than was present in the original whole wheat. A few slices of bread can supply all the iron you need for an entire day.

Almost all white flour has been enriched with iron in the form of *ferrous sulfate*. This is the name of iron you will mostly commonly see on ingredient labels. So any product made with white flour is also enriched with ferrous sulfate. Think about it. How many items do we eat every day that are made from refined wheat flour? We usually just think of bread and rolls but must include bagels, cookies, crackers, pretzels, pancake mix, breakfast cereal, flour tortillas, burritos, pizza, macaroni, spaghetti, frozen dinners, pot pies, cake, and donuts—the list can go on and on. These are the types of foods most people live on!

Almost all hot and cold breakfast cereals are "fortified" with additional iron. Many of the cold cereals are predominantly sugar, and sugar has no nutritional value other than providing calories. Some breakfast cereals are as much as 60 percent sugar. So in effect, when you eat these products, you are eating fortified sugar. The worst cereals, in terms of iron content, are those that appear to be the healthiest, such as Total and Product 19. These cereals have 100 percent of the RDA with each serving. One serving will supply all the iron you need for an entire day, but everything else you eat during the day will supply additional iron, all of which will be stockpiled in your body. With all the iron we get, it's no wonder why iron-induced free-radical destruction has been identified as a major source of concern.

As if this weren't enough iron, many of us intentionally add more to our body's stores by taking multiple vitamin and mineral supplements and enriched drinks. Most multiple vitamins contain iron. However, now that people are becoming aware of the iron problem, some manufacturers are making multiple vitamins with reduced amounts of iron or with no iron at all. You should avoid all dietary supplements that contain iron. Even women who are premenopausal should avoid iron-containing supplements unless told otherwise by their doctor.

There is one more major source of iron that affects a few people: cookware. Using cast iron pots to cook foods not only increases the amount of this metal in our bodies but also destroys vitamin C and other antioxidants in the food.[24] It's safer to use stainless steel or glass.

Now that you are aware of the iron problem, how do you protect yourself from overload? If you're an adolescent or a premenopausal woman you have little to worry about. The young have not had time to build up iron stores to any great amount and women of child-bearing age continually lose iron with their periods. Some women may lose so much iron that they may even develop an iron deficiency. Those who should be most concerned about excess iron are adult men and postmenopausal women.

For those who are at risk, the best way to avoid iron overload is to avoid eating enriched foods—primarily breakfast cereals and white flour products. Look for the words "ferrous," "ferric," or "iron" on the ingredient label.

One of the benefits of eating whole wheat products, brown rice, and other whole grains is that they contain fiber, which is removed in the process of making white flour or polished white rice. The fiber is beneficial because it binds to toxic metals, including iron, and pulls them out of the digestive tract so the amount of iron absorbed into the bloodstream is reduced. Whole grains and beans are the richest dietary sources of fiber.

Regular aerobic exercise also helps to reduce iron stores. A small amount of iron is excreted in sweat. A vigorous workout can help unload extra iron, but a single bowl of breakfast cereal can replenish the iron lost in two hours of strenuous exercise. You can't depend on exercise alone to reduce iron reserves.

Alcohol increases iron absorption. A number of studies have shown that drinkers have higher iron levels than nondrinkers.[28-29] Alcohol damages the intestinal lining, disrupting the body's ability to regulate nutrient absorption, including iron. When this self-regulating mechanism goes awry, iron absorption can be increased.

Oral contraceptives partially rob younger women of the protection they get through menstruation. Oral contraceptives decrease menstrual blood flow in most women to a third or half the normal rate. This reduces the amount of iron that would normally be lost. Those who use oral contraceptives are more likely to build up their iron stores earlier in life. This has been confirmed in studies which show that the amount of stored iron in women who use oral contraceptives for two years or more is roughly double that of nonusers.

Any loss of blood will reduce iron loads. Donating blood has been suggested as a means to lower iron reserves. Donating blood a couple of times a year is sufficient for most people to keep iron reserves within bounds as long as iron intake is kept moderate.

Periodic fasting is also an effective way to reduce body stores of iron. While fasting, the body continues to lose small amounts of iron daily without it being replenished in the diet. Total body iron reserves decline. In traditional fasts you refrain from all foods and beverages except water. Juice fasts include vegetable and fruit juices, but the juices need to be low in iron. Milk can also be used in a fast. It provides a full spectrum of nutrients but essentially no iron. If you are unfamiliar to fasting, I suggest you get assistance from someone who is experienced before fasting longer than a couple of days.

MERCURY

Mercury is the most toxic non-radioactive metal known to science. Just inhaling the vapor can cause brain damage. Animal studies show that mercury exposure causes changes in the brain that are identical to those seen in Alzheimer's patients.[30] Of all the toxic metals, mercury has been shown to be the most damaging to nerve and brain tissue.

In addition to brain damage, mercury poisoning may cause kidney failure and liver damage that can ultimately lead to death. Symptoms of acute mercury poisoning include tingling or pricking sensations in the skin (a sign of nerve damage); loss of coordination, unsteady movements, and staggering gait; difficulty speaking and pronouncing words; vision loss; and deafness.

One of the most famous outbreaks of acute mercury poisoning occurred in Iraq in the early 1970s. In response to a famine in 1971-1972 the United States, Mexico, and other nations shipped wheat grain, intended for planting, to Iraq. The seeds had been treated with a methylmercury-containing fungicide to hold down mold growth and preserve the viability of the seeds. The seeds were dyed red to indicate that they had been chemically treated. In addition, warnings were placed on the sacks in Spanish and English that the seed was poisonous. Unfortunately, the Iraqis couldn't read either language. Instead of distributing the wheat to farmers for planting, Iraqi officials sold it for food. The people milled the seeds into flour and consumed the contaminated bread. Over a period of several weeks 6,530 persons were hospitalized and almost 500 died.

Chronic low-level mercury poisoning can cause tremors, impaired cognitive ability, memory loss, sleep disturbances, depression, and personality changes. In the 1800s mercury was used in the manufacture of felt hats. Workers who inhaled the mercury vapors over a period of time eventually became insane. This was the origin of the phrase "as mad as a hatter" and may have been the inspiration for the loopy mad Hatter character depicted in the story of *Alice's Adventures in Wonderland.* Mercury poisoning is even now sometimes referred to as "mad hatter's disease."

Mercury is found in organic and inorganic forms. The inorganic form can be divided into elemental mercury and mercuric salts. The mercury in a thermometer is elemental mercury. Organic mercury is formed when elemental mercury combines with organic compounds. Methylmercury and dimethylmercury are two common and deadly examples. Mercury in any form is toxic, but organic mercury is usually more toxic than the inorganic. Mercury poisoning can result from vapor inhalation, ingestion, injection, or absorption through the skin.

Mercury has many industrial and manufacturing uses. It is used in bronzing, electroplating, paper manufacturing, photography, silver and gold production, embalming, taxidermy, vinyl chloride production, wood preservation, and in the making of fluorescent lamps, neon lamps, paint, batteries, explosives, fungicides, insecticides, and many other products.

The most common dietary source of mercury is from eating fish contaminated by industrial pollution. Because of pollution, almost all fish contain mercury to some degree. Generally, fish higher up on the food chain are more likely to have greater concentrations of mercury, so it is best to avoid or limit consumption of large predatory fish. The table on the following page lists fish and shellfish with the least and the greatest levels of mercury. This data is from the FDA, which tests fish for mercury, and the Environmental Protection Agency (EPA), which determines mercury levels that it considers safe or unsafe to eat.

Another major source of mercury comes from medicine. For centuries mercury has been used as an essential ingredient in the formulation of medicines. Despite its well-known toxic properties, it was used extensively in diuretics, purgatives (strong laxatives), antiseptics, and antibiotics. Although toxic, it did work for these conditions because of its toxicity. When used as a laxative and diuretic, the body responded by purging the system to rid itself of the poison, causing diarrhea, increased urination, and sometimes vomiting. In the 18th and 19th centuries, many illnesses were believed to be caused by unspecified "impurities," and the cure was to purge them from the body. Increased bowel movements and urination were seen as a way to accomplish this. Up until the early 20th century, mercury-containing drugs were the most effective

Mercury Levels in Fish and Shellfish

LEAST MERCURY

Anchovies	Butterfish	Catfish
Clam	Crab (domestic)	Crawfish/Crayfish
Croaker (Atlantic)	Flounder	Haddock (Atlantic)
Hake	Herring	Mullet
Mackerel (Atlantic, Chub)	Oyster	Perch (ocean)
Plaice	Pollock	Salmon (canned)
Salmon (fresh)	Sardine	Scallop
Shad (American)	Shrimp	Sole (Pacific)
Squid (calamari)	Tilapia	Trout (freshwater)
Whitefish	Whiting	

MODERATE MERCURY

Bass (striped, black)	Carp	Cod (Alaskan)
Croaker (white Pacific)	Halibut (Atlantic)	Halibut (Pacific)
Jacksmelt (silverside)	Lobster	Mahi Mahi
Monkfish	Perch (freshwater)	Sablefish
Skate	Snapper	Tuna (skipjack)
Tuna (canned chunk light)	Weakfish (sea trout)	

HIGH MERCURY

Bluefish	Grouper	Sea Bass (Chilean)
Mackerel (Spanish, Gulf)	Tuna (albacore)	Tuna (yellowfin)

HIGHEST MERCURY

Mackerel (king)	Marlin	Orange Roughy
Shark	Swordfish	Tilefish
Tuna (bigeye, ahi)		

Source: Natural Resources Defense Council http://www.nrdc.org/health/effects/mercury/guide.asp.

diuretics and continued to be used. Mercury also killed bacteria, viruses, fungi, and parasites, so mercury-containing medications were used to treat intestinal parasites, skin infections, and systemic infections. One of the most common uses was in treating syphilis. Its usefulness may have been questionable, but until the discovery of antibiotics in 1939, there were few alternatives.

Because mercury was efficient in purging the impurities that were seen as the cause of so many ills, mercury-containing drugs were used to treat a wide variety of illnesses including consumption (tuberculosis), depression, child-bearing diseases, toothaches, eczema, psoriasis, liver disease, irregular menstruation, inflammation, conjunctivitis, and all manner of infectious diseases. It seemed that any health problem could be treated with mercury-containing medicines. Some medicines combined mercury with cyanide, aluminum, iodine, and other poisonous substances to "improve" their effectiveness. One of the most popular medicines of the 19th century was calomel—mercurous chloride. It remained popular even into the early 20th century.

Mercury-containing medicines were often administered to patients in such great quantities that their hair and teeth fell out.[31] Many patients died from their physicians' overzealous ministrations, and those that survived did so despite the "cure." Symptoms of mercury poisoning were often attributed to the disease rather than the treatment. Mercury-containing teething powders caused widespread mercury poisoning called pink disease, characterized by pinkish coloration of the palms and soles accompanied by fever, insomnia, lethargy, loss of appetite, and pain. These symptoms were believed to be simply effects of teething. The disease had a high mortality rate, killing 1 in 10 infants. Once it was discovered that mercury poisoning was the cause, mercury-containing teething powders were promptly taken off the market.

Over time, as the danger of the mercury in these products became better understood, mercury-containing medicines were replaced with safer and more effective alternatives. Yet modern medicine still uses mercury in some treatments. Vaccines often contain thimerosal, a mercury-containing preservative. Here the mercury is injected straight into the bloodstream. Some convincing studies have suggested that childhood vaccines containing thimerosal cause brain damage leading to autism. However, this issue is hotly debated. Yet, in response to public concern and due to the available scientific evidence, thimerosal use in childhood vaccines has been reduced, although it is still common in flu, hepatitis B, and diphtheria-tetanus vaccines. If you get a yearly flu shot, you are probably getting mercury injected into your bloodstream. In addition to mercury, vaccines often contain aluminum as well, so you get a double whammy with each vaccination.

A remnant of 19th century medicine that still survives today is the use of amalgam dental fillings. In the early 1800s when mercury was commonly used in the medical profession, dental surgeons (dentists) began using a mixture of mercury, tin, copper, zinc, and silver to make amalgam tooth fillings. These "silver" fillings offered a cheaper alternative to the more expensive gold fillings. The unique feature that made mercury so valuable in dentistry is the fact that it is the only metal that is liquid at room temperature. When mixed with other, harder metals the resulting amalgam is soft and pliable, thus allowing it to be molded snugly into the cavity of a tooth. Although mercury was recognized as a deadly poison at the time, those who used mercury amalgams claimed that by mixing the mercury with other metals, the mercury was bound tightly in the alloy and posed no threat to health. Despite the common use of mercury-containing medicines, most dental surgeons at the time did not accept the use of mercury amalgam as ethical and refused to use it. In 1859 the National Dental Association (now called the American Dental Association) was established. The founders of the organization favored the use of amalgam fillings and encouraged its members to use them. New dentists were taught that amalgams were safe, although there was no evidence to prove it. Dentists accepted the word of the dental association and amalgams became a standard in dental practice. The safety

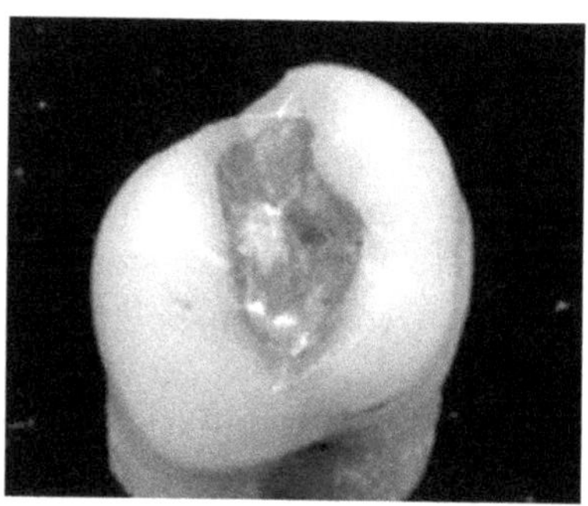

Our greatest exposure to mercury comes from amalgam dental fillings.

of amalgam fillings has been debated off and on for the past 150 years. The American Dental Association (ADA) takes the stand that they are completely safe, while a number of researchers have raised serious concerns that they are not.

If the amount of mercury used in amalgam fillings was small, maybe it wouldn't be such an issue. But amalgams consist of a whopping 50 percent mercury! The amount of mercury in a single filling is more than enough to cause brain damage and even death. As the filling sits in the tooth, mercury vapor is constantly released and absorbed into the body. Once the filling is put into the tooth, mercury vapor will continually be emitted as long as it stays in the mouth. Fillings as old as 50 years have been shown to still give off mercury vapor. No immediate effects are felt, but over time the continual absorption of mercury vapor into the mouth and lungs will have an effect.[32]

Animal studies show that exposure to mercury vapor at concentrations known to be released by dental amalgams in people produce brain lesions identical to those seen in Alzheimer's disease.[33] Mercury also erodes the myelin covering around nerve cells, suggesting a connection to multiple sclerosis.[34]

Elemental mercury, the type in amalgam fillings, emits mercury vapor at room temperature. In the warm and acidic environment of the mouth, mercury vapor is released at a much higher rate. When food is consumed, abrasion to fillings by chewing along with exposure to hot and acidic foods accelerate mercury release. Even the American Dental Association acknowledges the release of mercury vapor into the mouth (admitting mercury isn't tightly bound as they once claimed); but they contend that the amount absorbed is only harmful to a small number of highly sensitive people and that for most people there is little to worry about. What they fail to acknowledge is that mercury is toxic at *any* level! There is no safe limit on mercury. Small doses of mercury tend to collect in brain tissue. Continuous exposure to mercury vapor 24 hours a day, day after day, year after year for 10, 20, 30 years or more will have an accumulative effect. Every breath you take funnels mercury directly into the brain, where it accumulates and causes irritation and inflammation. This disrupts normal cellular function, promoting senile plaque and neurofibrillary tangle formation and brain cell death.

In a 2006 FDA hearing on the safety of amalgam fillings, dental experts testified of the deleterious effects of amalgam fillings on health. Among other things, it was brought out that in human autopsy studies the amount of mercury in the brains of the subjects studied were directly proportional to the number of fillings in their teeth. It was not proportional to any other factors, including fish consumption. Thus there is a direct relationship between amalgam fillings and brain levels of mercury. The hearing also revealed that babies whose mothers have amalgam fillings are born with higher mercury levels in the bodies. In fact, the amount of mercury found in baby's hair is proportional to the number of fillings in the mother's teeth.[35]

The ADA Council on Dental Materials advises dentists on how to protect themselves against the hazards of handling scrap amalgams. Amalgams from extracted teeth need to be treated as hazardous waste. Among the many precautions, dentists are told to prevent contact with skin. The fumes coming off amalgam fillings are so toxic that they are instructed to avoid breathing the unseen vapors and to store the amalgam by submerging it under water in unbreakable, tightly sealed containers. The work area must be well ventilated and all employees must be thoroughly advised on the proper way to handle this hazardous material. It is also advised that all employees in dental offices get checked yearly for mercury levels. Despite these precautions, dental workers are at high risk of mercury poisoning.[36]

This same toxic waste that must be handled with so much care is exactly the same material that is placed in your mouth. Yet, the ADA says that when it is in your tooth it suddenly loses its toxicity and becomes safe. This just doesn't make sense. With all the evidence against the use of amalgam fillings and with the ADA's own precautions to dentists, it makes one wonder if the royalties* the ADA receives from amalgam filling placed in patients' mouths has anything to do with their position on the matter. Another reason may be that they have been denying the danger of mercury fillings for so long that if they suddenly admitted that they were wrong, it would be extraordinarily embarrassing: they would lose credibility in the scientific community and among their own membership.

With the naked eye you cannot see the mercury fumes coming off the amalgam in a tooth. However, against a phosphorescent screen the vapor becomes readily visible. An excellent demonstration of this is shown on youtube.com using a 25-year-old amalgam filling at www.youtube.com/watch?v=9ylnQ-T7oiA. Another amalgam filling, this one over 50 years old, emits just as much mercury vapor: www.youtube.com/watch?v=jN5QVL4N9oU. No matter how old a filling is, mercury continues to be released. Once in your mouth, you will be constantly exposed to mercury until you die or have the amalgam removed. When these fumes are absorbed into the body, they go to the brain. A remarkable demonstration of how mercury kills brain cells is graphically illustrated in this video of a neuron cell culture: www.youtube.com/watch?v=XU8nSn5Ezd8&NR=1. If you have access to the Internet, these videos are worth watching.

All amalgam fillings leak mercury. There is no such thing as a safe amalgam filling. All metal or "silver" fillings are made from mercury amalgam. If you have amalgam fillings, you need to decide if you want to continue being poisoned by the mercury or if you want to do something about it.

---

*The ADA receives royalty payments from amalgam manufacturers, as well as from makers of toothbrushes, mouthwashes, dental floss and other products through its "seal of acceptance" program. While receiving funding from manufacturers, the ADA in turn agrees to promote the product to both its members and the public. The ADA claims through its "seal of acceptance" that it has researched the safety of mercury amalgam and found it to be safe. In truth, they have never done a peer-reviewed study demonstrating the safety of mercury fillings, instead relying on the belief that it must be safe because it has been in use for over 150 years.

The best choice is to have the amalgam removed. Nowadays, there are many other nontoxic dental filling materials available. They are called composites. Composites are made using synthetic resins combined with a hard filling material such as silica. They are made to match the color of your teeth so when they are placed, they become indistinguishable from the rest of the tooth. You can't tell you have a filling. Composites are just as strong and durable as amalgams, so there is no need to ever have an amalgam filling placed in your mouth.

Most any dentist can give you a composite filling, however, not any dentist can remove an amalgam filling safely. The proper removal of amalgam fillings takes special precautions and skills that most dentists are not trained for. Since dentists are taught in dental school that amalgams are harmless to patients, they are not inclined to take the safety precautions necessary to protect the patient from mercury toxicity during removal. In fact, the only time they would ever remove an amalgam is when they extract the entire tooth or drill most of it away to do a root canal procedure, so they have little experience in amalgam removal.

The proper methods of amalgam removal are generally taught in special courses after graduating from dental school. Those dentists who are properly trained in amalgam removal, who understand and know the dangers of mercury fillings and don't ever use them in their practice, are called *biological* or *holistic* dentists or sometimes *mercury-free* dentists. They use these terms to set themselves apart from other dentists who have no qualms about putting poisonous metals in patients' mouths.

Proper amalgam removal will involve placing a rubber dam in the patient's mouth to prevent particles of amalgam from going down the throat. Suction under the rubber dam is used to remove mercury vapor that accumulates underneath the dam. The rubber dam does not stop mercury vapor, but it slows it down so that the vapor produced by drilling will not be absorbed into oral tissues. A respirator is used for breathing so the patient does not inhale any of the toxic vapor that is being released during the process. Other considerations the dentist will take into account is the order in which amalgams are removed from the teeth and how much to do in one session.

Any dentist can claim to be able to remove amalgam fillings, but if he or she uses amalgams, find another dentist. This is very important! Dentists that do not understand the danger of amalgam fillings also do not understand the dangers of amalgam removal. Do *not* have your amalgam fillings removed by any dentist who puts amalgam into patients' mouths!

To find the right dentist, look for those who advertise themselves as practicing biological, holistic, or mercury-free dentistry. Any dentist can claim to practice this type of dentistry. Before making an appointment, ask them if they use amalgam fillings. If they do, look elsewhere. They may give you a song and dance about only using it on certain people or that some people do better with amalgams or that amalgams are perfectly safe. Don't argue, find someone else and ask if they can remove amalgam fillings and replace them with composites.

Ask them if they can do compatibility testing. Compatibility testing is to test you against hundreds of dental materials and identify those that you may be allergic or sensitive to and those you are compatible with. You do not want to place a composite in your mouth that will give you problems. The compatibility test requires that a blood sample be taken. Your blood is then tested against the materials used in a variety of composites. A report is compiled that lists all the materials you are sensitive to and should not be put into your mouth, as well as all the materials that are safe to put into your mouth. You must have a compatibility test done before you allow the dentist to put any composite into your teeth. A properly trained biological or holistic dentist will understand this and provide the test or refer you to a lab that will do the test. Most dentists don't do their own compatibility tests but will refer you to another service to take care of this step. If the dentist tells you the compatibility test is unnecessary, find another dentist.

You can locate biological dentists in your area though the Holistic Dental Association, phone (619)923-3120, or visit www.holisticdental.org. Another referral service is Huggins Applied Healing, phone (866)948-4638 or visit www.hugginsappliedhealing.com. The International Academy of Oral Medicine and Toxicology (IAOMT) also maintains a referral list at www.iaomt.org/testfoundation/hgfreedentists.htm. This last resource lists dentists who have requested to be included on the IAOMT registry of mercury-free dentists. The list includes dentists in North America, Europe, Australia, and New Zealand. The only thing worse than having a mouth full of mercury fillings is having them removed improperly. Regardless of who you choose to replace your mercury fillings, insist that your dentist follow the IAOMT-approved protocol for the safe mercury amalgam removal.

Prevention, of course, is the best weapon against mercury poisoning. If you have already been exposed, you need to prevent all future exposure. This would include avoiding eating fish that are known to have a moderate to high mercury content and avoidance or removal of all amalgam fillings.

The next thing you can do is protect yourself against the damage mercury in your tissues may be causing and try to remove as much as possible. Removing mercury from the brain is a difficult and slow process. Taking antioxidant supplements can help temper the flames of inflammation and reduce the damage mercury and other toxic metals can do. The major antioxidant nutrients include Vitamins A, C, and E, beta-carotene, alpha-lipoic acid, flavonoids and the trace minerals zinc and selenium. These can all be found in a good multiple vitamin and mineral supplement. However, the best source of these nutrients comes directly from foods, mostly fresh vegetables and fruits. Dietary fiber (whole grains, legumes), garlic, citrate (citrus fruits), and various flavonoids (curcumin, hesperidin, quercetin, catechins, rutin), and alpha-lipoic acid (red meat, organ meats, brewer's yeast) act as chelators that help remove mercury from the body. This topic will be discussed in more detail in a later chapter.

10 Infections

Infectious microorganisms have long been associated with neurodegenerative disease. Medical literature contains an enormous number of studies linking Alzheimer's, Parkinson's, ALS, and other neurodegenerative diseases with infections. Of all the factors known to affect neurodegeneration, infection may be the most common, and consequently the most important. While not all cases of neurodegeneration are associated with infection, the number of cases that are is vastly under-recognized. There are four primary reasons for this: 1) Some cases are clearly influenced by other factors such as drugs or toxins, with infection possibly being an unrecognized contributing factor; 2) Microorganisms are not always easily detectable or even looked for in autopsies or studies; 3) After an acute infection has done its damage, it may be eradicated from the brain, leaving no evidence of its presence; 4) An active infection can cause neurodegeneration without being present in the brain. This last one is very important because an infection can cause neuronal damage without ever directly infecting the brain and without leaving a trace of evidence that it was involved.

INFECTION AS A CAUSE OF PARKINSON'S DISEASE

In the 1970s, Dr. David Poskanzer, an associate professor of neurology at Harvard Medical School, and colleague Dr. Robert S. Schwab found that the number of Parkinson's patients diagnosed at Massachusetts General Hospital where they worked increased exponentially from the 1920s into the 1960s. Then they noticed something intriguing: with each passing year, the average age of the new patients increased by a year. Poskanzer believed this observation provided a clue to the elusive cause of Parkinson's disease.

Poskanzer and Schwab reasoned that, except for a few cases caused by chemical poisoning, the great epidemic of Parkinson's disease they had witnessed over the preceding few decades resulted from something that happened years ago and then ceased. What was that something? Poskanzer believed it was a brain infection that caused encephalitis or brain inflammation. There are many causes of encephalitis—bacterial and viral infections are the most common. The two neurologists evolved the hypothesis that encephalitis could have damaged brain cells when the infection was active. If the patient survived, then years later, as the effects of aging began to take its toll on the brain, the signs of Parkinson's disease would gradually appear.

The most likely infection was an illness called lethargic encephalitis (also called encephalitis lethargica). The illness was initially thought to be caused by a virus, but more recently a form of streptococcal bacteria has become the prime suspect.[1] From 1916 to 1926 a lethargic encephalitis outbreak caused a worldwide epidemic of brain inflammation. The name included the word "lethargic" because the disease was characterized by severe sleepiness and was commonly referred to as the "sleeping sickness." (This is not to be confused with African trypanosomiasis, a parasitic disease that is also known as the "sleeping sickness.") The illness started off with a sore throat, fever, headache, and nausea, then within days developed into uncontrollable drowsiness that would cause the sufferer to fall asleep almost anywhere or in any situation, even while they were eating. Severely stricken victims spent days or weeks almost comatose and immobile. During the epidemic over 5 million people—about 40 percent of those who developed the disease—died. Examination of the brains of those who died showed pronounced inflammation and cell death in and around the substantia nigra, the same area involved in Parkinson's disease.

Millions of people were infected with lethargic encephalitis. Some seemed to recover completely, but almost half of the survivors experienced brain damage that left them with Parkinson's disease. Some of those who initially appeared to recover developed Parkinson's disease months or even years later. Doctors distinguished this form of parkinsonism from those of unknown origin with the name postencephalitic Parkinson's disease. Poskanzer believed that the majority of Parkinson's patients he saw up through the 1970s were victims of the encephalitis lethargic epidemic. While some of his patients knew they had encountered the infection decades before, others did not. In the latter case, the patients may have misidentified their illness as a simple case of the flu and thought nothing more of it. The influenza pandemic of 1918-1920, which killed some 20 to 40 million people worldwide, overlapped the lethargic encephalitis epidemic, so many of the victims of encephalitis epidemic may have thought they had survived the flu.

By 1928 the lethargic encephalitis epidemic was over. However, thousands of the survivors now suffered with Parkinson's disease. Over the next several decades as survivors aged, new Parkinson's cases surfaced. Alive but trapped in useless bodies, many were institutionalized. In 1969, over 40 years after the disease had disappeared, some catatonic victims were treated with the newly developed anti-parkinson drug Levodopa (L-dopa). A number of patients improved dramatically. They became conscious, responsive, and aware of their surroundings, even getting up out of their wheelchairs. Tragically, the miraculous recovery was short-lived. Most patients slipped back into a catatonic state within days or weeks. Repeated dosages proved useless. This event was documented by Dr. Oliver Sacks in a book titled *Awakenings,* published in 1973.

Knowing what we do now about the effects of L-dopa, the failure of the drug was predictable. While L-dopa can bring almost immediate improvement in Parkinson's symptoms, it damages the surviving dopamine neurons.[2] Over time, it accelerates the rate of neuron degeneration and the progression of the disease. That is why it eventually stops working. The number of dopamine neurons that survive are so few that the drug becomes useless.

There have been no further epidemics of lethargic encephalitis since the 1920s, although sporadic cases have continued to be reported. What we learn from all this is that certain infections can cause neurodegenerative brain damage that may not become evident until years later and may not be readily associated with an infection.

George L. was in his late 40s, a college graduate and an accountant for a National Guard Unit. One day he developed severe burning sensations in his face and head accompanied by mental confusion. He was admitted to a hospital where he stayed for several days. He was diagnosed with a fever of unknown origin and received symptomatic treatment until the fever abated. At home he was not his old self. He often became confused and mostly sat in his chair, seemed to be in poor contact with his surroundings, responded only to simple commands, and most importantly, could no longer perform the mathematical calculations required by his job. By all accounts he was suffering from the early stages of dementia.

He was later treated with a variety of drugs without success. Over the years, in addition to his declining mental state of mind, his movements became slow and deliberate, he developed tremors, slurred speech, anxiety, and depression—all characteristic of Parkinson's disease. He eventually digressed to a bed-and-wheelchair existence. Occasionally he suffered from relapses of high fevers and received symptomatic treatment as he had previously.

Eight years after the onset of the illness he suffered again with a relapse of fever and was taken to the hospital. This time, however, he was diagnosed with relapsing encephalitis caused by herpes simplex type 1 (HSV-1) infection. HSV-1 is the same virus that causes cold sores or fever blisters on the lips. He was given antiviral drug therapy and within three weeks, his health was miraculously restored, including his ability to do mathematics. At the time he was discharged, his doctor reported that he was well oriented, had good focus of attention, good abstracting ability, a pleasant sense of humor, and interestingly, no Parkinson's symptoms.

After the initial infection, the herpes virus can lie dormant in the body indefinitely. During an active infection, HSV-1, otherwise known as oral herpes, invades the trigeminal nerve where it finds a safe haven from the immune system. The trigeminal nerve connects to the brain stem and branches out over the face, controlling muscle movement and picking up sensations to relay back to the brain. The virus can remain alive indefinitely within the roots of the trigeminal nerve. It is kept from spreading outside the nerve by the immune system. Whenever the immune system is compromised or becomes overburdened (due to excessive stress, fatigue, infection, depression, etc.), the virus may be allowed to spread out beyond the trigeminal nerve roots, causing fever blisters on the lips. In time, the immune system pushes the virus back into hiding. In some cases, the virus can spread from the trigeminal nerve into the brain, where it sets up residence. Poor immune function can lead to attacks of acute encephalitis. Antiviral drugs have limited use because they are only effective against active infections when the virus spreads beyond the nerve cells. They cannot rid the body of viruses hiding within the nerve cells.

The patient described above likely had a continual low-grade infection that periodically flared up, causing a systemic fever. His immune system was probably ineffective in controlling the chronic infection. If his immune system comes under stress again, he may still experience another acute encephalitis infection.

While the herpes virus can infect any part of the brain, it appears to have an affinity for the substantia nigra that controls motor movement.[3] Since herpes is a very common infection, it is possible that many cases of Parkinson's disease could be herpes-related. One tell-tale sign of infection are periodic outbreaks of cold sores, indicating the presence of the herpes virus. Most people are infected with this herpes virus—more than 70 percent of the population over age 50. About 70 percent of those who are infected, do not experience periodic outbreaks or cold sores, so most individuals aren't even aware they are infected.

Researchers have discovered that at least one strain of the avian (bird) flu leaves survivors at significantly increased risk for Parkinson's and possibly Alzheimer's disease. The virus travels from the stomach, through the nervous system, and into the brain. Animals infected by the virus have demonstrated acute neurological symptoms ranging from mild encephalitis to motor disturbances to coma.

Researchers report that mice which survive infection with the avian flu are more likely than uninfected mice to develop brain changes associated with neurological disorders. The researchers found that avian flu destroyed neurons in the substantia nigra and caused the accumulation of protein deposits commonly found in both Parkinson's and Alzheimer's diseases.[4]

Researchers examined the longer-term neurologic consequences of the virus among survivors. Mice were infected with a strain of the avian flu virus called H5N1. After three weeks there was no evidence of the virus in the nervous systems of the surviving mice, but the inflammation the infection triggered within the brain continued for months afterwards. Although the tremor and movement problems disappeared as flu symptoms eased, investigators reported that 60 days later the mice had lost 17 percent of their dopamine-producing cells.

The researchers point out that neither the avian flu nor any infection that activates the immune response in the brain directly causes Parkinson's disease but rather increase *susceptibility* to the disease. We all lose some brain cells as we age, but most people die before they lose enough neurons to get Parkinson's or Alzheimer's. Infections that affect the brain can change that curve. This study supports a hit-and-run mechanism at work with Parkinson's disease. In this case, the avian flu sparks an immune response that persists long after the initial threat is gone, setting patients up for further divesting losses from another infection, drugs, or environmental toxins. The hit-and-run mechanism would also explain the absence of microorganisms in some brain tissues from Parkinson's and Alzheimer's patients. Infections could be a very significant factor in initiating the neurodegeneration yet leave little evidence they were ever involved.

Other viruses known to induce parkinsonism include Coxsackie, Japanese encephalitis B, St. Louis encephalitis, West Nile, and HIV.[5-6] In addition, there also appears to be a possible association with the bacteria *Mycoplasma pneumoniae*, *Borrelia burgdorferi* (Lyme disease), *Helicobacter pylori* (gastric ulcers), and others.[7-8] There is even evidence that the yeast *Candida albicans* may contribute to the disease.[9]

INFECTION AND AMYOTROPHIC LATERAL SCLEROSIS

Dr. Christopher Martyn at the University of Southampton, England believes that ALS, like Parkinson's disease, may originate from infections that occur earlier in life. Martyn and colleagues found a correlation between the incidence of ALS in the UK during the 1960s and the incidence of polio in the 1930s. He believes that ALS is a delayed consequence of an infection with poliovirus that affects the central nervous system and causes loss of motoneurons but is not usually severe enough to cause motor symptoms or paralysis at the time of the acute illness.[10]

The polio virus is not the only infection that can lead to ALS, just as all Parkinson's cases are not the result of encephalitis lethargic. Any number of viruses, bacteria, fungi, and parasites could be responsible for initiating neuro-inflammation and brain cell loss that set the stage for neurodegeneration. ALS has been linked to a number of infectious organisms, including mycoplasma, *Treponema pallidum* (syphilis), HIV, echovirus, herpes simplex 1 virus, human herpesvirus-6, *Chlamydia pneumoniae*, and *Borrelia burgdorferi.*[11-17] Of these, *Borrelia burgdorferi,* the cause of Lyme disease, may be the most significant.

Borrelia burgdorferi is a member of the spirochete family of bacteria. Spirochetes are a troublesome group with the various species causing Lyme disease, syphilis, yaws, periodontal disease, and leptospirosis, among others. Spirochetes are long, thin, corkscrew- or spiral-shaped bacteria, thus the term "spiro" in the name. Several species of spirochetes can and do infect the brain.

The spirochete that causes Lyme disease is carried by deer ticks. It is passed on to humans through the bite of an infected tick. Since the ticks are small, bites often go undetected. The infection usually starts off with the development of a circular rash at the site of the tick bite; later, flu-like symptoms develop. Often the infection is believed to be caused by the flu and little is done for it. Left untreated, the disease can affect the joints, heart, and central nervous system. In most cases the infection is eliminated by antibiotics, especially if the illness is treated early. Late or inadequate treatment can lead to more serious symptoms which can be difficult to treat and may require months of intense antibiotic therapy. Even after the acute infection is over, chronic symptoms may persist indefinitely. Acute neurological symptoms appear in 15 percent of inadequately treated patients, with about 5 percent experiencing chronic disorders.[18] Among those disorders is ALS.[19]

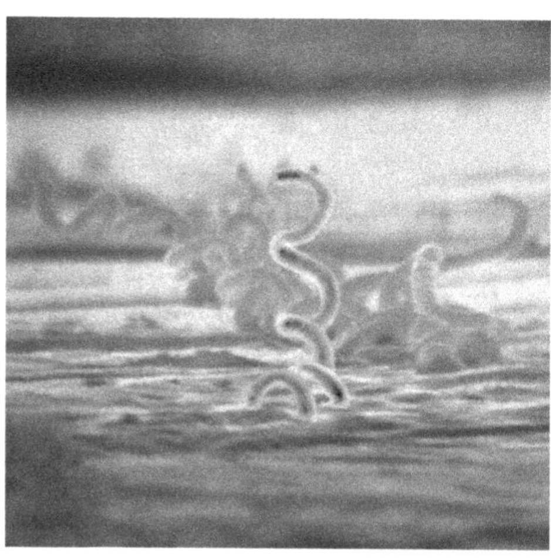

Spirochetes (Treponema pallidum).

Dr. David Martz of Colorado Springs, Colorado, who has become a specialist in treating chronic Lyme disease, says about 15 percent of his ALS patients substantially improve and another 20-30 percent stop declining with intensive antibiotic treatment. His interest in Lyme disease was ignited in 2003 after he was unknowingly stricken with the disease and afterwards developed ALS. He deteriorated rapidly to the point where he was unable to drive, dress himself, or walk, which forced him to retire from his medical practice at the age of 62. At this point, he was unaware that he had been infected with Lyme disease. Eight months later, while bedridden and confined to a wheelchair, he learned from a friend, who sent him a newspaper clipping, that it was possible his ALS may have resulted from a tick bite.

Six times he was tested for Lyme disease and six times the tests came back negative (late-stage Lyme is notoriously difficult to detect). Finally a seventh, more accurate test showed he was positive for Lyme Borrelia. Based on this new information, Dr. Martz began intensive antibiotic therapy to treat his ALS. He noticed dramatic improvement in his symptoms and within 12 weeks was walking again without assistance. Although he suffered some damage that will likely never heal, he was fully mobile and improved to about 60 percent of his health before the infection. His recovery was so remarkable that the case was reported in an international medical journal.[20] Inspired by his own success, he opened a new clinic specializing in Lyme disease. Although in his mid-60s, he put in 50 hours a week until his second retirement a few years later.

INFECTION AND HUNTINGTON'S DISEASE

Many health conditions can be influenced by genetics. It is believed that a small number (5 percent) of Alzheimer's disease cases are caused by genetic factors; the same is basically true for Parkinson's and other neurodegenerative diseases. While Huntington's disease is generally considered a genetic disease, it too can be influenced by infection.

We now know that environmental factors can activate genes associated with certain health conditions. If conditions are not right, these genes remain dormant and their associated diseases never become a problem. Exposure to toxins or infections that promote inflammation and oxidative stress create an environment in the central nervous system that turns on the huntingtin genes, allowing them to be expressed. Environmental conditions play a huge part in determining if and when those with the huntingtin gene develop the disease. Infections are known to accelerate the onset and progression of Huntington's disease.

INFECTION AND MULTIPLE SCLEROSIS

Data from studies of twins imply that MS is an environmentally caused disease. The most likely environmental factor is infection. MS has been associated with a number of viruses and bacteria, most notably Epstein-Barr virus, herpes simplex virus (oral and genital herpes), human herpesvirus-6, varicella zoster virus (chicken-pox virus), *Chlamydia pneumoniae*, and spirochetes. Of these, Epstein-Barr virus, which causes infectious mononucleosis, appears to have the strongest connection, but any of them may play a contributing role.

Epstein-Barr virus is known to infect the central nervous system and cause demyelination—the characteristic feature of MS. Once infected, the virus remains in the host for life. The virus usually remains dormant but can be reactivated. The periodic flare-ups associated with MS are believed to be associated reactivation of the virus. Although the majority of adult MS patients do not have an active mononucleosis infection at the time of diagnosis, nearly 100 percent demonstrate evidence of having been infected by the Epstein-Barr virus at some time before developing MS.[21]

Epstein-Barr virus does not infect animals; humans are its exclusive natural host. This may explain why MS is unique to humans.[22]

Perhaps the most convincing study to demonstrate the connection between the Epstein-Barr virus and MS was conducted by researchers at the Walter Reed Army Institute of Research in Washington, DC. Investigators had access to a massive database that included blood samples of 3 million US military personnel. Rarely do studies have anywhere near this many human samples for comparison, giving the results of this one an extraordinarily high degree of credibility. The study demonstrated a strong positive association between Epstein-Barr infection and the development of MS.[23] Their results indicated a lag time of several years between the initial infection and subsequent development of MS. Although infection is strongly associated with MS, that does not exclude other factors from possibly being involved, such as a high-sugar diet, mercury dental fillings, vitamin D deficiency, etc.—the combination of such events may be the trigger that ignites the disease.[24]

INFECTION AND ALZHEIMER'S

It has been known for a century that dementia, brain atrophy, and amyloid plaque can be caused by chronic infections. In fact, Alois Alzheimer, for whom Alzheimer's disease is named, suggested infection as the underlying cause of the disease. A number of microorganisms associated with Alzheimer's have been found, including spirochetes, herpes virus (HSV-1), *Chlamydia pneumonia*, Epstein-Barr virus, human immunodeficiency virus (HIV), picornavirus, Borna disease virus, *Helicobacter pylori*, and cytomegalovirus.[25-29]

The three most common suspects are spirochetes, herpes (HSV-1), and *Chlamydia pneumonia*. The evidence linking these three microorganisms to Alzheimer's is so compelling that researchers are now beginning to accept them as major contributors, if not the primary causes, of the disease.

Dementia has long been known to be associated with the syphilis spirochete *Treponema pallidum*. Another troublesome spirochete that has gained notoriety as a cause of dementia is the Lyme disease bacterium *Borrelia burgdorferi*.

Once an acute Lyme infection is over, it has generally been believed that the Borrelia bacterium has been completely eradicated from the body. However, health problems associated with the bacterium often linger for months or years afterwards. Some researchers have interpreted this as an autoimmune response initiated by the infection, but it is becoming evident that a low-grade infection can persist indefinitely, causing chronic health problems. Evidence for this is found in the brains of Alzheimer's patients who have previously been infected with Lyme disease. The bacterium is found in Alzheimer's brains in association with amyloid plaque.[30]

Herpes virus, too, has often been found in the brains of Alzheimer's patients. The virus is believed to be directly involved in the aggregation of amyloid beta protein in brain tissue. When the virus is added to cultured brain cells, it results in a dramatic increase in amyloid beta. Likewise, in rat brains the virus causes the proliferation of amyloid beta.[31]

In human studies, evidence of herpes virus has been found in 90 percent of the plaque examined in Alzheimer's brains, strongly implicating a connection between the virus and Alzheimer's disease.[32] It is apparent that herpes plays a major role in the development of Alzheimer's disease. Preliminary experiments have shown that the antiviral drug acyclovir reduces amyloid deposition, strengthening the connection even further.

Herpes is insidious. It can hide within the nerve cells safe from the effects of immune defenses, yet when immune strength dips due to stress or infection, the virus can come out of hiding, ignite inflammation, and further the progression of neurodegeneration and brain cell death. Reactivation causes repeated damage and the accumulation of amyloid plaque. The virus plays this cat and mouse game throughout the host's life, slowly eating away at the brain.[33]

The virus is absent in the brains of most young people, but infection rates increase in older individuals.[34] Carrying the herpes virus is no guarantee a person will develop Alzheimer's. The virus is frequently found in the brains of normal elderly individuals as well.[35] This suggests that herpes infection is not the only cause of the disease but combines with other factors.

Herpes doesn't need to be present in the brain to cause neurodegeneration. Any microorganism that infects the arteries, causing plaque buildup and strokes, can potentially promote dementia. Herpes is one of these. This was demonstrated by researchers from Columbia University. The researchers studied 1,625 adults whose average age was 68.4 years living in the multi-ethnic urban community of northern Manhattan, New York. Blood was obtained from all participants—none of whom had a history of stroke—and was tested for antibodies indicating prior exposure to herpes simplex virus type 1 (oral herpes) and type 2 (genital herpes) as well as three other common pathogens: *Chlamydia pneumonia*, *Helicobacter pylori*, and cytomegalovirus. A weighted composite index of exposure to all five pathogens was developed. Participants were followed up annually over a median of 7.6 years. During this time period, 67 had strokes. Although herpes simplex type 1 was common, all five of the infections were positively associated with stroke risk.[36]

There were several reasons to investigate these five particular pathogens. First, each of these common pathogens may persist after an acute infection and thus contribute to perpetuating a state of chronic low-level infection. Second, prior studies demonstrate an association between each of these pathogens and atherosclerosis. Studies examining several of these pathogens individually have shown that they can be involved in the process that leads to stroke and, consequently, vascular dementia and Alzheimer's.[37]

Chlamydia pneumoniae is perhaps the most common microorganism found in arterial plaque. As the name implies, this bacterium is a common cause of pneumonia. It is also associated with sinusitis, laryngitis, bronchitis, asthma, and other respiratory problems. While some of these infections can be serious, others are relatively minor and may produce little more than sinus congestion and coughing, which may be presumed to be a cold. Infection by *Chlamydia pneumoniae* is common and a person may be infected without realizing it. It is a common cause of what is termed *walking pneumonia*, so named because people are able to continue most normal daily activities during the infection. In the United States about 50 percent of adults have been infected by it, and reinfection throughout life appears to be common.

While primarily associated with respiratory infections, *Chlamydia pneumoniae* can enter the bloodstream, causing a variety of problems including arthritis, myocarditis (inflammation of the heart), Guillain-Barré syndrome (inflammation of the nerves), encephalitis, and atherosclerosis. In the bloodstream the bacterium attacks the arteries causing chronic inflammation and the formation of plaque (atherosclerosis), which can clog arteries and lead to heart attacks or strokes.[38-39]

Many researchers consider infection to be the primary cause of atherosclerosis and heart disease, instead of simply an accumulation of excess cholesterol. Most arterial plaque contains evidence of *Chlamydia pneumoniae* or other microorganisms even when little or no cholesterol is present, indicating that infection is more important to plaque buildup than cholesterol.[40-41] For example, in a group of 90 heart disease patients, investigators found *Chlamydia pneumoniae* in the arterial plaque of 79 percent. In comparison, they found fewer than 4 percent in the artery walls of individuals who did not have heart disease. Animal studies provide more direct evidence. Rabbits infected with *Chlamydia pneumoniae* show measurably thickened arterial walls.[42]

Not only can *Chlamydia pneumoniae* induce atherosclerosis that can lead to strokes and neurodegeneration, but it can also directly infect the brain. In fact, studies have repeatedly shown the presence of the bacterium in Alzheimer's brains. In one study, investigators found the bacterium in the brain tissue of 17 out of 19 Alzheimer's patients, while in age-matched non-Alzheimer's brain tissue it was found in only 1 out of 19 cases.[43]

In another study, investigators analyzing brain tissue from deceased Alzheimer's patients found *Chlamydia pneumoniae* in 90 percent of the subjects studied. In comparison, only 5 percent of non-Alzheimer's brains contained this bacterium.[44] Apparently, *Chlamydia pneumoniae* not only causes plaque formation in the arteries but does the same in the brain. The bacterium in the above study was found within the amyloid plaques that are characteristic of Alzheimer's disease.

In addition, when mice were exposed to a nasal spray containing the bacterium, they developed the same senile plaques in their brains, providing further proof that the bacterium triggers amyloid plaque formation.[45]

When you look at the various forms of neurodegeneration you repeatedly find the usual suspects: spirochetes, herpes, and *Chlamydia pneumoniae*. These appear to be the principle instigators. Yet, an assortment of other nefarious microorganisms may also on occasion be involved.

DRUG THERAPY

Since infections are often associated with neurodegeneration, it might be assumed that antibiotic or antiviral therapy would provide an easy solution. This, however, is not the case. Drug therapy is not always successful because most drugs cannot cross over the blood-brain barrier. In addition, antibiotics work only against bacteria; they are ineffective against viruses, fungi, and drug-resistant bacteria. Antiviral drugs have also proven to be generally ineffective in eradicating viruses in the brain.[46] Some infections are transitory: they hit-and-run, causing damage and inflammation before being ousted by the body's immune defenses, or, as in the case of herpes, go into hiding within the nerve cells.

Since any number of microorganisms can be involved, and may or may not even be actively present, drug therapy is generally impractical.

For the most part, we must rely on the immune system to keep the brain clear of infection and running smoothly.

THE IMMUNE SYSTEM AND SENILE PLAQUE

The immune system protects against infectious organisms and toxins; recycles old, diseased, or renegade cells (cancer); and promotes tissue repair and healing. The backbone of the immune system is the army of white blood cells which constantly patrol the body and of which there are many varieties with various functions. Some white blood cells phagocyte (eat) the invader and others secrete lethal substances on them. Others produce antibodies—proteins created to neutralize specific microorganisms.

The immune system is normally capable of providing adequate protection against infection. However, due to the blood-brain barrier, the central nervous system is generally inaccessible to the white blood cells and antibodies. Therefore, the brain must rely on another form of defense to fight infection.

As you recall from Chapter 2, the brain consists of two primary types of nerve cells: neurons that relay messages and store memories and glia that function in a supporting capacity. There are different types of glia, each with specific functions; one type, called the *microglia,* acts as the brain's defense against infection and toxins.

Normally, microglia cells are in a resting state and rather inconspicuous. When activated by an intruder or injury they spring into action, quickly proliferating, enlarging, becoming mobile, and going on the attack engulfing foreign substances and removing damaged cells. They take on the duties and character of white blood cells. In the process, they send signals that increase blood flow, stimulate inflammation, and rally various substances to their aid. After the crisis is over, the microglia gradually return to a docile existence as they were before the insult.

Ordinarily, this process protects the brain from insults due to infections, injury, and toxins while stimulating cleanup and repair. But repeated insults to the brain can lead to a chronic heightened level of activity, causing further damage leading to neurodegeneration. Deposits of heavy metals, frequent drug use, toxic exposure, or chronic infection can keep the microglia activated, stoking the flames of inflammation and tissue degeneration.

Inflammation disrupts the blood-brain barrier, causing it to become leaky. White blood cells, blood proteins, bacteria, and other substances that were once locked out of the central nervous system are now allowed to enter, stirring up more trouble and activating more microglia and producing more inflammation, resulting in a vicious cycle.

In addition to the white blood cells, the immune system incorporates a number of specialized proteins called antimicrobial peptides (AMPs) that are synthesized in various cells and present in the blood. AMPs specifically target invading microorganisms but also defend against cancerous cells and various toxins. AMPs were originally discovered in white blood cells after activation by bacteria, viruses, and fungi. Their action kills these invading organisms, moderates inflammation, and promotes healing.[47]

One of the most extensively studied AMPs is known by the name LL-37. This particular AMP is produced in various cells, among which are a number of white blood cells. When faced with an intruder, white blood cells secrete LL-37 into the blood. LL-37 is attracted to the outer membrane of the invading microorganism where it hooks in, causing the invader to rupture and die. LL-37 is also synthesized and secreted in significant amounts by cells in the mucous membranes of the mouth, tongue, esophagus, lungs, intestines, cervix, and vagina. In addition, it is produced by salivary and sweat glands, testis, and mammary glands. LL-37 is secreted into wounds, sweat, airway surface fluids, seminal fluid, and milk.

The central nervous system also has resident AMPs. Its version of LL-37 is amyloid precursor protein (APP). This is the same protein transformed in amyloid beta that builds up to form the characteristic plaque of Alzheimer's disease. For years the prevailing theory has been that amyloid beta plaque was one of the chief villains in Alzheimer's disease. It was believed to be nothing more than a sticky waste product that interfered with normal brain function, and much research has focused on reducing amyloid beta buildup.

New research has demonstrated that instead of being part of the problem, it is one of the means by which the body fights off infection and other insults and thus preserves brain function.[48-49] The discovery was made by researchers at Harvard Medical School. Rudolph E. Tanzi, a neurology professor who is also director of the genetics and aging unit at Massachusetts General Hospital, was looking at genes of senile plaque from Alzheimer's patients. To his surprise, the genes looked just like those associated with antimicrobial peptides of the immune system, particularly LL-37.

That evening, Dr. Tanzi wandered into the office of another faculty member, Robert D. Moir, and mentioned the strange similarity in the genetic code of amyloid beta and LL-37. Dr. Moir turned to him and said, "Yeah, well, look at this." He handed Dr. Tanzi a spreadsheet. It was a comparison between amyloid beta and LL-37. Among other things, the two proteins had similar structures. Like amyloid beta, LL-37 tends to clump into hard little plaques. Both induce pro-inflammatory activities, stimulating the immune system. The likenesses were uncanny. Was it possible that amyloid beta was actually part of the immune system?

The scientists could hardly wait to see if amyloid beta, like LL-37, killed microbes. They mixed amyloid beta with microbes that LL-37 is known to kill—candida, listeria, staphylococcus, streptococcus, E. coli, and others. It killed 8 out of 12.[50]

In most cases the amyloid beta was just as potent and, in some cases, more potent than LL-37. The pathogen that was most sensitive to amyloid beta was the yeast *Candida albicans*—a major cause of meningitis. Amyloid beta was far more effective in killing candida than was LL-37.

The researchers then compared the antimicrobial effects of Alzheimer's and non-Alzheimer's brain tissues. Samples of brain tissue containing amyloid beta from an Alzheimer's brain demonstrated strikingly higher antimicrobial activity against Candia compared to similar tissue without amyloid beta from an age-matched non-demented brain. However, when tissue samples without amyloid beta from the Alzheimer's brain were compared to those of an amyloid-free normal brain, there was no difference in antimicrobial potency. Whether the brain was affected by Alzheimer's didn't matter; it was the presence of the amyloid that gave the tissue the antimicrobial effect. They found that the higher the amyloid beta content, the greater the activity against candida. Clearly the amyloid beta present in the Alzheimer's brain is not a mistake or incidental debris but is there as a means of defense. It is a product of the body's immune system.

If the normal function of amyloid beta is to act as an AMP, then the absence of the peptide may result in an increased vulnerability to infection. In animal studies, this appears to be the case. Mice bred with a genetic deficiency of the enzymes needed to generate amyloid beta have an increased susceptibility to infections.[51] These mice have mortality rates of 40 to 60 percent higher than normal when exposed to infectious microorganisms in the environment. The same thing occurs in humans. In a clinical trial, Alzheimer's patients given medication to reduce the formation of amyloid beta developed increased rates of infection.[52]

When the brain is exposed to herpes, *Chlamydia pneumoniae*, Lyme Borrelia, and other pathogenic microorganisms, the body responds by producing amyloid beta in its defense.[53-56] Amyloid beta isn't restricted to just infections; it is also produced in response to traumatic brain injuries, stroke, and chemical toxins.[57-59]

Amyloid beta may not be the only AMP that is active in the brain. Other protein deposits associated with neurodegenerative disease, such as alpha-synclein in Lewy body deposits—a common feature in Parkinson's disease—also appear to be products of our immune defense. Richard Smeyne and colleagues from St. Jude Children's Research Hospital have reported that mice infected with the avian flu virus develop extensive alpha-synclein deposits throughout their brains, including the substantia nigra area associated with Parkinson's disease. The avian flu virus triggers the alpha-synclein build-up just as other infections activate amyloid beta formation.[60] The reason for the different types of protein deposits may be that different microorganisms activate different AMPs. In some cases, a microorganism or toxin may trigger several AMPs, leading to the accumulation of various protein deposits often seen in neurodegenerative disease. For example, LL-37 is more effective in combating *Streptococcus pyogenes*, but amyloid beta is more potent against *Candida albicans*. Only the most relevant AMPs would be activated to fight each pathogen.

Just as *Chlamydia pneumoniae* and herpes are found within amyloid plaques, Borrelia burgdorferi have been found in Lewy bodies of Parkinson's patients, providing further evidence that alpha-synclein functions as a AMP.[61]

It might be that other protein deposits found in the various neurodegenerative diseases are also products of the immune system. Future research will have to verify this.

SYSTEMIC INFLAMMATION KILLS BRAIN CELLS

Prior to the 1990s, the brain was regarded as an immune privileged organ, meaning it was not susceptible to inflammation or immune activation and was thought to be largely unaffected by systemic inflammatory and immune responses. This view has changed considerably.

We now know that the brain can mount a robust response to acute insults with the activation of microglia, AMPs, and other immune defense factors, along with releasing inflammatory mediators to stimulate blood flow and loosen the blood-brain barrier to allow peripheral white blood cells into the central nervous system to assist in the battle.

Although the blood-brain barrier shields the central nervous system from many infectious organisms and other potentially harmful substances, the brain is not as isolated from the rest of the body as is commonly believed. What goes on elsewhere in the body can have a profound effect on the brain. Even minor infections such as a seasonal flu or a cold can have a direct influence on the brain.

It is well known that people suffering from systemic infections can experience delirium—a temporary state of mental confusion accompanied by anxiety, hallucinations, disturbed speech, and impaired cognition. This disruption in mental function is more common in the elderly and in those with neurodegenerative disease.[62]

Systemic infections of any type, whether from the flu, food poisoning, bladder infection, yeast infection, pneumonia, or even periodontitis (gum infection), can release inflammatory mediators—special proteins manufactured by the immune system to activate inflammation. One of these mediators is called *tumor necrosis factor-alpha* or TNF-alpha. Blood levels of TNF-alpha are increased by infections or physical trauma and indicate higher levels of inflammation in the body. An injury or infection causes the release of TNF-alpha into the bloodstream to stimulate inflammation. As TNF-alpha crosses over the blood-brain barrier, it activates microglia, triggering an inflammatory response in the brain. Neuroinflammation triggered by systemic infection or trauma can cause a rapid decline in cognitive and motor function, which in turn, is followed by an accelerated rate of neurodegeneration.[63]

Any infection or injury can adversely affect the brain, igniting the onset of neurodegenerative disease or accelerating its progression. When the brain is already crippled with disease, the decline can be observed and measured. For example, a Huntington's disease patient, whose mental test and function scores had been stable for more than a year, received a flu and pneumonia vaccine. As a result of the vaccination he developed a high fever accompanied by delirium. After his recovery, he scored significantly poorer on his mental and functional tests. Over the next few years he experienced a steady decline in mental and functional ability with a rapid progression of his disease.

This same thing occurs in Alzheimer's patients. This was documented in a study published in the journal *Neurology*, which showed that even a minor infection, such as a cold, could double the rate of memory loss. This study involved 222 patients with mild to severe Alzheimer's. Over the course of six months, blood samples were taken periodically from each patient. During the study period, about half of the patients had one or more colds (or other respiratory or gastrointestinal infections) or experienced falls that led to increased levels of TNF-alpha. Those who experienced increased TNF-alpha levels had *twice* the rate of cognitive decline than those with normal levels.

Some of the patients had high levels of TNF-alpha at the start of the study, an indication they may have been suffering from chronic inflammation. Chronic inflammation could be due to such things as arthritis, irritable bowel syndrome, hemorrhoids, and such, which are common with older people. These patients had *four* times greater cognitive decline than those who did not have elevated TNF-alpha levels, even when they did not experience colds or other transitory infections. Interestingly, those who had both beginning high levels of TNF-alpha and experienced an infection had *10* times the memory loss.[64]

Illnesses that we normally consider to be of little consequence such as a cold or urinary tract infection need to be taken much more seriously in seniors with neurodegenerative disease. Acute illnesses or injuries that increase inflammation, even outside the central nervous system, may have serious consequences on cognitive and motor skills. The authors of the study stress the point that the decline in mental function is not a temporary effect but remains even after the illness and inflammation have long gone.

The authors conclude that quelling inflammation with medications may help stem mental decline but noted that studies using nonsteroidal anti-inflammatory drugs, like Celebrex and Aleve, have so far proven to be ineffective.[65-66] Maintaining a healthy immune system capable of keeping infections and inflammation at bay through diet, lifestyle, and other natural means is a better option.

11 The Dental Connection

ORAL HEALTH AND THE BRAIN

Researchers have found evidence of a number of different bacteria and viruses in the brains of Alzheimer's patients and others with neurodegenerative diseases. As noted earlier, the most common microorganisms associated with Alzheimer's disease are spirochetes, herpes simplex virus type 1 (HSV-1) and *Chlamydia pneumonia*, but others, such as *Helicobacter pylori* and cytomegalovirus, may also become involved.

Where do all these infectious organisms come from? Some may come from the bite of an infected insect or from unprotected sex. Some may even enter through a cut or an ulcer on the skin. But most come from the mouth. All of these microorganisms are common inhabitants of the mouth and sinuses. Any cut, ulcer, or other opening inside the mouth allows these microorganisms access to the bloodstream, which can carry them to the brain.

Wayne, age 54, was admitted to hospital after suffering from a sudden weakness on one side of his body accompanied by a series of epileptic fits. He underwent a succession of tests and brain scans to determine the cause. The diagnosis: cerebral abscess—an infection in his brain. The doctors then began to look for the source of the infection. Radiograph images of his mouth revealed the presence of periodontal disease and multiple dental cavities. Believing his condition was caused by his dental infections, treatment involved the removal of his decayed and diseased teeth along with antibiotic therapy. The patient made a complete recovery and over a period of 2½ years has remained healthy.

The health of our teeth and gums has long been known to affect the health of the rest of our bodies, including the brain. It is not unusual for oral bacteria to infect the brain, causing acute and chronic illness.[1-8]

Darrel had a history of repeated episodes of memory loss with increasing severity and duration, extending over a period of four years. During these episodes his mentality was so void that he would eat when things were put before him but lacked judgment regarding eating. His attacks would come on with at first a sense of excitement, then extreme nervousness followed by a period of crying. During the onset of his last attack he drove his car 35 miles on dirt roads and could not recall the trip or any incident in connection with it. He would have to stop to think to answer simple questions such as "How much is two plus two?" When crossing the street, he would have to stop and study what the crossings were and where they were. When these attacks first started, his brain seemed go into slow motion.

Some years previously he had several infected teeth that were cleaned and covered with gold crowns. Afterwards he began developing these serious symptoms. The first symptom was a slight and transient disturbance of memory. His symptoms grew progressively worse over time.

Suspecting the teeth may still be harboring infection, the gold crowns and the infected teeth were extracted. Within days of their removal his memory returned to normal and the appearance of his face changed from that of confusion and emptiness to one of mental alertness. The change was permanent and he did not experience any relapses in memory loss.

Poor oral health can give you more than just cavities or aching teeth—it can cause dementia and motor disturbances. In other words, your teeth can give you Alzheimer's or Parkinson's disease. Poor oral health has been linked to a number of health problems including atherosclerosis, stroke, heart failure, kidney disease, pneumonia, diabetes, low birth weight, and premature deliveries; now Alzheimer's has been added to the list.[9-13]

The danger of oral bacteria spreading to other parts of the body is very real and potentially serious. Dental patients who have certain health conditions, especially prosthetic limbs or artificial heart valves, are given antibiotics whenever they receive dental treatment. Dentists know that even routine dental work can cause cuts or tears in the patients' gum tissue that can allow oral bacteria to enter their bloodstream and cause an infection elsewhere in the body.[14]

While antibiotics are usually prescribed for those with obvious health problems, they are not generally given to otherwise healthy individuals. It is believed that healthy people are capable of fighting off the bacteria that get into the system during dental treatment. This isn't always the case. Emmy-winning actor Peter Falk, who starred in the hit television series *Columbo* for many years, slipped rapidly into dementia after receiving a series of dental operations in 2007. Falk was 79 at the time and was still mentally sharp and active in his career, which required him to memorize pages of script in a matter of days. After the dental work his memory quickly faded. In less than two years he digressed into an advanced stage of Alzheimer's and could no longer remember his role in *Columbo*, for which he earned four Emmys.

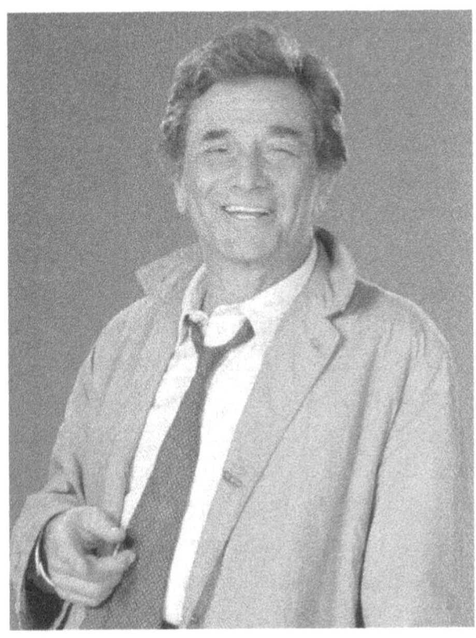

Actor Peter Falk suffered from Alzheimer's soon after receiving a series of dental operations.

BREEDING GROUND OF INFECTION

We have billions of bacteria, viruses, fungi, and parasites living in our mouths. There are over 600 species of bacteria alone that make our mouths their home. Many of these bacteria produce toxins as by-products, which damage the teeth and irritate the gums, causing inflammation and bleeding. An overgrowth of these bacteria leads to tooth decay, gum disease, and eventually tooth loss.

Periodontal or gum disease starts with dental plaque—a sticky film that grows on the teeth due to the interaction of bacteria with starches and sugars in the foods we eat. Plaque is made up of colonies of bacteria growing on and around the teeth. Brushing removes most of the plaque, but it quickly reforms over the course of a few hours. If plaque stays on the teeth, it can harden into a calcified deposit called tartar or calculus. Brushing and flossing cannot remove tartar. It can only be removed by professional cleaning. Plaque and tartar act as breeding grounds for bacteria. As bacteria colonies grow, they and their toxic byproducts irritate gums and teeth, breaking them down.

The longer plaque and tartar remain on the teeth, the more damage they cause. When infection is restricted to the topmost layers of the gum tissue, it is called gingivitis. Gingivitis is the first stage of periodontal disease and is characterized by red, swollen, and bleeding gums. Usually there is little to no pain or discomfort, so those with the infection often don't realize they have a problem.

Periodontitis extends deeper into the gums and is a much more serious condition—and very difficult to treat. Chronic inflammation causes pockets to develop between the gums and teeth and fill with bacteria, plaque, and tartar. In time, the pockets become deeper and more bacteria accumulate, eventually burrowing under the diseased gum tissue and extending down into the bone. Deep infections can destroy underlying bone and connective tissues, leading to tooth loss.

Among the oral bacteria that live in the mouth are a number of spirochetes, relatives to the spirochetes that cause Lyme disease and syphilis. Essentially everyone has oral spirochetes in their mouths. Like their well-known cousins, oral spirochetes are also the cause of disease, most notably periodontal disease.[15]

Oral spirochetes are exceptionally resistant to disinfectants (mouthwashes), detergents (toothpaste), and antibiotics, which makes them difficult to control. Antibiotics, or any other unfriendly environmental condition, can trigger a survival mechanism, transforming the corkscrew shaped bacterium into a more protective spore-like or spherical body. In this form they can survive harsh conditions and resurface at a later time.

There are numerous species of oral spirochetes, some of which have yet to be identified and named. Most of those that have been identified are closely related to *Treponema pallidum*—the spirochete that causes syphilis.

Oral spirochetes can burrow down beneath the gum line, causing infection. This infection can fester deep into the gums and even extend down into the underlying bone.

An overgrowth of oral spirochetes along with other normal mouth bacteria can lead to acute necrotizing ulcerative gingivitis, otherwise known as trench mouth—a severe form of gum disease that causes painful, swollen, bleeding gums, and ulcerations. The gums between the teeth erode and become covered with gray decaying tissue accompanied by a foul odor. Trench mouth received its name from soldiers fighting in the trenches during World War I. The disease became epidemic among soldiers who were stuck in trenches for long periods of time without being able to take proper care of their teeth. Regular dental hygiene has made trench mouth uncommon nowadays, but the bacteria that cause trench mouth are still very much alive and well, even in the cleanest of mouths.

Lyme disease and syphilis spirochetes are well documented causes of Alzheimer's and other neurodegenerative diseases.[16-19] More recently, oral spirochetes have proven to be just as destructive. In fact, the danger from oral spirochetes is much greater than that from Lyme and syphilis spirochetes because infections by these latter two bacteria are relatively rare. Yet virtually everyone has oral spirochetes in their bodies, waiting for the opportunity to cause infection. Several studies have now linked oral spirochetes as a cause or a contributing factor in Alzheimer's disease.[20-25]

For example, in postmortem examinations of brain tissues, researchers from Oregon Health and Sciences University School of Dentistry looked for evidence of two species of oral spirochetes known to cause periodontal disease. They detected evidence of these spirochetes in brain tissue in 88 percent (14 of 16) of samples from subjects with Alzheimer's disease, but only 22 percent (4 of 18) in samples from control subjects.[26] Oral spirochetes do not belong in the brain—ever! In the mouth, they cause inflammation, ulcers, pus, and tissue decay. They do the same thing in the brain. The researchers only looked for two species of spirochetes out of perhaps two dozen species that inhabit the mouth. If they looked for all known species (and many are yet to be identified) they undoubtedly would have found an even higher percentage of spirochetes in the Alzheimer's brains. The fact that these researchers found two species in 88 percent of the Alzheimer's subjects examined strongly suggests their involvement in the disease.

In another study, researchers found spirochetes in all 14 autopsy cases of Alzheimer's examined, but failed to find them in any of the 13 age-matched subjects who did not have the disease,[27] providing further evidence to the strong involvement spirochetes may play in Alzheimer's disease.

Spirochetes are not the only oral microorganisms that can find their way into the brain. *Chlamydia pneumoniae* is another. Most of us have *Chlamydia pneumoniae* living in our sinuses and mouths. Like spirochetes, it too is a common cause of periodontal disease. Approximately 50 percent of young adults and 75 percent of elderly persons have antibodies showing evidence of an infection with *Chlamydia pneumoniae* at some time in their lives. As stated earlier, *Chlamydia pneumoniae* has been found in the brain tissue of 90 percent of Alzheimer's cases examined.

Herpes simplex type 1 (oral herpes) infects the vast majority of the population, up to 90 percent of the elderly.[28] It can also be actively involved in periodontal disease, but most frequently lies relatively dormant in the trigeminal nerve in the face. When the infection is active and cold sores erupt on the lips, the virus is most easily passed to other people and spread to other parts of the body. Ulcerations and bleeding gums caused by periodontal disease allow the virus a doorway into the bloodstream, where it can travel to the brain. However, it can also reach the brain through the trigeminal nerve.

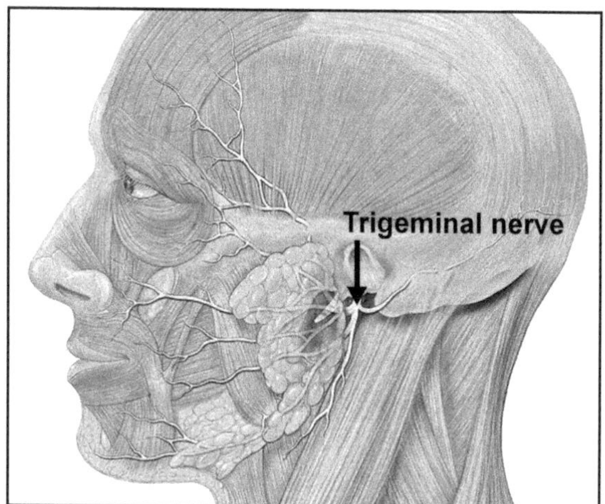

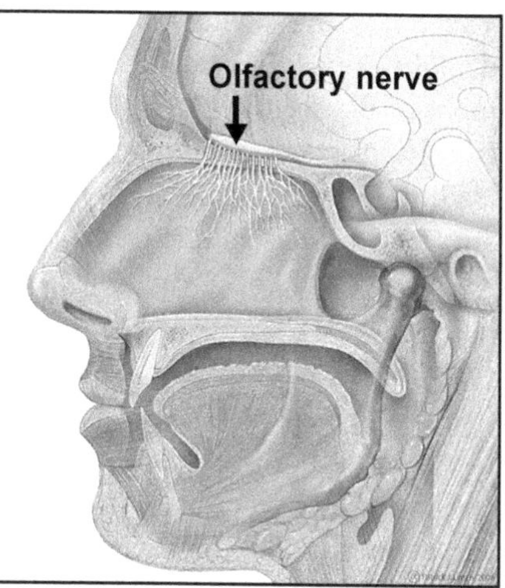

Bacteria and viruses can enter the brain through the trigeminal or olfactory nerves.

Bacteria can also enter the brain through the same nerve pathway. Spirochetes have been known to sometimes travel this route to the brain.[29] In like manner, *Chlamydia pneumoniae* may invade the brain through the olfactory nerve in the sinus cavity.[30] The olfactory nerve is responsible for our sense of smell and is directly attached to the brain.

Helicobacter pylori is another bacterium commonly found in the mouth and is better known as the primary cause of gastric ulcers. *Helicobacter pylori* is frequently found in dental plaque and in periodontal pockets at the base of the teeth, where it often contributes to gum disease.[31]

Helicobacter pylori infection is more common in those with Alzheimer's disease than those without. A study showed the bacterium was detected in the digestive tract of 88 percent of Alzheimer's disease patients but in only 47 percent of age matched controls without the disease.[32] The fact that *Helicobacter pylori* populations are greater in Alzheimer's patients suggests they are likely to also infect the brain. Studies do show that cerebrospinal fluid from Alzheimer's patients have a higher than normal percentage of antibodies to *Helicobacter pylori*, indicating a past or current infection in the brain.[33]

It is interesting that several oral microorganisms have been found to be associated with Alzheimer's disease and other forms of neurodegeneration. Judith Miklossy, MD, PhD, of the University of British Columbia and author of numerous studies on infectious causes of Alzheimer's states that "co-infection of spirochetes with other bacteria, including Chlamydia and Herpes, is frequent."[34] That makes sense. A person with a history of dental problems would have an overgrowth of many types of microorganisms in their mouths and consequently, several of these would likely escape from the mouth and find their way in the brain. It would be reasonable to assume that the type of organisms and their location in the brain would greatly influence whether a person develops Alzheimer's disease or Parkinson's disease or some other neurodegenerative condition.

Multiple sclerosis has also been linked to oral health. Bacteria that cause gum disease can trigger inflammation in the brain that contributes to axon demyelination.[35]

There is also evidence that those with MS also generally have a higher incidence of dental cavities.[36] The link between dental cavities and MS may be due to any one or more of the following: oral infection or toxins entering the brain; oral inflammation triggering neuroinflammation and accelerating disease progression; a high sugar diet leading to tooth decay, which may also influence nerve cell health; or mercury from amalgam fillings in decayed teeth migrating into the brain.

ORAL HEALTH AS AN INDICATOR OF BRAIN HEALTH

A number of studies have shown that Alzheimer's and dementia patients have, in general, poor oral health. This is evidenced by decayed, missing, and filled teeth and the presence of periodontal disease.[37-42] Patients suffering from dementia have twice the number of caries (dental cavities) as age-matched people with normal mental function. While Alzheimer's or dementia itself may accentuate the lack of dental hygiene due to neglecting to take proper care of one's teeth, generally poor dental health exists prior to the onset of the disease.

Parkinson's patients, who are generally not handicapped by poor memory, also suffer from an increased incidence of tooth decay, periodontal disease, and tooth loss.[43-44] In some cases, the onset of Parkinson's disease has been linked directly to bacteria overgrowth and periodontal disease.[45]

Periodontal disease is the most common cause of tooth loss in adults. Except for wisdom teeth and damage due to accidents, teeth are usually extracted because they are diseased. Generally, missing teeth indicate a history of poor oral health and bacteria overgrowth. The fewer teeth a person has, the greater the likelihood of developing neurodegenerative disease. Therefore, oral disease is a risk factor for neurodegeneration.

A team of researchers from the University of Kentucky College of Medicine and College of Dentistry investigated the relationships between tooth loss, dementia, and Alzheimer's in what is known as the Nun Study. The study included 144 Catholic nuns ranging in age from 75 to 98 years. The researchers analyzed dental records and the results of annual cognitive examinations over a period of ten years. Autopsy findings were also used for 118 of the participants who died during the study period. The researchers found that those with the fewest teeth at the beginning of the study were the most likely to develop dementia. This study demonstrated that the more teeth removed due to poor dental health, the greater the risk of dementia.[46]

In a similar study, researchers monitored 686 elderly subjects aged 65 or over who did not have dementia. Dental status was evaluated at the beginning of the study. Two and a half years later dental health was compared between those who remained free from dementia with those that developed dementia by the end of the study. Those with fewer teeth had a significantly higher incidence of dementia and Alzheimer's disease.[47]

The number of teeth a person has reflects overall health and risk of dementia. Investigators interviewed and surveyed all centenarians living in Japan to evaluate their health and activities of daily life. A total of 2,649 centenarians completed the survey. Those who were in good health physically and mentally retained most of their natural teeth. Those who were in poor health and often suffering from dementia had few or no teeth.[48]

In another Japanese study investigators looked at 60 cases of Alzheimer's disease and 120 matched controls without the disease. Five significant risk factors associated with Alzheimer's disease were identified: psychosocial inactivity, physical inactivity, head injury, low education, and loss of teeth. The investigators then evaluated the risks numerically. Compared with those who had none of the risk factors, those who had all five were *935 times* more likely to develop Alzheimer's disease.[49]

To rule out possible genetic factors, researchers investigated the relationship between tooth loss and dementia among identical twins. Participants included 106 pairs of identical twins age 65 or older with one twin from each pair suffering from dementia. Investigators discovered that a history of tooth loss, particularly before age 35, was a significant risk factor for Alzheimer's disease.[50] This study not only showed that oral health is a risk factor for dementia, but that the processes associated with dental health that lead to dementia start earlier in life. A person's dental health in the prime of life can affect their mental health in their later years.

Most people consider their dental health to be far better than it really is. More than 75 percent of American adults currently have some level of active periodontal disease, but according to a major survey only 60 percent of those with the disease have any significant knowledge about the problem. That equates to some 90 million Americans who have periodontal disease and are unaware of it, and as a result are doing nothing to correct the problem.

Periodontal disease and tooth decay are among the most prevalent microbial diseases of mankind. According to a study in the British medical journal the *Lancet*, periodontal disease affects up to 90 percent of the population at some point in their lives.[51] In many cases the disease is treated and overcome, but in others it becomes chronic. In addition, nine out of ten of us have some level of tooth decay. The difference between gum disease and tooth decay is that in the former the infection starts in the gums, and in the latter, it starts in the teeth. As we age, dental health declines and teeth are lost. Poor dental health has become epidemic in our society. One in every 20 middle-aged adults have lost *all* of their teeth. By the age of 65 the chances of having lost all teeth are one in three. These are pretty grim statistics.

Periodontal disease can have a pronounced affect on neurodegeneration whether or not bacteria or viruses from infected teeth and gums actually find their way into the brain. Periodontal disease is a potent and often chronic source of inflammation. Inflammatory chemicals, such as TNF-alpha, are constantly being generated and, being only inches away from the brain, pass over the blood-brain barrier and ignite inflammation there as well. Any inflammation in the mouth will affect the brain. Oral bacterial and viral infections do not even need to be present in the brain to cause neurodegeneration.[52]

In addition to triggering inflammation in the brain, periodontal infections can promote insulin resistance. Pro-inflammatory chemicals released in response to infection or injury desensitize cells to insulin. Untreated periodontal disease causes chronic inflammation, which in turn can increase systemic insulin resistance, promoting diabetes or exacerbating the condition if it already exists.[53-54] Systemic inflammation increases the risk of brain insulin resistance, further promoting neurodegeneration. Treating periodontal disease and improving oral health has shown to improve systemic insulin resistance.[55]

HIDDEN DENTAL PROBLEMS

Having a bright white smile and no obvious problems is no guarantee that a person is free of infection. Modern dentistry can make a person's teeth appear to be healthy while harboring chronic infection. Some signs and symptoms of poor dental health are easy to recognize while others are less obvious.

Signs of poor dental health and increased risk of neurodegenerative disease include red, swollen gums that bleed easily; receding gums that make the teeth look longer than normal; spaces developing between teeth; ulcers; persistent bad breath; loose teeth; tooth or jaw pain; discolored teeth; hypersensitivity to heat or cold; tartar buildup; and cavities. The presence of crowns, bridges, fillings, and root canalled and missing teeth indicate a history of chronic poor oral health and bacteria overgrowth, strongly suggesting current ongoing problems.

When teeth are infected and begin to decay, the dentist will attempt to remove the rotting tissue and then replace it with a filling or a crown, or do a root canal procedure. In each of these cases it is assumed that the infection was completely removed before the restoration work is commenced. If the infection is not completely removed, covering it with filling material or a crown is not going to make it go away; it only hides the rotting tissue so that it is no longer visible. The infection continues and bacteria dig deeper into the teeth, seeping into the bloodstream.

Most fillings, which are fairly shallow infections, are generally free from infection. Crowns, which are put on teeth that are more decayed, occasionally remain infected. Root canals, however, *always* remain infected. Root canals are a major source of hidden infection.

A root canal procedure is performed when tooth decay is so advanced that the tooth cannot be saved. Instead of pulling it and replacing it with an artificial one, the dead tooth is allowed to remain in place. The soft pulp in the center of the tooth is drilled out, the inside is disinfected, and the hollow center (the root canal) is filled and capped. It is assumed that this process removes all of the infection.

However, it is impossible to remove infection that has become so virulent and so invasive that it kills the tooth. The reason for this is that the teeth are not solid blocks of hardened calcium, but living tissue filled with pores that allow circulation of fluids through them. The teeth are riddled with microscopic hollow tubes called tubules. Each tooth has millions of tubules running through it. If you could take all the tubules in one small front tooth and line them up end to end, they would extend for a mile.

When decay is so extensive that it eats its way down into the pulp where the nerve and blood supply are, the tooth eventually dies. Bacteria infiltrate into the tubules. Once bacteria infect the tubules, it is impossible to get them out. The tubules are so small that antibiotics and disinfectants cannot penetrate deep enough to kill the bacteria. Researchers have taken root canalled teeth and placed them in formaldehyde solution, completely soaking the teeth, yet bacteria hiding within the tubules still survive.[56] It is impossible for a dentist to subject patients to antiseptic treatment that would come anywhere close to actually soaking the infected teeth in a container of formaldehyde. Harsh disinfectants easily damage surrounding soft tissue, so the disinfectants they use are mild in comparison. If strong disinfectants cannot remove the infection outside the mouth, weaker ones used inside the mouth certainly won't either.

After a root canal procedure, the bacteria inside the tubules thrive and multiply. They or their toxins continually seep out of the tooth, causing chronic but low-grade inflammation and potentially spreading infection to other parts of the body, such as the brain. From all outward appearances, the root canalled tooth may look normal, but the tooth is actually dead tissue swimming in a sea of bacteria inside the mouth. Teeth are, in essence, bone. If you had a bone, let's say in your finger, that was dead, what would happen to it? It would begin to rot and cause infection, just like any dead tissue would. A dead tooth is no different. Even if root canal treatment could manage to kill all the bacteria within the tooth, it would not last long. The mouth is a reservoir of bacteria, so the tooth would immediately become infected again. There is no way to keep a root canalled tooth germ-free.

If a tooth is so badly diseased that a root canal is recommended, your best option is to have the tooth extracted. If you already have a root canalled tooth, extraction is still the best course of action. Root canalled teeth are dead teeth and attract infection and disease. You don't want them in your mouth poisoning your body or your mind.

Chances are, if you ask your dentist if root canals are safe, he or she will tell you that they are. Approximately 40 million root canal treatments are performed in the US each year. The sad fact is that most dentists are unaware of the presence of bacteria in the tubules and are ignorant of the fact that these bacteria escape and spread throughout the body. Dentists are taught to believe that the disinfecting treatment used during root canal therapy kills all the infection in the diseased tooth.

However, biological or holistic dentists (see Chapter 9) are very familiar with the dangers of root canals. They would never perform this operation or recommend it. Although they were taught in school that root canal procedures are safe, they have continued their education beyond the dental school curriculum and have learned better, safer methods of dental treatment.

George E. Meinig, DDS, one of the founding fathers of The American Association of Endodontists (root canal specialists) states: "Bacteria in teeth act much like cancer cells that metastasize to other parts of the body. These bacteria inside the structure of teeth similarly metastasize, and as they migrate throughout one's system, they infect the heart, kidneys, joints, nervous system, brain, eyes, and endanger pregnant women and in fact may infect any organ, gland, or body tissue. In other words, root canal filled teeth always remain infected. Even worse, these infections are responsible for a high percentage of the degenerative disease illnesses (including neurodegenerative diseases), which are so epidemic in our country today."

Like most endodontists, Dr. Meinig initially believed root canal procedures benefited his patients and performed the procedure for many years. When he stumbled upon the research on root canals documenting the impossibility of sterilizing root canalled teeth and the fact that these teeth act as breeding grounds of infection, he said he was in "utter shock." He hadn't learned about this in dental school. "I became very concerned about the millions of people who are suffering illness from the infection still present in their root canal-filled teeth." He immediately stopped performing root canal procedures and began intently researching the safety of the procedures and looking for alternative therapies. His research led him to write a book on the topic titled *Root Canal Cover-Up*. Dr. Meinig explains in detail the science and research that opened his eyes to the consequences of root canal therapy. Anyone who is considering getting a root canal procedure done or is concerned about what to do with existing root canalled teeth, should read his book!

THE CAUSES OF GUM DISEASE AND TOOTH DECAY

The destructive cycle that starts with the accumulation of plaque is the most common cause of periodontal disease; a number of other factors can contribute to or aggravate the condition. These include:

Tobacco use. Smoking and chewing tobacco are major contributors to periodontal disease. Tobacco use in any form depresses the immune system, putting a person at greater risk of dental infections. It also creates an environment in the mouth which promotes the growth of harmful bacteria and interferes with the normal mechanisms that limit bacterial growth.

Drugs. There are hundreds of prescription and over-the-counter drugs—antidepressants, cold remedies, antihistamines, anti-seizure medications, calcium channel blockers, and immune-suppressing drugs that decrease the body's production of saliva. Adequate saliva secretion is essential for good oral health. Saliva helps to keep teeth clean and inhibit bacterial growth. When saliva production decreases, risk of bacteria overgrowth and infection increases dramatically. Anticholinergic drugs, which are used to treat a myriad of ills ranging from sinus congestion to insomnia, are among the most potent salivary gland inhibitors. Anticholinergics also have a direct antagonistic effect on brain function. A listing of these drugs can be found in Appendix C.

Diabetes. Those people with diabetes or insulin resistance are plagued with elevated blood glucose levels. Glucose is a form of sugar. When the blood sugar levels are high, so is the glucose content in the saliva. The bacteria in the mouth feed on this sugar, promoting their growth even when no food is being eaten. The sugar-enriched saliva acts like fertilizer for the oral bacteria. Diabetics also suffer from impaired circulation to the gums and other tissues in the body, reducing their ability to fight off oral infections. Consequently, diabetics have a much higher risk of gum disease than non-diabetics.

Poor diet. A diet that is deficient in essential vitamins and minerals weakens the teeth and promotes gum disease and tooth decay. Eating too many refined carbohydrate-rich foods also promotes bacteria overgrowth and dental decay. Oral bacteria thrive on carbohydrates—sugar, starch, bread, candy, soda, pastry, chips, cookies, and such. People who eat these types of foods have a very difficult time controlling bacteria growth and are bound to have serious dental problems.

12 Cholesterol is Good for You

THE CHOLESTEROL MYTH

Cholesterol—the mere mention of the word sends shivers up the spine with thoughts of clogged arteries and an ailing heart on the verge of collapse. To most people cholesterol has become synonymous with poison. It is generally believed to be the major cause of heart disease, our number one killer, and the less cholesterol we have in our bodies, the better. Consequently, we do everything we can to reduce our cholesterol levels in hopes of avoiding a heart attack or stroke.

So far it hasn't worked. Heart disease is still the number one cause of death. Doctors have been on a campaign to lower cholesterol for over five decades. We have been eating less cholesterol and fat and taking cholesterol-lowering drugs, exercising more, and doing everything imaginable to reduce our cholesterol. Cholesterol levels have come down, but it hasn't done any good. Despite sales of over 20 billion dollars in cholesterol-lowering statin drugs each year, the benefit of lowering blood cholesterol has been a miserable failure. Yet the drug companies continue to push cholesterol therapy as the most effective way to fight heart disease. With billions of dollars a year at stake, you bet they are very actively campaigning for the continued use of cholesterol-lowering drugs.

There are many diseases that affect the heart, but the one that we hear most about and the one that is of greatest concern regarding cholesterol is coronary heart disease. Coronary heart disease occurs when the coronary arteries that supply blood to the heart become narrowed by a build-up of plaque. When the plaque accumulates to an extent that blood flow to the heart is completely blocked, a heart attack occurs. Likewise, when arteries feeding the brain become blocked, it leads to a stroke. Thus, coronary heart disease affects both the heart and the brain. The arterial plaque consists of a mixture of cholesterol, fat, protein, and calcium. When plaque forms in the arteries, it is called atherosclerosis, or hardening of the arteries. The hardening is due primarily to the calcium deposits that stiffen the arteries. When people talk of heart disease, they are usually referring to coronary heart disease, the type that leads to heart attacks and strokes.

The idea that diet, and specifically cholesterol and fat, is connected to heart disease was proposed by Dr. Ancel Keys in 1953. Using data from six countries Keys showed that the populations that consumed the most fat had the highest death rates from heart disease and that those who ate the least fat had the lowest. Using this data as evidence, he proposed the idea that cholesterol in the blood, for some unknown reason, tends to stick to the inside of artery walls causing a buildup of plaque. The higher the cholesterol levels in the blood, the greater the chances that some of it would end up sticking to the artery walls. Eating a diet high in meat and fat raised blood cholesterol levels. His idea was called the cholesterol hypothesis of heart disease.

Although not immediately recognized, Key's study was seriously flawed. It was later discovered that Keys had access to data from at least 22 countries, but he only used the figures from six in his paper. If he had used all the data that was available to him, the correlation between dietary fat consumption and heart disease would have disappeared. He apparently believed his cholesterol hypothesis so much that he selectively chose only the data that would support his idea and conveniently ignored the contradictory evidence.

The cholesterol hypothesis provided an answer to one of medical science's most baffling mysteries—the cause of coronary heart disease, the nation's number one killer. The cholesterol hypothesis was simple and seemed to make sense. It was immediately accepted by many in the medical community. Others, however, had their doubts.

Dr. Paul Dudley White was one of them. Dr. White is known as the founder of American cardiology (the study of the heart and its diseases). He graduated from medical school in 1910 and served as President Dwight D. Eisenhower's physician during his terms in office. As a young man, White wrote that he had an interest in a rare new disease that he had read about in the European medical literature. It wasn't until 1921, 11 years after he began his practice, that he saw his first heart attack patient. At that time, heart attacks were extremely rare. By the 1950s, when he served as Eisenhower's physician, heart disease had become the nation's leading cause of death. Later in his career, and as the foremost authority in the United States on cardiology and, consequently, heart disease, he was asked for his opinion about the theory that cholesterol and saturated fat caused heart disease. He stated that he couldn't support the theory because he knew it didn't fit the history of the disease.[1]

Prior to 1910, heart disease was extremely rare. Beginning around 1920, the incidence of heart disease suddenly began to skyrocket. From 1910 to 1920 only 10 out of every 100,000 deaths per year were attributed to heart disease. By 1930 the death rate jumped to 46 per 100,000 and by 1970 the rate reached 331 per 100,000.

According to the cholesterol hypothesis, the rise in heart disease rates was caused by an increase in cholesterol and saturated fat consumption. However, during this time period cholesterol and saturated fat consumption remained relatively constant. Historically then, there is absolutely no correlation between saturated fat and cholesterol consumption and heart disease, just as Dr. White indicated.

It is interesting to note that the consumption of trans fatty acids, which are found in margarine and shortening, increased dramatically from 1920 through 1970. Trans fatty acids are artificial fats created when polyunsaturated vegetable oils are hydrogenated. Trans fats have long been known to be associated with heart disease. The rise in heart disease is more closely related to trans fat consumption than it is to cholesterol or saturated fat.

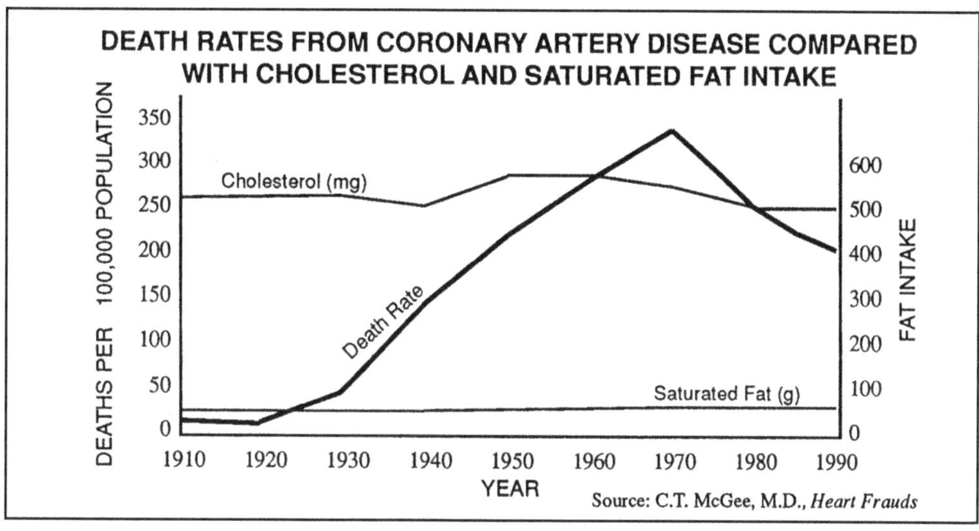

From 1910 to 1970 deaths from heart attacks due to coronary artery disease increased an incredible 3,010 percent, then began to decline. During this time, cholesterol and saturated fat intake remained fairly constant, indicating no correlation between cholesterol or saturated fat with heart disease.

Despite these facts, many studies were carried out to try to prove the cholesterol hypothesis. After more than five decades of research, there has yet to be a study that proves that eating saturated fat and cholesterol causes heart disease.[2] Most of the studies show no correlation between elevated blood cholesterol and heart disease. In only a handful of studies has a relationship been found, and that evidence has been so small that it borders on being nearly statistically insignificant—in other words, the result may have occurred simply by chance.

In some cases, the correlation between high blood cholesterol and heart disease vanished over time. For example, one study that seemed to support the cholesterol hypothesis was a Finnish trial published in 1975. In the five years that the trial ran, cholesterol levels were lowered significantly with positive results, and the study was hailed as a success. However, a 10-year follow-up study reported in 1991 found that those people who had lowered their cholesterol and continued to follow the low-fat cholesterol-lowering diet were *twice* as likely to die of heart disease as those who didn't.[3]

Despite numerous studies, the only correlation between elevated blood cholesterol and increased incidence of heart attacks have been found in men between the ages of 35 and 59 who have already suffered at least one heart attack. In middle-aged men who have *not* suffered a heart attack, there is no correlation. There is also no correlation between men under the age of 35 or over the age of 59 or women of any age.[4] In other words, for the vast majority of the population there is no relationship between elevated cholesterol and increased risk of heart disease.

Approximately 90 percent of those who die from heart attacks and strokes are over the age of 60. There is no evidence that high cholesterol in older men is harmful. One of several studies to prove this fact was headed by Dr. Harlan M. Krumholz from Yale University School of Medicine. His team monitored 997 people

70 years of age and older for four years. They found "no evidence that an elevated level of cholesterol increased the risk of death or heart disease among this group."[5]

Similar results were reported by researchers at the University of Hawaii following the Honolulu Heart Program study. In this study 3,572 participants over the age of 70 were followed for 20 years. The researchers warned that *reducing* cholesterol in the elderly population *increases* risk of death. They state: "Our data accord with previous findings of increased mortality in elderly people with low serum cholesterol, and show that long-term persistence of low cholesterol actually increases the risk of death. Thus, the earlier that patients start to have lower cholesterol concentrations, the greater the risk of death."[6]

While studies have indicated that men over the age of 59 who have high cholesterol are not at any increased risk of developing heart disease, that age may be much lower. In a 30 year follow-up report from the Framingham Study researchers could find no correlation between high cholesterol and heart disease in men above the age of 47.[7] It seems that high cholesterol has importance to only a very small number of people, namely middle-aged men between the ages of 35 and 47 who have already suffered a heart attack. In the rest of the population there is no correlation between elevated cholesterol and heart disease. Even in this narrow age group, the benefit of lowering cholesterol is doubtful.

Having low blood cholesterol appears to provide no protection from heart disease regardless of age. A study headed by Dr. Michael DeBakey at Baylor University found that out of 1,700 patients who had atherosclerosis severe enough to require hospitalization, only 1 patient out of 5 had high blood cholesterol.[8] That means out of a random population of heart disease patients four out of five had normal or

An 86-year-old woman came running into my office one day waving a lab slip in her hand, and I do mean running. She had been in good health all of her life and was still living alone in a self-sufficient manner. Her internist had just presented her with a copy of her blood tests. He had told her she was at a high risk for a heart attack because her blood cholesterol was 360 mg/dl (9.3 mmol/l). She caught me in the hall between patients and asked me what she could do to bring her cholesterol level down.

I asked her, "What do you think your cholesterol has been running all of your life?"

She replied, "Well, I suppose it has been about this high for many years, probably most of my life."

I said, "That is a safe assumption. How much damage do you think it has done to you?"

She was forced to answer that no apparent damage had been done. I went on to tell her not to worry about the high cholesterol level and that there were steps she could take to protect herself from a heart attack. However, I assumed it would be hard for her to forget about the test because of all the brainwashing and media hype about cholesterol.

—Charles T. McGee, MD, *Heart Frauds*

low cholesterol. In other words, about 80 percent of the heart disease cases serious enough to require hospitalization do not have high cholesterol.

Lowering high blood cholesterol through diet or drugs does not save lives. A team of researchers led by Dr. Gregg Fonarow, Professor of Cardiovascular Medicine at the UCLA School of Medicine, published a study in 2009 that showed that 75 percent of patients hospitalized for heart attacks have normal to below normal cholesterol levels.[9] This study confirms Dr. DeBakey's earlier study.

In this study, Dr. Fonarow's team analyzed data from 136,905 patients hospitalized for heart attacks nationwide between 2000 and 2006 where lipid levels upon hospital admission were documented. Twenty-one percent were taking cholesterol-lowering medication. The drugs apparently didn't help; despite lowering their cholesterol to within a "healthy" range, they still suffered heart attacks. Eighteen percent had cholesterol levels that would be considered "ideal" or lowest in risk, yet they still suffered heart attacks. Having low or very low cholesterol did not save them.

Another study published the same year by researchers at the Henry Ford Heart and Vascular Institute in Detroit came up with the same result and conclusion. Patients who survived their heart attacks at the beginning of the study were followed for three years. During that time the death rate was twice as high among those who had the lowest cholesterol.[10]

If you use a little logic you can see the fallacy of the cholesterol hypothesis. If high blood cholesterol were the cause of heart disease, then *all* people who die from heart attacks and strokes must have high cholesterol—but they don't. As you have seen from the above studies, just as many or more people with normal or low cholesterol die of heart disease as those with high cholesterol. Using cholesterol-lowering drugs or low-fat diets will not reduce the risk of heart disease.

Over the past decade, a large and convincing body of evidence has emerged showing that atherosclerosis is not simply an accumulation of fat and cholesterol but is an inflammatory disease influenced by many factors.[11-13]

YOU MAKE YOUR OWN CHOLESTEROL

It is assumed that a diet high in cholesterol and saturated fat leads to high blood cholesterol. Saturated fat is included because it can be converted into cholesterol by the liver. The fat we eat, according to the cholesterol hypothesis, is directly responsible for the amount of cholesterol in our blood. The problem with this argument is that dietary consumption of fat has only a minor affect on blood cholesterol levels. The reason for this is that the vast majority of the cholesterol in the blood does not come from the diet, but from the liver. More than 80 percent of the cholesterol in our blood is manufactured in our own bodies.

Cholesterol is not the evil villain it has been made out to be. It is a natural and normal component of our bodies with many useful purposes. Without cholesterol you would not be alive. It is so important that our bodies produce about 1,000 milligrams of cholesterol per day. Less than 20 percent of the cholesterol in your blood comes from your diet.

The body has a genetically determined level of cholesterol it prefers and it will always try to maintain this level. In some people the preferred level may 185 mg/dl (4.8 mmol/dl), while in others it may be 260 mg/dl (6.7 mmol/l) or more, although some disease conditions may also affect these levels up or down. On average, cholesterol levels run between 180 mg/dl to 240 mg/dl (4.7-6.2 mmol/l). But it may be perfectly normal for someone to have a cholesterol reading upwards of 300 mg/dl (7.8 mmol/l) or more.

The cholesterol hypothesis makes the assumption that the more cholesterol and saturated fat a person eats, the higher the blood cholesterol will climb. Since the liver produces most of the cholesterol in our bodies, it is depicted as an inept machine that blindly cranks out as much cholesterol as it possibly can—the more saturated fat we eat, the more cholesterol it cranks out.

Such a scenario is inconsistent with human physiology. The liver produces and carefully regulates a balance of hundreds of compounds essential for growth, digestion, and protection. Blood cholesterol is not an accident that is easily influenced by diet. The liver doesn't just crank out products, like cholesterol, for the fun of it. It does it for a specific reason. The amount is carefully controlled and monitored to achieve and maintain homeostasis or chemical equilibrium. The liver carefully regulates the amount of cholesterol in our bodies, so it doesn't really matter how much saturated fat or cholesterol we eat; the liver will only manufacture the amount we need to maintain homeostasis. Everyone's body is different, so everyone has a different level of cholesterol with which their bodies are happy.

The liver doesn't need saturated fat to make cholesterol. It can make it from other fats and even from sugar or carbohydrate.[14] So the claim that saturated fat and cholesterol raises blood cholesterol, while ignoring other fats and sugar, is illogical and inaccurate. If insufficient cholesterol is eaten, the liver will make it from other dietary sources. This is why even drastic decreases in dietary cholesterol and saturated fat intake often produce only small changes in blood cholesterol levels.

Low-fat, low-cholesterol diets can only reduce cholesterol levels by about 5 to 15 percent. To reduce cholesterol further requires medication. Cholesterol-lowering statins can reduce blood cholesterol as much as 40 percent. Forcing cholesterol levels down by drugs or drastic dieting can upset cholesterol homeostasis, leading to some very serious consequences, particularly in regards to brain function.

Most cholesterol researchers now admit that high blood cholesterol does not cause heart disease. Yet, you will still see the media broadcasting information suggesting that it does. This is due primarily by the aggressive marketing efforts of the pharmaceutical industry. Their cry that high blood cholesterol leads to heart disease has been so loud and so frequent that we've been brainwashed into believing it. If you tell a lie often enough and loud enough, eventually everyone will accept it as truth, no matter how preposterous it may be. That is what has happened with cholesterol and heart disease.

Paul Addis and Gregory Warner, professors in the Department of Food Science and Nutrition at the University of Minnesota state: "The prevailing opinion, that atherosclerosis is simply an accumulation of cholesterol on arteries, has clearly shown to be erroneous. Therefore, the 'lipid hypothesis' has become less well accepted by serious researchers and has been replaced by a competing hypothesis, i.e. response-to-injury hypothesis."[15] Because of the many inconsistencies with the cholesterol or lipid hypothesis, it is often referred to as the cholesterol myth.

YOUR BODY NEEDS CHOLESTEROL

Cholesterol is one of the most important substances in your body. It is vital for the proper function and regulation of all body systems. You have cholesterol in every cell in your body. It is there for an important reason.

The cells of our body are encased in a lipid (fat and cholesterol) membrane. Even the individual organelles (cell organs) inside the cell are encased in a lipid coat. Cholesterol is a vital element of the cell and organelle membranes. Cholesterol is uniquely able to influence the structure, thickness, permeability, deformation, and other characteristics of the cell membranes. Cholesterol is needed to regulate the entry and exit of certain hormones, fats, and proteins. Cholesterol typically makes up about 20 percent of the membrane. In certain areas of the membrane, cholesterol concentration increases to 30 to 40 percent. Some cells, such as the nerve cells, contain even more.

For the cells to function properly, an ample amount of cholesterol needs to be available. Cholesterol must be continually supplied to form new cells and repair damaged tissues. For example, when an injury occurs within a blood vessel, cholesterol is used to repair the damage. If the injury becomes chronic, as in the case of an artery beset by chronic inflammation, cholesterol, along with protein and calcium, is laid down repeatedly. This can lead to the formation of the plaque characteristic of atherosclerosis. Promoters of the cholesterol hypothesis of heart disease claim that since cholesterol is present, that it must be the cause the clogging in the artery. But according to the newer and more widely accepted response-to-injury hypothesis, the cholesterol didn't cause the plaque, it was part of the repair process that is trying to fix the problem. It is the chronic inflammation that caused the cholesterol, as well as the protein and calcium, to be deposited and the amount of plaque deposited has absolutely no relationship to the amount of cholesterol in the blood.

Cholesterol also functions as the precursor for a number of vital hormones. All of the steroid hormones start out as cholesterol, including pregnenolone, aldosterone, estrogen, progesterone, testosterone, cortisol, and others. These hormones regulate sexual differentiation and behavior; mediate menstrual cycle and pregnancy; regulate the excretion of salt and water by kidneys; affect carbohydrate, protein, and lipid metabolism; and influence a wide variety of other vital functions including inflammatory reactions and the capacity to cope with stress. It is cholesterol that makes you who you are and keeps your body running smoothly.

Bile, too, gets its start as cholesterol. Bile is secreted by the liver and stored in the gallbladder. When we eat a meal, bile is released into the digestive tract to emulsify dietary fats and fat soluble nutrients and facilitate their digestion and assimilation. Without bile we could not digest fats, which are necessary for proper health.

Vitamin D is manufactured in our bodies as sunlight interacts with the cholesterol in our skin. Vitamin D has a multitude of functions, including immune system support and the building of strong bones and teeth. It is also needed for healthy brain function and helps lower risk of diabetes, heart and kidney disease, high blood pressure, and cancer.

Cholesterol is essential for proper immune function. When blood cholesterol is low, white blood cells, the workhorse of our immune system, are under-produced, and the body is less capable of fighting off infections, neutralizing toxins, and removing cancerous cells.[16] Cholesterol also acts as a detoxifying agent by neutralizing toxins secreted by disease-causing bacteria.[17-18]

The toxins secreted by infectious bacteria do more harm than the organisms themselves. It is the toxins that poison the body and cause the majority of symptoms associated with the bacterial infections. Cholesterol works with the immune system to neutralize these harmful toxins. *Staphylococcus aureus* is a common bacterium that causes a variety of infections including skin infections (impetigo), connective tissue infections (cellulitis), breast infections (mastitis), blood infections (sepsis), lung infections (pneumonia), bone infections (osteomyelitis), heart infections (endocarditis), toxic shock syndrome, and food poisoning, among others. Cholesterol helps protect against these infections by aiding the immune system in neutralizing the toxins secreted by this and other organisms.[19]

Cholesterol is needed for building strong bones and protects against osteoporosis. Bone tissue is continually being broken down and rebuilt. As we grow older, the process of breaking bone down occurs more rapidly than rebuilding. Consequently, bone density declines with age. Higher blood levels of cholesterol is associated with greater bone density and fewer fractures in the elderly.[20] Lowering cholesterol weakens the bones and increases risk of osteoporosis.

Cholesterol is found as a structural component in every cell but most prominently in the nerve cells. It constitutes a major component of the myelin sheath that coats the long axons of the neurons and forms a substantial part of the cell membrane. As a major component of nerve tissue it is the most common molecule in the brain.

Cholesterol is absolutely essential for the transmission of nerve impulses and the communication between neurons. It is needed for storing and retrieving memories. The synapses—the highly specialized contacts that sits between adjacent neurons in the brain—depend on cholesterol for their function.[21]

New synaptic vesicles are continually being formed in order to maintain multiple nerve transmissions. In order to accomplish this, there must be ample cholesterol available to construct the vesicles. If adequate cholesterol is not available, the vesicles are not manufactured and nerve transmission stops. If the nerve is involved in creating a memory, then the memory will not be formed. If the nerve is involved in retrieving a memory, the memory will not be found. If the nerve is involved in producing or controlling physical movement, the action will not occur as desired. If the nerve is involved in making rational decisions and thinking, then bizarre or uncharacteristic behavior may result. Cholesterol availability can affect any and all brain functions. Cholesterol is the key to our ability to learn and remember. It is the key to all mental functions. Not only must it be present, but it must be present in sufficient enough quantities to fulfill its role in normal brain function.[22]

While the brain accounts for only 2 percent of the mass of the body, it contains almost 25 percent of the body's cholesterol.[23] In fact, the brain's need for cholesterol is so great that it manufactures its own cholesterol to supplement what is produced by the liver. The cholesterol in the brain is produced by the glial cells—the supporting tissue of the brain.

As cholesterol research continues, the importance of cholesterol in human health is becoming increasingly evident. Many medical professionals are questioning the sanity of prescribing cholesterol-lowering drugs. Some investigators are even suggesting that a time may come when doctors will be prescribing cholesterol-*raising* medications to patients to take advantage of the many benefits rendered by this essential substance.[24]

THE DANGERS OF LOWERING CHOLESTEROL

Behavioral Changes

In the mistaken belief that high blood cholesterol contributes to heart disease, cholesterol-lowering drugs are prescribed. Statins are the drugs of choice since they can lower blood cholesterol by as much as 40 percent. They do this by blocking the action of enzymes in the liver needed to produce cholesterol.

Since this process disrupts normal liver function, these drugs can cause serious damage. Liver damage is one of the most well-documented and recognized side effects of statin use. Therefore, those who take statins must be monitored closely by their doctors. Patients are given liver function tests periodically to make sure the drugs are not destroying their livers. Those patients who already have liver problems or have a history of moderate to high alcohol consumption are usually discouraged from taking statins.

Another problem with statins is that they also interfere with the production of cholesterol in the brain. The same enzymes needed to make cholesterol in the liver are also present in the brain. If the disruption of cholesterol synthesis in the liver can lead to liver damage, what can it do to the brain? Think about it.

Cholesterol is constantly being formed to maintain, replace, and repair the cells and tissues, especially nerve tissue. Any interference with normal cholesterol synthesis can impair nerve tissue maintenance and repair, leading to neurodegeneration through neuron loss.[25] Even a small depletion of cholesterol—less than 10 percent—in the neuron endings at the synapse has been shown to be enough to inhibit the release of neurotransmitters and block nerve transmission.[26]

Drug-induced cholesterol lowering causes a loss in brain function.[27-28] A decrease in brain cholesterol is known to contribute to neurodegeneration and Alzheimer's disease.[29] The effects of cholesterol-lowering drugs on brain health have been reported for decades. In the early studies that compared cholesterol-lowering drugs with placebos (dummy pills), an unexpected phenomenon quickly surfaced. While fatal heart attacks in some middle-aged men slightly declined, deaths from suicide and violence, as well as cancer, increased. The overall results showed a total *increase* in deaths among the drug users compared to those without.

Those subjects who were taking cholesterol-lowering drugs reported a significant increase in depression, irritability, and aggression that apparently led to increased incidences of suicides and violent deaths. Researchers brushed these findings aside, claiming they were simply the result of chance. The studies were repeated with larger numbers of subjects. The results were the same: increased deaths due to suicide and violence.[30-31] In none of these studies was the difference significantly large, but all pointed in the same direction—lowering cholesterol disrupted normal mental processes.

Dr. Matthew Muldoon, assistant professor of psychiatry at the University of Pittsburgh, did not believe these deaths were just a coincidence. He and colleagues at the university analyzed all the studies that reported violent deaths and found that they were indeed very significant.[32] They also showed that the rate of death from violence and suicide in the control groups were identical with the rate of the country in general, while in the group taking the cholesterol-lowering drugs the rate was *twice* as high. This was a heavy blow to the drug industry, who continued to downplay the significance of these side effects to lowering cholesterol.

The conclusions of Muldoon and colleagues were strengthened by a large investigation in Sweden headed by Dr. Gunnar Lindberg. They measured blood cholesterol levels in more than 50,000 men and women and then kept track of them for 20 years. During the first six years, 20 men with cholesterol below 207 mg/dl (5.4 mmol/l) committed suicide. Yet only five with cholesterol above 296 mg/dl (7.7 mmol/l) committed suicide.[33]

The suicide rate was much higher early in the study when the drop in cholesterol levels was the greatest. The authors concluded that the increased risk of suicide may be associated with reducing cholesterol too far below the subject's normal or genetic set point. They pointed out that if a person's natural cholesterol level is low then there is little risk of suicide, but the risk is great if the low cholesterol is induced by extreme dieting or drugs.

Cognitive Decline

In addition to behavioral changes, a number of studies have shown a link between drug-induced cholesterol lowering and a decline in cognitive ability.[34-37] Not everyone who takes statins complains of memory loss, depression, or other neurological symptoms. However, *everyone* who uses statins is adversely affected to some degree. This was demonstrated by researchers at the University of Pittsburgh School of Medicine. The investigators took 209 healthy adults and randomly assigned them to one of two groups. The treatment group was placed on statins and the control group on placebos. At the beginning of the study cognitive performance and psychological well-being of each participant was carefully assessed. After six months, all of the patients on placebos showed a measurable increase in cognitive function, while 100 percent of the statin patients showed a measurable decrease in cognitive function in one or more areas.[38] So apparently, *everyone* who takes cholesterol-lowering drugs is adversely affected to some degree.

Researchers have also found that depriving the brain of cholesterol sets into motion chemical changes that lead to the formation of abnormal proteins and neurofibrillatory tangles characteristic of damage seen in Alzheimer's and other neurodegenerative diseases.[39]

Ironically, drug companies have touted statins as a novel means to *lower* the risk of Alzheimer's disease. This move appears to be a ploy by the drug companies to counter negative publicity surrounding statins' detrimental effects on the brain. Their position is based primarily on the idea that high blood cholesterol clogs arteries going to the brain, thereby increasing the possibility of stroke. Reducing blood cholesterol, they contend, would reduce this risk. Preliminary animal studies sponsored by the drug companies seem to support this theory. However, the experiences of many people who have suffered cognitive problems suggest this is not the case in humans. This has been backed up by several studies on human subjects that have demonstrated that statins provide absolutely no protection against Alzheimer's disease or dementia in general.[40] Even autopsy studies—the most definitive in regards to the changes occurring in the brain—have shown no protective benefit whatsoever in taking statins.[41]

Despite the negative findings in human studies, the drug companies continue to support research to back their position. In one study with elderly African Americans, researchers stated that "Initial use of statins resulted in less cognitive decline in individuals, but continued use of a statin resulted in more cognitive decline."[42] It is believed that the initial improvement was due to the anti-inflammatory effect of the drug, but in the long run the damaging effects of cholesterol depletion overshadowed this positive effect. Depending on how a study like this is reported, it can be made to appear to support statins if the long term effects are ignored. So you might still run across news articles now and then about statins reducing risk of Alzheimer's as part of the drug industry's effort to divert attention away from this troublesome side effect.

Perhaps the most vocal advocate for educating people about the dangers of statins on brain health is Duane Graveline, MD, MPH. His passion stems from his own experience using these drugs. Dr. Graveline is a former United States Air Force Flight Surgeon and Astronaut.

As a NASA astronaut he was required to be in tip-top shape both mentally and physically. During a routine medical exam, Graveline was told his cholesterol was too high, so he began taking 10 mg of Lipitor daily. Six weeks later he began to lose his mind.

One day Graveline seemed fine, but then his wife spotted him walking aimlessly about their driveway and yard. When she confronted him, he acted confused and gave no evidence of recognizing her. He refused to come into the house or get into the car to see the doctor. She had to call an old friend of his to convince him to go see the doctor. A neurological examination that included an MRI found no abnormalities. He remembers nothing of this incident. About six hours after his wife first noticed his condition he slowly began to come to his senses. He was completely bewildered by the experience. Over the next few days his mind began to function normally again. He questioned neighbors and asked them if they saw him walking about on that day. One of them said he saw Graveline walk past his house and that he stopped to talk to another neighbor for a few minutes. Graveline had no memory of it.

During this recovery period he had neglected to take the medication. He experienced no further memory problems. He began to wonder whether the cholesterol medication was at the bottom of it all. In researching statin side effects he found only slight references to possible cognitive problems. He questioned several doctors and pharmacists if Lipitor could cause memory loss. They all assured him it didn't. He was not so sure.

A year later at his next astronaut physical, he was again advised to take cholesterol-lowering medication. When he expressed concern about the drug's effect on his memory the doctor replied, "Statins don't do that." The doctor convinced him to get back on the drug but reduced his dose to only 5 mg a day. Six weeks later he experienced a second episode of sudden amnesia, this time more severe than the first. He lost all memory of his wife and children, his career as an astronaut, his medical school training, and his college life. He could recall his early teenage years and before, but nothing of his entire adult life. He remained in this stupor for 12 hours.

Again the examining doctors chorused that "Statins don't do that" but he was convinced they do. No one seemed to believe him. Desperate to find out more about the connection between statins and memory loss, he sent an e-mail describing his problem to the *People's Pharmacy,* a newspaper column that is syndicated throughout the country. His letter was printed in the column. The authors of the column were immediately bombarded with hundreds of letters from readers reporting similar experiences. Graveline, too, started receiving similar correspondence.

One letter read: "My husband had been taking Zocor for about 6 weeks. One day he got up from bed and couldn't remember what day of the week it was. As the morning progressed, he couldn't remember the month and date. He could not remember how many stocks we had and numerous other things. He nearly drove me crazy asking the same questions over and over. He became very frustrated as he basically has total recall and is known for having a very sharp mind. He could not understand how I could know the date, etc. and he could not remember at all. I thought he had some kind of stroke so I insisted that he go to the doctor. The doctor admitted him to the hospital and had numerous tests run on him including a CAT scan. A neurological doctor also did some testing. The diagnosis was transient global amnesia. The episode had lasted about eight hours. My husband took himself off Zocor and has been doing great!"

Another stated: "Four months ago I was put on Lipitor to reduce my bad cholesterol to 100. Suddenly I found I could not handle basic math or remember how to spell. It became so bad that I was in a constant fog. I should tell you I spent most of my career in Silicon Valley writing specifications for software and hold a patent on expert system technology. I had an MRI to rule out a brain tumor or stroke. Since the only thing that had changed was the addition of Lipitor I stopped taking it. Five weeks later I am still having problems spelling and frequently forget things."

After receiving hundreds of reports similar to these and uncovering studies linking cognitive problems with statin use, Dr. Graveline wrote a book titled *Lipitor Thief of Memory*. He also set up a website at spacedoc.com to further explain the dangers of statins.

Anyone who is taking cholesterol-lowering drugs should seriously consider the consequences. If you need further convincing, I suggest you read Graveline's book. It has helped many others. For instance, one woman writes, "After taking statins for several years, my mother-in-law suddenly became very forgetful—repeating the same question four times in less than 15 minutes, forgetting that she had gone shopping or to the doctor that morning, etc. It was quite frightening for all of us. The battle to persuade my parents-in-law that she needed to stop taking the statins went on for months until, with the help of [Graveline's] book and *The Great Cholesterol Con* by Dr. Malcolm Kendrink, they finally agreed that she should stop—just for a few days, mind you—this so-called 'medication' (it's clearly just a poison by another name). Within 10 days of coming off simvastatin (Zocor), she was noticeably better, but we're still not sure she will recover completely. I believe these two books helped to save her life—and certainly the quality of her life."

Motor Neuron Degeneration

Since the publication of his book in 2006, Dr. Graveline has received thousands of letters describing a variety of disabling neurodegenerative conditions associated with statin use, including ALS and Parkinsonism. This has led him to write another book titled *The Statin Damage Crisis*.

Joe and Teresa Graedon authors of the syndicated column *The People's Pharmacy* have received over a hundred reports of ALS among statin users. "My husband started on lovastatin for high cholesterol and soon began to notice weakness in his right arm," writes in one reader. "This weakness progressed, so he saw his doctor, thinking he had a pinched nerve. He was referred to a neurologist, who gave him a diagnosis of 'possible ALS.' On his 60th birthday, a second opinion confirmed the diagnosis of ALS. Since that time, my husband has progressed from weakness in his right arm to complete loss of function in his arms, very weak leg muscles and difficulty breathing. The doctors are now encouraging us to enter him into hospice care. This took only 10 months. We are still in a state of shock! It really bothers me that his cholesterol was not that high—239. Since then, we have heard that niacin and diet might have brought it down without a statin drug. The ALS specialist has told our daughter that she should never, ever take a statin."

Another woman reports, "My mom has been taking cholesterol medication for 15 years now. Recently the past couple months she has been showing signs of ALS. These symptoms include muscle weakening in the arms, tingling, twitching, slurred speech, fatigue, neck aches, and an overall mood change. She went to see a couple different doctors and they have taken her off her medication. One of the doctors told her that she has ALS...She is only 48 years old."

And still another writes, "My dad died on 6/1/06 at the age of 65 from a six-year battle with ALS. I said to my mom a million times that dad got ALS from taking Lipitor. When he was taking it he would wake up in the middle of the night from severe muscle pain and cramping. When he told his doctor about it, his doctor said, 'Hey, I get aches and pains too, but that's life'. Then he doubled my father's dosage.

"My dad finally was diagnosed with the ALS and kept taking the Lipitor because no one told him of any connection of his aches and pains and the Lipitor.

He went from stumbling, to falling down, to walking with arm braces, to a walker, to a wheelchair, to total paralysis except for his hands. I watched him die from a disease that took away every bit of his pride and dignity because he needed help eating and going to the bathroom, to being completely paralyzed and helpless. He was a proud, strong hard working carpenter and this disease turned him into a sobbing, completely petrified paralyzed person.

"My dad worked for an extremely wealthy man who finally sent him to and paid for him to see one of the United States' top neurologists after he was diagnosed. After seeing this doctor for awhile I said to him that I thought my dad might have gotten ALS from taking Lipitor and the doctor said, 'You see all of those folders behind me?' There were hundreds. He said, 'Those are all cases that pharmaceutical companies have sent me of people who are in lawsuits because they think they got ALS from their cholesterol-lowering medications and they want me to read them all over and decide if I think that is the case or not.' He said, 'In your father's case, honestly I'm just not sure.' Well I know Lipitor gave my dad ALS...Maybe if someone told my dad this from the beginning he would have opted to lower his cholesterol in another way."

The Food and Drug Administration (FDA) has been receiving numerous reports of ALS associated with statin use as part of their Adverse Event Reporting System. Concerned, they contacted all the drug companies that make statins and requested copies of studies each of them conducted regarding the side effects of these drugs. The drug companies happily sent the FDA some 41 placebo-controlled studies. Their studies showed no statistical difference between the occurrence of ALS among those taking statins and those taking placebos. The FDA was satisfied with the data and announced to the public that "statins are not linked to a higher risk of ALS." This announcement pleased the drug companies. Since this statement came from the FDA, most people have taken it as fact and refer to this report to back up their position. The problem here is that the studies supplied to the FDA came from a very biased group who would do anything to hide the effects of statins on mental health and have, in fact, been working very hard to discredit any claims between statins and neurodegeneration.

Data from the World Health Organization conflicts with that of the FDA report. After hearing of Dr. Graveline's accounts of ALS associated with statin use, Ralph Edwards, MD, went to his computer database to look for a possible link. As the director of the World Health Organization's drug-monitoring center, Dr. Edwards has amassed about four million reports of medical problems experienced by people taking prescription drugs. His job is to sift through reported adverse events, looking for unrecognized side effects. He found something that concerned him. Of 172 people in his database who developed ALS while taking prescription medicines, 40 had been on statins. This was 5 to 10 times higher than what he anticipated. He would have expected a number in the single digits, judging from how often other drugs in the database were linked to the disease.[43]

In Edwards' database a total of 5,534 cases of peripheral neuropathy (damage to nerves radiating from the spine to the arms and legs) were reported. Out of that number, 547 were associated with statins, another strong as destroy peripheral nerves, it stands to reason they can destro brain and spinal cord as well.

Parkinson's disease is another concern. Dr. Xuemei Huang, an assi of neurology at the University of North Carolina's School of Medicine, b people taking cholesterol-lowering drugs may be at a much higher risk of de this disease. Her studies have shown an unsettling link between low chole and Parkinson's disease.[44] Researchers are not certain if the disease is promot by the lower cholesterol or if it is a consequence of the drugs used to reduce the cholesterol. Statins have now been in common use for well over a decade. If they do contribute to Parkinson's, researchers say we will be seeing a big surge in cases in the coming years. In fact, we are seeing the increase already.

Diabetes

One of the concerns now being identified with statin use is the drug's adverse effect on the body's ability to properly regulate glucose and insulin. Evidence shows that statins increase a persons' risk of developing type 2 diabetes. This is bad news for those with Alzheimer's or other neurodegenerative conditions. Diabetes can accelerate the onset and progression of neurodegeneration.

The report was based on an analysis of the major clinical studies of statins, including previously unpublished data. This study analyzed 13 studies encompassing 91,140 participants. According to this data, statin use is associated with an increased risk of developing diabetes.[45]

Stroke

Strokes, especially mini-stokes which can affect cognitive and motor abilities, are often associated with dementia and other forms of neurodegeneration. Evidence from observational data and randomized trials show higher hemorrhagic stroke risk with low cholesterol.[46] In the Stroke Prevention with Aggressive Reductions in Cholesterol Levels (SPARCL) trial, patients with high cholesterol were aggressively treated with Lipitor and compared with controls receiving placebos. The Lipitor group was associated with a 66 percent increase in hemorrhagic stroke compared to the control group.[47]

In the Heart Protection Study a similar increase in risk of hemorrhagic stroke during follow-up was demonstrated.[48] The evidence seems to point to an increase risk of hemorrhagic stroke with statin use.

Statins cannot be blamed for all cases of stroke, Alzheimer's, ALS, Parkinson's, and dementia, but it is clear that they can play a significant role in contributing to the problem.

In older people, who may also have experienced previous brain trauma or sustained damage from other drugs, toxins, or infection, the symptoms may become pronounced. In fact, those who don't experience noticeable neurological symptoms may simply have had fewer assaults on their brain cells over the years and, therefore, are better able to handle the statins' harmful effects. One of the problems with statins on the drug, the patient is supposed to take it ardless of the brain's health, is going to have

L FOR BRAIN HEALTH

in. In recent years a number of studies have higher blood cholesterol are at lower risk of s such as Alzheimer's, ALS, Parkinson's, and

lesterol in our brains declines,[49] increasing the as 1991, researchers suggested that increasing delivery of cholesterol to the brain may help Alzheimer's patients and recommended increasing fat consumption.[50]

Researchers from Boston University added support to this view when they examined the relationship between total cholesterol and cognitive performance.[51] In this study 1,894 men and women who were free of dementia were given cognitive tests and cholesterol screenings. The researchers found a significant association between blood cholesterol levels and cognitive skills. Participants with so-called "desirable" cholesterol levels of less than 200 mg/dl (5.2 mmol/l) performed significantly poorer than participants with cholesterol levels higher than 240 mg/dl (6.2 mmol/l), the level at which cholesterol-lowering drugs are often recommended.

Several studies have found that Alzheimer's patients have lower total blood cholesterol, lower LDL cholesterol, and lower triglyceride levels than age matched controls with normal mental function.[52]

Analyzing brain tissues from deceased Alzheimer's patients, researchers have found that the diseased portions of the brains were deficient in cholesterol.[53] This finding is consistent with the observation that the hippocampus (the memory center of the brain) of some Alzheimer's patients presents a moderate yet significant reduction in membrane cholesterol.[54]

In addition, decreasing brain cholesterol through the use of drug therapy promotes the production of amyloid proteins that clog the brains of Alzheimer's patients.[55] They state: "Our data…imply that lowering central nervous system cholesterol would be deleterious to neuronal function."

Higher blood cholesterol seems to protect against Alzheimer's. It may also protect against ALS and other neurodegenerative diseases. Recent research has demonstrated that hyperlipidemia (high blood cholesterol) significantly improves the survival of patients with ALS. Investigators found that when ALS patients have what is normally considered high cholesterol (over 240 mg/dl) their survival is much better than those with low cholesterol (below 200 mg/dl).

This study, conducted at Hopital de la Pitie-Salpetriere, Paris, involved 369 patients with ALS. The patients with relatively low cholesterol had a 35 percent increased risk of death. The median survival time in those with higher cholesterol was 49.2 months compared with 36.7 months in those with lower cholesterol levels. This study was preceded by animal studies that showed similar results. According to Dr. Vincent Meininger, one of the investigators in the study, "The relationship between survival and lipids was previously shown in a mouse model of ALS, with the mice living longer when they are fed a high fat diet." The investigators concluded that consuming a high fat diet would be protective against the disease and cautioned against the use of cholesterol-lowering drugs.[56]

Scientists are also beginning to investigate why people with low cholesterol are more likely to develop Parkinson's disease. The link between low cholesterol and Parkinson's is not new,[57] but the results of recent studies provide the strongest evidence to date.

This interest was stimulated by concerns that statins may increase the number of people with this disease. Dr. Xue Mei Huang, an assistant professor of neurology at the University of North Carolina's School of Medicine, sounded warnings after discovering that patients with low levels of cholesterol (particularly LDL, the so-called "bad" cholesterol) were three and a half times more likely to have Parkinson's disease than those with high cholesterol levels.

Dr. Huang's initial study compared 124 Parkinson's disease patients with 112 controls. This study sounded an alarm about the implications of using statins to lower cholesterol in Parkinson's patients.[58] Huang repeated the study the following year, increasing the number of subjects to 3,233. The results were the same.[59]

Depression, irritability, mood swings, aggression, anger, memory loss, confusion, disorientation, and movement disorders are all documented effects of lowering cholesterol. It is apparent that reducing cholesterol too much below its normal set point can have dramatic effects on brain health. Although cholesterol-lowering drugs may have some direct effect on the brain, it is more likely that the side effects associated with brain health are caused by interference with cholesterol synthesis.

Maintaining natural cholesterol levels may help protect against neurodegeneration. Keep in mind that everyone's cholesterol level is different. Some people naturally have what is generally considered to be low cholesterol while others have higher cholesterol. Higher cholesterol isn't bad if it is the level that has been set by your genetic blueprint and is not a consequence of some rare inherited defect or illness. Forcing your cholesterol level down with drugs will only cause problems.

BUILD BETTER BRAIN CELLS

If you are going to build a house with brick, you will need an ample supply of bricks and mortar for the job. If the supply company delivers only half the bricks needed, your house cannot be completed and will not function as designed. The same is true with your brain. When you reduce your cholesterol with extreme dieting or drugs, the brain is deprived of the building blocks it needs to function properly.

Higher cholesterol helps protect against neurodegenerative disease, as researchers at Johns Hopkins University discovered. The investigators measured cholesterol levels and conducted cognitive tests on 392 elderly subjects. They found that those with the highest blood cholesterol levels scored highest on cognitive tests.[60]

These results were supported by another study from Mount Sinai School of Medicine, in New York. In this study 185 subjects over the age of 84 and without

Pilots Perform Better on High-Fat Diets

If the type of food we eat can affect our mental abilities, then the diets of people whose jobs affect the lives and safety of others must be of the best quality to assure top mental performance. This was the focus of a study commissioned by the U.S. military.

Unlike many studies financed by the food and drug industries, there was no preconceived prejudice involved in this study. The government demanded the facts, without bias from political correctness or financial influences. They simply wanted the truth; lives depended on it.

The study tracked 45 student pilots to assess how different foods affected the pilots' mental performance. Every three weeks, each pilot spent one week on one of four different diets: high-fat, high-carbohydrate, high-protein, and a control diet. The menus were similar so the type of diet wouldn't be obvious to the participants.

The study used a flight simulator that required students to navigate and descend in cloudy weather when the runway wasn't visible and using only the plane's computers. They also took tests that required memorizing and repeating numbers and comparing shapes. Although the pilots did not know the difference in the foods, they did notice the difference in their own performance. "I could tell the difference on how well I was doing on the different diets," said Jeremy Ternes, who participated in the study. "There were times I thought, "Wow, I was a lot more on today as compared to last week.'"

Based on the pilots' test scores, the researchers found that those who ate the fattiest foods, such as butter and gravy, had the quickest response times in mental tests and made the fewest mistakes when flying in challenging conditions. The pilots' mental performance was significantly better with the high-fat diet over the other diets. This was an important finding because it may help decrease the number of aviation accidents due to pilot error, which is especially important for the combat fighter.

It is also important for the non-pilot as well. It means that getting adequate fat into the diet is important for proper mental function.

Source: Dave Kolpack. Study shows high-fat diet might help pilots. Associated Press, October 7, 2009.

dementia were assessed. Higher total cholesterol and higher LDL cholesterol (the so-called bad cholesterol) was associated with higher memory scores on tests. The researchers' conclusion: "high cholesterol is associated with better memory function."[61]

Researchers at Seoul National University in South Korea came to similar conclusions. For three years they followed 106 elderly subjects with possible dementia. As with the other studies, those with the highest cholesterol readings performed the best on neuropsychologic tests. Those who eventually digressed into Alzheimer's disease had lower cholesterol readings.[62]

The Journal of Biological Chemistry published a study showing that dietary cholesterol, the type found in foods such as eggs and meat, can protect the brain from the physiological changes that are associated with Alzheimer's disease. This study provided evidence that dietary cholesterol improves brain cholesterol status and helps protect against the formation of amyloid beta proteins.[63] This study showed that dietary measures can be taken to help protect against developing neurodegenerative disease. It also suggests that the wrong type of diet (i.e., low-fat, low-cholesterol) can promote neurodegeneration.

If you want your brain to be healthy, one of the things you should do is to make sure you get enough meat, eggs, dairy, and good fats in your diet. These foods provide the basic building blocks the body needs to manufacture and maintain proper cholesterol levels. Keep in mind that eating foods rich in cholesterol and fat will not raise your blood cholesterol over its genetic set point. You do not have to worry about high cholesterol. Ignore the cholesterol-lowering propaganda from drug companies and the doctors who are educated by them. As you have seen in this chapter, high cholesterol is not harmful.

Low-fat and low-protein diets, however, are dangerous. They can lower cholesterol levels enough to have a significant impact on brain function and overall health. These types of diets should be avoided. You need to supply the body and brain with the nutrients it needs.

The good fats are saturated and monounsaturated fats from both animal and vegetable sources. Meat, eggs, and dairy are good animal sources of both of these fats. Vegetable sources include olive oil, coconut oil, and palm oil. Cholesterol-rich foods are also important. These include meat, eggs, and dairy. Plant foods and vegetable oils do not contain cholesterol.

Taking statins to lower your cholesterol is dangerous. Often doctors recommend statins even for patients who don't have high cholesterol just as a precaution. If you are taking statins now, you should seriously consider getting off them. They do absolutely no good and have the potential to do great harm. If you are not totally convinced yet about the dangers of statin use and the uselessness of lowering cholesterol to prevent heart disease, I highly recommend reading *Fat and Cholesterol Are Good for You* by Uffe Ravnskov, MD, PhD, or *Good Calories, Bad Calories* by Gary Taubes.

13 The Ketone Miracle

THE BRAIN DISORDER CURED BY A "MAGIC" DIET

"On March 11, 1993, I was pushing my son, Charlie, in a swing when his head twitched and he threw his right arm in the air," recalls Jim Abrahams. "The whole event was so subtle that I didn't even think to mention it to Nancy, my wife, until a couple of days later when it recurred. She said she had seen a similar incident. That was the beginning of an agony I am without words to describe."

Charlie suddenly went from being a normal, active one-year old to a toddler racked with multiple violent seizures. He was diagnosed with Lennox-Gastaut Syndrome, a severe form of epilepsy. Charlie's attacks became so extreme that his parents padded the walls of his room and had him wear a football helmet to protect himself.

Over the next nine months Charlie experienced thousands of epileptic seizures, an incredible array of drugs, dozens of blood draws, eight hospitalizations, a mountain of EEGs, MRIs, CAT scans, and PET scans, and one fruitless brain surgery. He was treated by five pediatric neurologists in three cities, two homoeopaths, and even a faith healer. Despite all this, Charlie's seizures remained unchecked and his mental development delayed. His prognosis was that of continued seizures and progressive retardation.

At 20 months of age Charlie weighed only 19 pounds. He was taking four medications, but still suffered hundreds of seizures daily. The side effects to the drugs he was taking were nearly as bad as his disease, compounding his agony.

Refusing to believe that nothing more could be done, Jim went to the library to research the disease. There, he found a book by John Freeman, MD, a professor of neurology at Johns Hopkins University, which contained references to a dietary treatment for epilepsy called the ketogenic diet. Jim learned that the ketogenic diet had been used successfully for over 70 years in treating severe cases of epilepsy.

Jim took Charlie to see Dr. Freeman at Johns Hopkins Hospital in Baltimore, Maryland, the only place in the country at the time that was prescribing the ketogenic diet. The ketogenic diet is like a low-carb diet on steroids—high in fat with adequate protein, a little carbohydrate, and no sugar. Charlie began the "magic diet" and within two days his violent seizures miraculously stopped.

"Charlie has been virtually seizure-free, completely drug-free, and a terrific little boy ever since," says Jim. "He has had to remain on a modified version of the ketogenic diet after being on the full diet for two years, but he goes to school and leads a normal, happy life." Charlie was successfully weaned off the diet at the age of seven. Despite worries about developmental delays and retardation, the diet corrected the problem in his brain and allowed him to develop normally, physically and mentally.

Inspired by Charlie's success, his parents founded the Charlie Foundation to Help Cure Pediatric Epilepsy to support medical research and education about the ketogenic diet. Jim Abrahams, Charlie's father, was a successful movie producer and director in Hollywood. In 1997 Jim wrote and directed a movie based his son's experience titled *...First Do No Harm* starring Meryl Streep and Fred Ward. The movie also included a cast of several bit players who had, in real life, been cured from epilepsy using the ketogenic diet. Millicent Kelly, a dietitian who helped run the ketogenic diet program at Johns Hopkins, played herself in the movie.

Seizures can be as dramatic as violent, uncontrollable thrashing movements and loss of consciousness, or as mild as a brief loss of awareness to one's surroundings. Doctors are not completely sure why they occur or how to stop them. Although there are many anticonvulsive drugs available to treat the symptoms, none are completely effective or without adverse side effects, and none of them can even remotely be called a cure. The most successful treatment for epilepsy is the ketogenic diet. Not only can it reduce the occurrence of seizures, but in many cases it can bring about a complete and lasting cure. Generally, patients stay on the diet for a period of two years. In some very severe cases, a modified ketogenic diet may be continued for a longer period of time to allow the brain adequate time to heal. After that time a large percentage of patients can resume eating normally again without ever experiencing another seizure.

Bryce suffered his first seizure shortly after his fourth birthday. "I still remember the day vividly," says his mother Dr. Deborah Snyder, DO, "I was at work when the director of his preschool called to tell me. I ran to my car, leaving an office full of patients behind and barely stopping at traffic lights."

When she arrived, Bryce was in a state of mental confusion that typically follows seizures. At the hospital he had an MRI of his brain and many laboratory tests, all of which appeared to be normal. Snyder clung to the hope that this was an isolated incident and would never recur. She was wrong.

Three weeks later Bryce had another seizure at daycare and was placed on medication. He suffered many side effects from the medications, including abnormalities with his blood counts and behavioral issues such as biting, kicking, and spitting. His cognitive ability began to decline. He was slow to find his words, his writing and drawing regressed, and he even fell asleep in the middle of his cousin's birthday party. To make matters worse, the seizures didn't stop.

"The first time I actually witnessed a seizure myself was one of the most horrific events I've ever experienced," says Snyder. "To see your little boy writhing on the floor, muscles contracted, eyes deviated, drooling, and unresponsive is like having someone reach into your chest and rip out your heart. As a parent, even as a doctor-parent, you are helpless."

Two months into his illness, his seizures began to spiral out of control. Five different anticonvulsive medications proved fruitless, even when he took three at once. His physicians thought he had Lennox-Gastaut Syndrome. Most children with this condition become mentally retarded.

The Snyders received new hope after watching a Dateline NBC television special featuring Charlie Abrahams and his success with the ketogenic diet. "I had heard mention of the ketogenic diet in passing in medical school, but really knew nothing about it," says Snyder. "So I read some more. The more I learned about the diet, the more I believed it was our best option." She made an appointment for Bryce to be admitted to the hospital to start the ketogenic program, but had to wait three weeks for an opening. In the meantime, his mother began to reduce the carbohydrates in his diet and started to introduce foods that were on the diet, such as macadamia nuts, heavy whipping cream, and blueberries. His seizures improved. Bryce had up to 25 seizures daily before he started the ketogenic diet. Within three weeks, he was seizure free. He was maintained on the diet and one medication for a year, then the diet alone for another year. He was weaned completely off the diet in the summer of 2005.

"The ketogenic diet gave me my son back," says Snyder. "Bryce has been seizure free, medication free, and on no special diet for four years and counting. Rather than becoming mentally retarded as was his prognosis, he just completed third grade with straight A's. Bryce is a true modern day miracle!"

Gathering together what she learned during her two years working with what is often referred to as the "miracle diet," Dr. Snyder wrote a book to help other parents succeed with the diet, titled *The Keto Kid: Helping Your Child Succeed on the Ketogenic Diet.*

In April, 1971, three-year-old Tim Intermittee had his first grand mal seizure. Over the next four months he went to six hospitals, saw 21 doctors, and received 38 drug combinations, yet he was still experiencing between 150 and 200 seizures a day.

He spent two and a half months in intensive care at Presbyterian St. Luke's Hospital in Chicago. "I was almost praying Tim would die instead of living his life as a grossly impaired person with this problem," says his mother Connie.

Seeking answers, she spent weeks pouring over books at the University of Illinois library. Then she stumbled on a book that talked about the research on the ketogenic diet at Johns Hopkins University in Baltimore. "I called Baltimore and they told me to come right away," she says. "I tried to take him out of the hospital, but they would not let me transfer him from Presbyterian St. Luke's. He was on valium IV and eight other drugs. With the help of a nurse and a retired doctor I stole him from the hospital. We got on a commercial flight to Baltimore. I wasn't sure if he'd live to see Baltimore. He was seizing every half to three quarters of an hour."

They made it to the clinic and began the ketogenic diet. "A pure Miracle," exclaims Connie. Tim's seizures quickly ceased. He stayed on the diet for two years. Tim is now 41 years old and has not had another seizure since that trip to Baltimore. "He is a smart, handsome, successful man," says Connie proudly.

Many thousands of children as well as adults have found the ketogenic diet a godsend. For many years the ketogenic diet was used out of desperation, a last resort after medications failed. This diet has proven successful with even the most severe cases of epilepsy. Because of its success, the ketogenic diet is gaining wider acceptance as a standard form of treatment rather than an alternative to drug therapy.

THE KETOGENIC DIET

The ketogenic diet has been around since the 1920s. Its origin stems from therapeutic fasting, which in the early 20th century was a popular form of treatment for many chronic health problems. Patients would fast, consuming nothing but water, for up to 30 days and sometimes even longer. Fasting therapy was used to treat a wide variety of difficult to treat health problems including digestive problems, arthritis, cancer, and diabetes. In many instances prolonged fasting proved beneficial.

Some health problems responded very well to fasting therapy. One of these was epilepsy. One of the most outspoken proponents of fasting therapy for the treatment of epilepsy was Dr. Hugh Conklin. He recommended fasting for 18 to 25 days. He treated hundreds of epilepsy patients with his "water diet" and boasted of a 90 percent cure rate in children and a 50 percent cure rate in adults.

Dr. H. Rawle Geylin, a prominent New York pediatrician witnessed Conklin's success first hand and tested the therapy on 36 of his own patients, achieving similar results. His patients ranged in age from 3.5 to 35 years. After fasting for 20 days, 87 percent of the patients were free of seizures. Geylin presented his findings at the annual meeting of the American Medical Association in Boston in 1921, ushering in fasting therapy as a mainstream treatment for epilepsy.

In the 1920s when only phenobarbital and bromides were available as anticonvulsant medications, reports that fasting could cure epilepsy were exciting. These reports set off a flurry of clinical investigations and research activity.

As a result of fasting therapy, many epileptic patients would remain seizure free for years, if not for life. For others the cure was only temporary, lasting only a year or two. In children, long-term freedom from seizures occurred in about 18 percent of cases. Repeating the fast would stop the seizures again, but there was no guarantee for how long. Longer fasts seemed to produce better results, but for some patients the length of time required to bring a lasting cure seemed impractical. Researchers began looking at ways to mimic the metabolic and therapeutic effects of fasting while allowing the patient to consume enough nourishment to sustain life and maintain health for extended periods of time, and hopefully bring about a higher cure rate. The result was the development of the ketogenic diet.

Under normal conditions, our bodies burn glucose for energy. During fasting when no foods containing glucose are consumed, fat is utilized to supply the body's need for energy. Some of this fat is converted by the liver into water-soluble compounds (beta-hydroxybutyrate, acetoacetate, and acetone) collectively known as ketone bodies. Normally the brain uses glucose to satisfy its energy needs. If glucose is not available, one of the only other sources of fuel it can use is ketone bodies or ketones. Other organs and tissues in the body can utilize fat for energy, but not the brain—it must have either glucose or ketones. Ketones actually provide a more concentrated and efficient source of energy than glucose. They have been described as our body's "superfuel," producing energy more efficiently than either glucose or fat.[1] It is like putting high grade gasoline into your car—the engine runs smoother and cleaner, with better fuel efficiency. Ketones have a similar effect on the brain, they allow the brain to function more efficiently. They are also neuroprotective. As a consequence, the dysfunction or short circuit caused by epilepsy is overridden and the brain is allowed to gradually rewire and heal itself.

The elevated level of ketones produced in the blood during fasting can be duplicated by simply restricting the consumption of carbohydrate (starch and sugar)—the primary source of glucose in the diet. Starch and sugar are found in all plant foods but are most abundant in grains, fruits, and starchy vegetables. Meat and eggs contain only a very small amount of carbohydrate.

The ketogenic diet consists of eating a high proportion of fat, adequate protein, just a little carbohydrate, and absolutely no sugar. High fiber carbohydrate foods are preferred over those rich in starch or sugar. The diet provides just enough protein and sufficient calories to maintain growth and repair.

The classic ketogenic diet contains a 4:1 ratio (3:1 for infants and teens) by *weight* of fat to combined protein and carbohydrate. So each meal contains four times as much fat as it does a combination of both protein and carbohydrate. There are 9 calories in 1 gram of fat and 4 calories each in 1 gram of protein and 1 gram of carbohydrate. An unrestricted, ordinary diet consists of about 30 percent fat, 15 percent protein, and 55 percent carbohydrate. The 4:1 weight ratio of the ketogenic diet equates to 90 percent of calories from fat, 8 percent from protein, and 2 percent from carbohydrate. So the ketogenic diet is a very high fat program.

Carbohydrate consumption is restricted to 10-15 grams per day. The diet excludes most high carbohydrate grains, fruits, and vegetables, such as breads, corn, bananas, peas, and potatoes. Total calorie consumption is reduced to 80-90 percent of estimated dietary requirements because this is believed to improve ketone levels. This hasn't been too much of a problem because ketones tend to reduce hunger so patients can feel satisfied without being hungry. Initially, fluid consumption was restricted to 80 percent of normal daily needs. This was done in the belief that it increased blood levels of ketones. But the lack of fluid resulted in an increased risk of developing kidney stones. Later it was found that restricting fluid intake had no benefit and the practice was discontinued.

Since every calorie of fat, protein, and carbohydrate is precisely calculated and measured, the patient is required to eat the entire meal without receiving any extra portions. Every meal needs to have the 4:1 ratio. Any snacks have to be incorporated into the daily total calorie allotment and must have the same ratio. Consequently, it takes a good deal of time and effort to prepare meals and snacks.

In 1921, Dr. Russel Wilder of the Mayo Clinic coined the term "ketogenic diet" to describe a diet that produced a high level of ketones in the blood through the consumption of a high-fat, low-carbohydrate diet. He was the first to use the ketogenic diet as a treatment for epilepsy.

Wilder's colleague, Mynie Peterman, MD, later formulated the classic 4:1 ketogenic diet. Peterman documented positive effects of improved alertness, behavior, and sleep with the diet in addition to seizure control. The diet proved to be very successful, especially with children. Peterman reported in 1925 that 95 percent of patients he studied had improved seizure control on the diet and 60 percent became completely seizure-free. That is an extraordinary cure rate for a disease that otherwise had been deemed incurable.

The diet was not without its drawbacks. A number of patients found the ketogenic diet too difficult to prepare and unappetizing. Consequently, many could not keep with it long enough to achieve satisfactory results. As many as 20 percent could not tolerate the diet and failed to follow through with it. In 1938 a new anticonvulsant drug, phenytoin (Dilantin), was developed. Taking a pill was much easier than worrying about preparing and eating a specific diet. The focus of research quickly turned to discovering new drugs. The ketogenic diet was mostly ignored by researchers and was used primarily as a last resort to treat very serious cases that did not respond to drug therapy. Publicity from the Charlie Foundation in the 1990s brought the therapy out of obscurity into the limelight where it has reemerged as an important treatment for epilepsy.

IS EATING A HIGH-FAT DIET SAFE?

As much as 90 percent of the calories in the ketogenic diet come from fat. The ketogenic diet is not just a high fat diet, but an *extremely* high fat diet. The American Heart Association and other organizations have recommended for years that we limit our fat intake to no more than 30 percent of our calories. They make this recommendation based primarily on the now outdated lipid hypothesis of heart disease, assuming that eating much more than 30 percent fat would cause heart disease. The high-fat ketogenic diet has been in use for 90 years. For most of that time, those on the diet ate primarily saturated fats, the kind that dietitians tell us to avoid. Yet after nearly a century of use with literally thousands of patients consuming a 60-90 percent fat diet for extended periods of time (years, in fact), there have been no heart attacks or strokes. Indeed, just the opposite has happened. People have been healed and have overcome an otherwise incurable disease, in the process experiencing many additional health benefits.

Many people worry that blood cholesterol levels would skyrocket on such a diet. This is really not an issue to worry about. As you learned in Chapter 11, cholesterol is not the enemy. Studies on cholesterol levels in patients following the ketogenic diet do show that, on average, total blood cholesterol levels often increase. But as you have seen, for optimal mental health this is actually a good thing. Lifespan as well as mental function improve with increased cholesterol levels, especially in the elderly. You would think that if the high-fat ketogenic diet was harmful, it would become clearly evident after nearly a century of clinical use.

As you learned in Chapter 11, total cholesterol is not an accurate predictor of heart disease risk because this number includes both the so-called "good" and "bad" cholesterol. Most of the increase is due to the good cholesterol—the type that is believed to protect against heart disease. Studies have consistently shown that those people who go on ketogenic diets generally have higher HDL (good) cholesterol and lower cholesterol ratio (both indicating a reduced risk of heart disease).[2-4]

Despite the rise in total cholesterol, there is no evidence that the high fat diet has a harmful effect on the heart or arteries. In the biggest analytical study on the safety and efficacy of the ketogenic diet to date, investigators failed to find any harm being done over time; the effects were all positive.[5] "We have always suspected that the ketogenic diet is relatively safe long term, and we now have proof," says Eric Kossoff, MD, a neurologist at Johns Hopkins who participated in the study. "Our study should help put to rest some of the nagging doubts about the long-term safety of the ketogenic diet."

The safety of high fat diets actually extends back thousands of years. A number of populations traditionally have survived and even thrived on diets supplying 60-90 percent of calories as fat. The most notable, perhaps, is the Eskimo. The Eskimo lived near the Arctic Circle from Alaska to Greenland where edible vegetation was scarce. The traditional Eskimo diet contained virtually no carbohydrate after weaning (milk contains some carbohydrate), relying totally on meat and fat for the rest of their lives. Yet, the primitive Eskimo was described by early arctic explorers as robust and healthy, free from the diseases of civilization such as heart disease, diabetes, dementia, and cancer, and living to an age equal to that of contemporary Americans and Europeans. The same can be said of the American plains Indians before colonization by white settlers, the native Siberians (Buryat Mongols, Yakuts, Tatars, Samoyeds, Tunguses, Chukuhis, and others) of northern Russia, and the Masai of Africa, all of whom thrived on an extraordinarily high fat diet. Their diet was not just high in fat but was high in saturated fat and cholesterol, yet heart disease was unheard of among them. Even today, those who continue their traditional high-fat diets are remarkably free from the degenerative diseases that are so common in Western society. High fat diets have withstood the test of time and have proven to be not only safe, but therapeutic.

THE MCT DIET

In the 1960s it was discovered that a certain group of fats known as medium chain triglycerides (MCTs) produce more ketones than normal dietary fats composed of long chain triglycerides (LCT). MCTs are more efficiently absorbed and preferentially used by the liver to produce energy in comparison to the more common LCT. In nature fats and oils are composed of fat molecules known as triglycerides. Most of these are classified as long chain triglycerides because they are built on a long chain of carbon atoms. Smaller triglycerides are known as medium chain triglycerides. A product was developed that consisted of 100 percent MCTs, and was appropriately named MCT oil.

The severe carbohydrate restrictions of the classic ketogenic diet made it difficult for parents to produce palatable meals for their children. In 1971, Peter Huttenlocher, MD developed a ketogenic diet in which about 60 percent of the calories came from

MCTs. This allowed more protein and up to three times as much carbohydrate as the classic ketogenic diet. Total fat consumption could be reduced from 90 percent of calories to about 70 percent (60 percent MCT, 10 percent LCT), with about 20 percent protein and 10 percent carbohydrate to round out the diet.

MCT oil is mixed with at least twice its volume of skimmed milk, chilled, and sipped during meals or incorporated into the food. Huttenlocher tested it on twelve children and adolescents with severe epilepsy and difficult-to-treat seizures. Most of the children improved in both seizure control and alertness, producing results that were similar to those of the classic ketogenic diet. The MCT ketogenic diet is considered more nutritious than the classic diet and allows patients the option to eat more protein and carbohydrate, providing a greater variety of foods and ways to prepare meals.

Despite all the positives with the MCT diet, there are some drawbacks. Consuming too much MCT oil can cause nausea, vomiting, and diarrhea. Many patients have had to abandon the MCT diet because they could not tolerate these side effects. A modified MCT diet, which is a combination of the MCT and classic ketogenic diets, is generally more tolerable and is currently being used in many hospitals.

MODIFIED ATKINS DIET

Dr. Robert Atkins is known for championing low-carb dieting for weight loss and better overall health. In his bestselling book *Dr. Atkins' New Diet Revolution,* he outlines four phases of his low-carb diet. The diet includes the induction phase, the ongoing weight loss phase, pre-maintenance phase, and the maintenance phase. The induction phase of the diet restricts total carbohydrate consumption the most, limiting it to 20 grams per day. The classic ketogenic diet restricts carbohydrates to 10-15 grams. Although Atkins induction phase allows a little more carbohydrate, it still produces ketosis (measurable levels of ketone bodies in the blood). In fact, ketosis can be produced by restricting carbohydrate to 40 to 50 grams a day, depending on how carbohydrate-sensitive an individual is.

Atkins encouraged those on the diet to get into ketosis. On a moderate fat, low-carb diet, as opposed to the high-fat ketogenic diet, ketosis indicates that body fat is being dissolved and utilized to meet the body's daily energy needs. As body fat is burned for energy, weight is reduced. In this case, ketosis is a sign the body is losing its excess fat and weight.

Even though the induction phase of the Atkins diet does not produce as high a level of ketosis as the ketogenic diet, people reported that it controlled their seizures. In response to these accounts, researchers at Johns Hopkins Hospital put people on the induction phase of the Atkins diet for extended periods of time, referring to it as a modified Atkins diet. The modified Atkins diet places no limit on calories or protein, and the lower overall ketogenic ratio (approximately 1:1) does not need to be consistently maintained in each meal of the day. Carbohydrates were initially limited to 10 grams per day in children, 15 grams per day in adults, and increased to 20-30 grams per day after a month or so, depending on the effect on seizure control.

The researchers reported that the modified Atkins diet reduced seizure frequency by more than 50 percent in 43 percent of patients and by more than 90 percent in 27 percent of the patients.[6] This and other studies have shown that seizure control with the modified Atkins diet compares favorably with the classic ketogenic diet. Although a higher level of ketosis may provide slightly better protection against seizures, the lower level is still highly effective.

THE NEUROPROTECTIVE EFFECTS OF KETONES

In the treatment of epilepsy, researchers have noted that patients on the ketogenic diet not only experience reduction in the incidence and severity of seizures but also show improved cognition, alertness, attention, and social interaction.[7-9] Brain function apparently experiences improvement in many areas.

Ketones possess potent neuroprotective properties that can ease inflammation, oxidative stress, disturbed glucose metabolism, and excitotoxicity, all of which are common in many neurological disorders. Investigators have reasoned that if ketones protect against seizures and improve mental function, they may protect against other neurological disorders as well.

Case reports have shown the ketogenic diet to be of benefit in the treatment of narcolepsy (a sleep disorder characterized by sudden, uncontrollable urges to sleep), cancer, autism, depression, migraine headaches, and disturbances in glucose metabolism such as type 2 diabetes, polycystic ovary syndrome, and some rare metabolic disorders.[10-20] Animal studies suggest that ketone bodies may be helpful in treating some forms of cardiovascular disease and male infertility.[21-22]

Ketones have been shown to have potent anti-cancer effects. Part of the reason for this is that cancer cannot live in an oxygenated environment. Ketones improve oxygen delivery to the cells throughout the body. A second reason is that cancer cells cannot use ketones to produce energy. Cancer cells burn glucose, but when ketones replace glucose in the bloodstream, cancer cells starve. Consequently, cancer cells have a difficult time surviving in an environment where ketones dominate. Studies show that in animals, ketones decrease tumor size and cancer-related muscle wasting.[23] Similar results have been reported in human cancer patients.[24-25] The anti-cancer effects of ketones are most pronounced in the brain.[26] In the absence of glucose, cancer cells can survive on fatty acids which are released from fat storage during a fast or when calorie consumption is restricted. However, non-esterified fatty acids cannot cross the blood-brain barrier. A person on a very low-carb or ketogenic diet depends on ketones to supply the vast majority of the brain's energy needs. Consequently, the brain gets very little glucose, essentially starving the cancer to death. This is exactly what has been seen in animal studies and in at least one human case study.[27-28]

Potentially the greatest benefit to ketone therapy may be in treating conditions affecting the brain. Oxygen is vital for proper brain function. The brain depends on oxygen so much that it consumes at least 20 percent of the body's oxygen. Consequently, brain cells are extremely sensitive to oxygen deprivation. Without oxygen, some brain cells start dying in less than five minutes, leading to brain damage or death. Ketones block the detrimental effects of hypoxia (lack of oxygen) by improving oxygen delivery. Ketones increase blood flow to the brain by 39 percent, improving circulation and oxygen availability.[29] A number of studies have demonstrated that ketones protect the brain against the damage caused by the interruption of oxygen delivery to the brain.[30-32]

Hospital patients who cannot eat for one reason or another are often given nutritional formulas administered intravenously. When patients who have suffered severe head trauma are given nutritional IV solutions containing the majority of fat in the form of MCTs, recovery is significantly enhanced.[33-34] In the body, the MCTs are converted into ketones which nourish the brain and speed healing.

Evidence from animal studies and human clinical trials suggest that the ketogenic diet can provide symptomatic relief and disease-mitigating effects in a broad range of neurodegenerative disorders including Alzheimer's, Parkinson's, Huntington's, ALS, traumatic brain injury, and stroke.[35-38]

Disturbance in glucose metabolism is an underlying problem common in neurodegenerative diseases. Ketones provide an alternative—and more effective—source of energy that bypasses the glucose metabolic pathways of energy production to give the neurons the life-giving energy they need to function properly and provide an environment in which healing can take place. Ketone bodies are actually the preferred substrates for the synthesis of neural lipids. In other words, ketones promote cellular repair and production of new brain cells.

In tissue cultures, ketone bodies have been shown to increase the survival of motor neurons—the neurons that control movement. This is important for those with ALS. In a mouse model of ALS, researchers fed a ketogenic diet to mice that were genetically modified to develop ALS. Physical strength and performance in these mice was preserved in comparison to mice that were fed a standard diet. On autopsy it was found that the ketogenic-fed mice had significantly higher numbers of surviving motor neurons than the control mice.

The mice that are used in Huntington's disease studies are bred to have the modified huntingtin gene. Dietary intervention that produces elevated levels of ketones has shown to delay the onset of the disease and extend the lives of the mice up to 15 percent longer. In humans, that would equate to an additional 10-12 years.

Tissue cultures from dopaminergic and hippocampal cells of the brain (areas affected by Parkinson's and Alzheimer's disease) are also protected by ketones.[39] MPTP, a neurotoxic drug that causes the destruction of dopamine neurons, is administered to animals to mimic Parkinson's disease. Ketones, however, protect the dopamine neurons in these animals from the harmful effects of MPTP, maintaining energy production and function.[40]

Ketones not only stop neurodegeneration but can restore lost function as well. This was demonstrated in a clinical study with Parkinson's patients by Dr. Theodore VanItallie and colleagues at Columbia University College of Physicians and Surgeons. "Ketones are a high-energy fuel that nourish the brain," says Dr. VanItallie. "Our study was very successful for our patients." The study involved five Parkinson's patients who were put on a ketogenic diet for 28 days. All of the participants' tremors, stiffness, balance, and ability to walk improved, on average, by 43 percent.[41]

The participants maintained a classic 4:1 ketogenic diet consisting of about 90 percent fat. Initially, seven subjects volunteered for the study, but one dropped out the first week because the diet was too difficult to maintain and the other dropped out for personal reasons. Three of the five participants who completed the study adhered faithfully to the prescribed menus. The other two participants did not adhere to the diet as strictly, but still achieved and maintained ketosis throughout the study. Each participant was evaluated using the Unified Parkinson's Disease Rating Scale at the beginning and at the end of the study. The scores were compared. In each case, the subjects showed marked improvement. Interestingly, the two participants who were not as strict with the diet and had slightly lower blood ketone levels improved the most. One improved by 46 percent while the other improved by 81 percent, indicating that a classic ketogenic diet may not be necessary, and a less restrictive diet such as the modified Atkins may be more effective.

The researchers monitored the participant's cholesterol levels closely because they were concerned about how the high fat diet might affect blood lipids. Total blood cholesterol levels in four of the five subjects showed no significant difference at the end of the study. The total cholesterol of the fifth participant, however, increased by 30 percent. Yet, she was the one who showed the greatest (81 percent) improvement in symptoms. The increased cholesterol certainly did not do her brain any harm and probably was part of the reason she improved so much more than the others.

In animal studies, ketones significantly reduce the amount of amyloid plaque that develops in mouse and dog models of Alzheimer's disease.[42-43] In dog models of the disease, ketones improve daytime activity, increase performance on visual-spatial memory tasks, increase probability of learning tasks, have superior performance on motor learning tasks, and increase performance in short-term memory.[44] A number of studies have shown that ketones protect the brain from injury and promote rapid healing after an injury occurs.[45-47]

Ketones improve the activity of *neurotrophic factors*—small proteins that exert survival-promoting and nourishing actions on neurons.[48] These factors play a crucial role in neuron survival. Neurotrophic factors regulate the growth, function, and the ability of neurons to make the neurotransmitters (e.g., dopamine, glutamine) that carry chemical signals which allow neurons to communicate with each other. They play a significant role in the maintenance of brain cell function throughout an individual's lifetime.

Ketones also supply the lipid building blocks for neurons.[49] Thus they aid in the regrowth or repair of damaged brain cells and the synthesis of new cells. This is exciting because it means that ketones potentially provide a means to reverse some of the damage caused by neurodegeneration.

One of the unfortunate consequences of converting glucose into energy is the production of destructive free radicals. It is like the exhaust expelled when a car engine burns gasoline, producing needed energy along with harmful exhaust. In the case of our cells, the exhaust is free radicals. Healthy, well-nourished cells, however, are prepared for this and carry with them a reserve of protective antioxidants that neutralize the free radicals, reducing the damage they may cause. When ketones are used to produce energy in place of glucose, much less oxygen is needed, which

Health Benefits Associated with Ketones

The following are some of the documented health benefits associated with ketones and low-carbohydrate ketogenic diets.

- Provides an alternative high-potency energy source that can be used by every organ in the body except for the liver.[51]
- Protects against brain damage caused by cerebral hypoxia and improves survival.[52-53]
- Reduces the formation of destructive free radicals.[21, 51, 54]
- Calms inflammation in the brain and throughout the body.[21]
- Protects brain cells from chemical toxins.[55]
- Protects against epileptic seizures, including difficult-to-treat drug-resistant seizures.[56]
- Protects against infantile spasms.[57]
- Protects against narcolepsy.[58]
- Mitigates symptoms of autism.[59]
- Prevents migraine headaches.[60]
- Acts as an antidepressant.[61]
- Protects the brain against damage caused by physical trauma.[62]
- Protects against neurodegenerative diseases including Alzheimer's, Parkinson's, Huntington's, and ALS.[63-66]
- Protects against symptoms of hypoglycemia.[67]
- Supplies the substrate from which new neurons can be synthesized.[68]
- Protects against diabetes. Reduces the liver's output of glucose and increases insulin production, thus improving blood sugar control and carbohydrate tolerance.[69-70]
- Mitigates the effects of insulin resistance by mimicking the acute metabolic effects of insulin.[71]
- Protects against cancer, especially brain cancer.[72-73]
- Enhances heart function by improving efficiency and strength while utilizing less oxygen. Ketones increase the hydraulic efficiency of the heart by 25 percent in comparison to glucose.[21, 74]
- Protects against brain damage caused by stroke.[75]
- Increases cellular resistance to stress and improves recovery after surgery.[76-77]
- Protects against polycystic ovary syndrome.[78]
- Increases sperm vitality and motility, important for successful fertilization.[79]
- Useful aid for weight management and obesity treatment.[80]
- May be helpful in alleviating the detrimental effects of almost every disease state due to the ability to calm inflammation and increase oxygen utilization.[81-82]
- Improves overall health and increases life span.[83]

greatly reduces the formation of free radicals and conserves precious antioxidants. Ketones act like a high-grade, clean-burning fuel that produces little exhaust and gives more power. In neurodegenerative states, antioxidant reserves are so depleted that free radicals generated from various sources run wild, promoting inflammation and degeneration.

Ketones can be utilized by every cell and organ in the body except the liver, where they are made.[50] Almost every disease state, whether it is in the brain or elsewhere, involves runaway inflammation and poor oxygen and glucose utilization. Ketones improve oxygen utilization and calm inflammation, thereby potentially providing protection against a large number of disease conditions.

As you see, the health benefits associated with ketones are numerous and varied. Dr. Richard Veech, MD, a senior scientist with the United States National Institutes of Health (NIH), calls ketones the body's "superfuel" for good reason. Ketones increase energy production by 25 percent while reducing oxygen consumption. This boost in energy has a stimulating effect on the cells and the body, transforming ordinary cells into super cells. Cell metabolism is revved up. Efficiency improves. Neurotrophic factors are activated. A mild-mannered Clark Kent of a cell is transformed into a Supercell. The cells' own mechanisms of self-preservation and healing kick into high gear. The Supercell's ability to fight off harmful influences such as toxins and stress are enhanced, and the cell's ability to survive under harsh conditions increases. The cell's productivity increases too. Just imagine two teams of workers who are given a challenge to build a structure. One team is composed of energetic workers (Supercells) while the other team is made up of lazy workers. Who do you think will complete the job first? The same is true with the energized cells in your body. It is no wonder that ketone bodies appear to be associated with so many health benefits.

KETONES AND COCONUT

"My husband Steve, age 58, has had progressive dementia for at least five years," says Mary Newport, MD, Director of the neonatology unit at Spring Hill Regional Hospital in Spring Hill, Florida. In May of 2008 he had an MRI showing significant brain shrinkage—a classic sign of Alzheimer's disease. He was often in a fog; he couldn't find a spoon or remember how to get water out of the refrigerator. Some days were not so bad; he almost seemed like his former self, happy, with his unique sense of humor, creative, full of ideas. "My gut feeling is that diet has something to do with the fluctuation, says Mary. "I knew that he was locked up in there somewhere, if only there was a key to open up the areas of his brain that he didn't have access to."

Just a few years earlier, Steve Newport worked as an accountant. He was a fast typist and loved computers. He could take them apart and repair them. He could fix practically anything without any special training. If he did not have a tool to do something, he would "invent" it and make a usable prototype. He was very intelligent.

In 2003, at the age of 53, he began to have trouble organizing his accounting work. Steve was unable to recall if he had carried out errands that were a daily part of his job and had difficulty completing accounting tasks accurately and on time. He often failed to keep appointments and frequently lost important items such as his wallet, keys, and shoes.

He knew that something was wrong and became depressed. After a year he went to a neurologist, who had Steve take the Mini Mental State Exam (MMSE)—a questionnaire to screen for cognitive impairment. The test has 30 questions; the lower the score, the more severe the dementia. Steve scored 23 out of 30, putting him into the mild range of dementia.

Steve's memory and cognitive abilities continued to decline. Beginning in summer 2005 he began taking the Alzheimer's drug Aricept to try to slow down the progression of the disease. It didn't seem to do much, so another drug, Namenda, was added. Eventually he replaced Aricept with Exelon; still no noticeable improvement.

By the fall of 2006 he was unable to perform any accounting or bookkeeping. By September 2007 he could no longer prepare simple meals for himself, discontinued driving, and required supervision to complete many other activities, such as digging a hole, replacing a light bulb, vacuuming, washing dishes, and dressing appropriately. He was easily distracted when attempting to complete such tasks and was no longer able to use a computer keyboard or calculator, or even perform simple arithmetic. He often wore just one sock or shoe and misplaced the matches to his pairs of shoes. He would have piles of the same sided shoes and no matches by the doors and in his closet. He also reported an inability to read because the words appeared to move about the page erratically. He had difficulty spelling simple words, such as "out" and "put," and when speaking had trouble recalling many common words.

Steve also experienced physical problems similar to those of Parkinson's disease. He had a moderate hand tremor that interfered with eating, and a jaw tremor that was most apparent while speaking. His gait was abnormal, walking slowly and pulling each foot up higher than usual with each step.

"It has been a nightmare to watch his decline and feel helpless to do anything but watch it happen," says his wife Mary. As a doctor, she continually searched for new treatments and drugs that might provide some help slowing down the progression of the disease. She was so desperate that she began looking for trials of new experimental drugs, thinking that Steve might be able to participate in some of these pilot studies.

In the early part of May 2008 she found a company looking for volunteers to test a new vaccine, but participants had to go through a screening first. Steve retook the MMSE test and scored a 12, a very poor performance indicating he had moderately severe dementia. This eliminated him from the study, which required a minimum score of 16. Investigators prefer to test drugs on mild to moderate cases, as these are the most likely to benefit from the drugs. Once the disease has progressed too far, there is little hope any drug would be of much help. Steve's condition was too far advanced. Mary was devastated.

She was still hopeful that Steve could be enrolled in another experimental study and continued looking for other drug trials. She came across a company with a new drug called AC-1202 that was recruiting people to test the tolerability of three different formulations of the drug. The drug appeared to be far more effective than any other Alzheimer's drug on the market. The most potent drugs available can only boast of a modest, at best, decline in the rate of deterioration. This new drug, however, not only stopped the progression of the disease, but even improved memory—something no other drug had ever done. "Most drugs talk about slowing the progression of the disease," says Mary, "but you never hear the word 'improvement.' Right then I knew I had to find out more."

She went online and began to search for everything she could find on this drug. During her research she located a copy of the patent application for the drug, 75 pages long, with a detailed description of the drug, the science behind it, and previous clinical studies. As she read the material and looked up many of the numerous studies referenced in the document, she was amazed.

Preliminary studies with 172 elderly individuals with dementia showed marked improvement within just 90 days. Some of the participants showed measurable improvement in cognitive ability after taking the drug only once!

In a similar study with 159 elderly subjects with normal memory impairment due simply to aging, not disease, those taking the drug performed significantly better on several memory tests than did subjects on a placebo. The results of these studies were published in the journal *BMC Neuroscience*.[84]

Although the drug was to be marketed for the treatment of Alzheimer's disease, the report suggested that it may also have potential in treating other conditions such as Parkinson's, ALS, Huntington's, multiple sclerosis, epilepsy, and diabetes.

As she pored over the report she discovered that this new drug contained only one active ingredient, a medium chain triglyceride called caprylic acid. Although this particular MCT was used, the report indicated that any MCT would give basically the same results. Mary was aware of the use of MCT oil in the treatment of epilepsy; it made sense. MCTs have been used safely for decades in the treatment of epilepsy and in hospital feeding formulas.

This was exciting news. Mary scheduled a screening for Steve in mid-May 2008 so that he could participate in the study. To help Steve with the tests, on the way to the screening she reminded him repeatedly the name of the city and county, what season it was, the month, day of the week, and other questions that are often asked. Unfortunately, Steve again scored too low on the MMSE test to qualify for participation in the study. In addition to the MMSE test, the doctor had Steve draw the face of a clock from memory. This is a standard test for Alzheimer's disease. Steve couldn't remember what a clock looked like, let alone draw it, and only managed to scribble a few figures (Figure 1). After looking at the drawing the doctor said Steve was leaning towards the *severe* stage of Alzheimer's.

"We were devastated,' says Mary, "and then it hit me." In the patent application, a statement was made that MCTs were extracted from coconut oil. Coconut oil is nature's richest source of MCTs, constituting up to 63 percent of the oil. Coconut oil is sold in most health food stores and in some major chain stores. "Why don't we just try coconut oil as a dietary supplement?" she thought. "What have we got to lose? If the MCT oil in it worked for them, why couldn't it work for us?"

On the way home, they stopped at a health food store and bought a quart of "virgin" coconut oil. Mary calculated the amount of coconut oil necessary to equal 20 grams of MCTs, the amount used in the studies. About 35 grams or just over 2 tablespoons (7 teaspoons) of coconut oil provided 20 grams of MCTs. "The following morning, around 9 am, I made oatmeal for breakfast and stirred two tablespoons, plus a little more for 'good luck,' into his portion," she says. "I had some as well, since I cannot expect him to eat something that I won't eat."

At 1:00 p.m. that day Steve had another screening in Tampa. Shortly after they arrived, Steve was whisked away for the test, about 4½ hours after consuming the coconut oil. When he returned, he was unhappy about his performance. Mary asked the research coordinator for his MMSE score. The answer floored her—he scored an 18! Steve remembered what season it was, the month, day of the week, and where he was, both city and county, all of which he had missed on the previous screenings. Just two weeks earlier, he had scored a 12. After a single dose of coconut oil he showed dramatic improvement in memory. "We were ecstatic!"

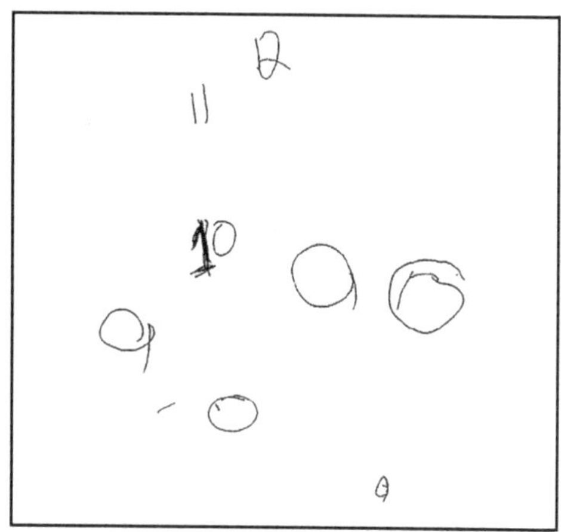

Figure 1. Clock face drawn one day before starting coconut oil.

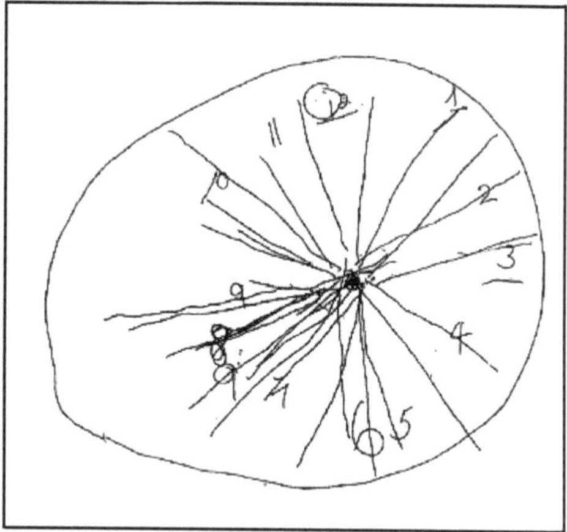

Figure 2. Clock face drawn 14 days after starting coconut oil.

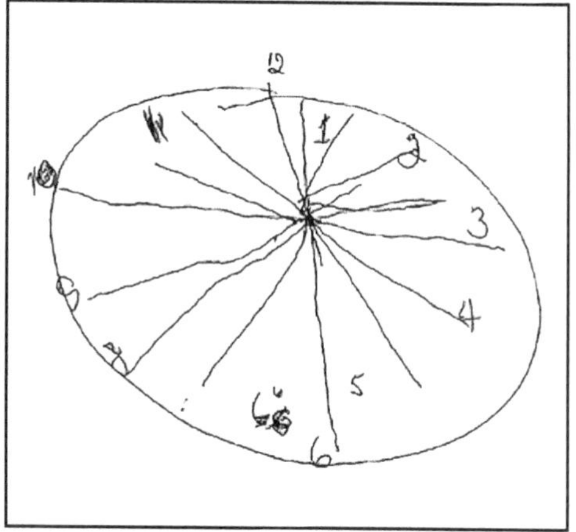

Figure 3. Clock face drawn 37 days after starting coconut oil.

From that day on coconut oil became a regular part of their lives. Two weeks after starting the coconut oil, Steve redrew the clock face (Figure 2). This time he could picture the clock in his mind, which he was unable to do before. He added the "spokes" to help align the numbers. He drew the clock a third time 23 days later (Figure 3). The differences between the first drawing and the latter two show remarkable progress. In June 2008 Steve retook the MMSE and scored

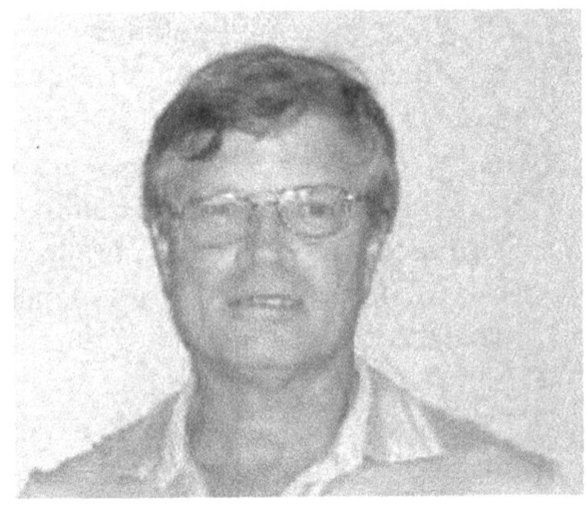
Steve Newport.

a 20, high enough now to be considered in the mild range for Alzheimer's.

At the end of June, the Newports visited Steve's family in Cincinnati. "They noticed a very significant difference in how he interacted with them socially compared to a year ago," says Mary. "Instead of looking lost, he was involved and interested in what they had to say. He recognized relatives by name immediately that were unfamiliar to him a year ago. His facial expression was more animated. He participated actively in conversations, understood jokes immediately and even came up with his own humorous comments. He still had difficulty finding some words, but he was talking in sentences and even stringing sentences together."

According to the MRI done before starting the coconut oil, Steve's brain has experienced serious atrophy that may never completely heal. But he is getting better. "He is a very different person than he was a year ago,' says Mary, "and perhaps even two or three years ago."

Prior to taking coconut oil Steve could not remember how to turn on a computer and was unable to recall how to use a "mouse," nor did he recall the concept of "left-" or "right-clicking." He had even lost his ability to type. By September 2008, about 18 weeks after beginning the coconut oil treatment, he was able to turn on the computer and open up an accounting program, using the mouse appropriately, without prompting. "I've gotten my life back," Steve exclaimed happily.

One year after starting the coconut oil, Steve has experienced the following improvements: absence of facial tremor, and minimal to no tremor involving the hands; gait has become normal; has a renewed interest in exercise and is able to run again; improved memory of recent and past events; is able to read again without the words moving about erratically on the page; ability to complete household and gardening tasks with minimal to no supervision and without distraction; libido has increased; wears both shoes and socks, and keeps the pairs of shoes together; can keep track of time and is wearing a watch after not wearing one for at least two years; is no longer depressed; his ability to initiate and continue a course of conversation has improved and his sense of humor has returned.

"Family members who talk to Steve every couple of months report that his conversational skills have improved each time they have contact with him," says Mary. "His memory for recent events continues to improve. He often brings up events that happened days to weeks earlier and relays telephone conversations with accurate

> "Ketones are a superfuel for the brain."
> —Richard Veech, MD, National Institutes of Health

Global Prevalence of Dementia

A study by researchers from Alzheimer's Disease International, a nonprofit federation of more than 70 Alzheimer's organizations worldwide, has determined the percentage of people with dementia in various parts of the world.

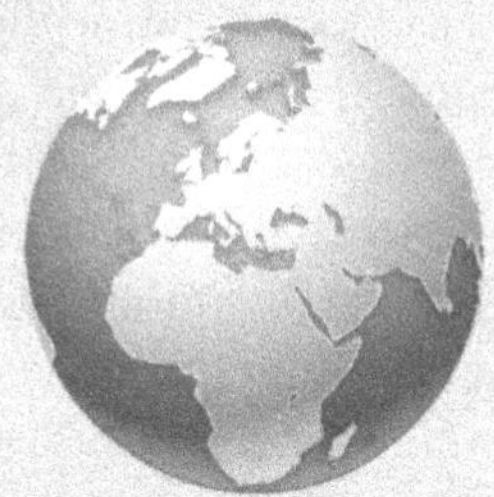

North America 6.4%
Western Europe 5.4%
Latin America 4.6%
Australia/New Zealand 4.3%
Eastern Europe 3.9%
North Africa 3.6%
Middle East 3.6%
Indonesia, Thailand, and Sri Lanka 2.7% ← Coconut eating
India and South Asia 1.9% ← populations

Southeast Asian countries and India have the lowest rates of dementia. Coconut is a traditional food in these countries. Many people in this part of the world still frequently eat coconut and use coconut oil in their cooking. Could this be one of the reasons why their incidence of dementia is so low?

Source: Ferri, C.P., et al. Global prevalence of dementia: a Delphi consensus study. *Lancet* 2005;366:2112-2117.

detail." Desiring to be more social and active, "He now volunteers twice a week at the hospital where I work, helping in the warehouse with boxes and stickers, and working with someone to deliver supplies around the hospital. He is very pleased with his new job and enjoys the people he is working with."

Inspired by Steve's early success, Mary increased the amount of coconut oil she gave him to 2 tablespoons at both breakfast and dinner. Later she added MCT oil and increased his dosage to 2 tablespoons three times a day. Mary discovered that when Steve was given 2 tablespoons of coconut oil for breakfast, the ketones in his blood peaked after about 3 hours and were nearly gone by dinner, lasting a total of about 8-10 hours. When Mary first started Steve on coconut oil, she was unaware that pure MCT oil was also available. She tried substituting MCT oil for the coconut oil and Steve's ketone levels peaked in half the time, at 90 minutes, but were gone after 3 hours. MCT oil raised the blood level of ketones faster than coconut oil, but coconut oil maintained the levels for a much longer time. Too much of the MCT also caused periodic episodes of explosive diarrhea. She now gives Steve a mixture of coconut oil and MCT oil, 2 tablespoons of the mixture at each meal. This way, ketones are maintained at a high level throughout the day and most of the night.

Because of the high amount of fat, especially saturated fat, added in this diet, some people have expressed concern about how it affects blood cholesterol levels.

Mary reports that Steve's cholesterol levels have actually improved. His HDL (good) cholesterol has gone up and his LDL (bad) cholesterol has gone down.

In March 2009, the experimental drug AC-1202, renamed Axona, was approved as a medical food by the US Food and Drug Administration for the treatment of Alzheimer's disease. "We don't use Axona," says Mary. "It costs $100 per month for just one dose a day, is a prescription, and Steve is doing well with what we are doing." The makers of Axona say they only recommend one dose a day because that is what they used in their studies. Another reason may be that when they did try a double dose it caused some of the users intestinal distress and diarrhea. Those who are using the drug report that its effects wear out after only a few hours and they have to take coconut oil to maintain ketone levels. Taking three doses spaced throughout the day to maintain ketone levels would cost $300 per month, compared to about $10 a month for coconut oil.

Coconut oil can be of benefit to anyone suffering from any neurological disorder. The ketones it produces provide energy to the brain and stimulate healing and repair. Coconut oil is especially important for people taking medications. For example, the symptoms of Parkinson's disease are diminished for a time with the drug L-dopa. Over time, the drug becomes ineffective due to destruction of dopaminergic neurons from continued free radical attack. Ironically, the drug itself causes an increase in free radical generation that ultimately accelerates the progression of the disease. Ketones decrease the formation of free radicals.[21] Anyone taking L-dopa should also be taking coconut oil to block the excessive formation of free radicals that damage dopaminergic neurons.

Dr. Mary Newport travels the country telling Steve's story and encouraging further research in the use of MCTs as a therapeutic aid in treating Alzheimer's disease as well as Parkinson's, Huntington's, ALS, multiple sclerosis, and other neurodegenerative disorders. You can visit her website at www.coconutketones.com. Following the Newports' example, many people with neurologic disorders are now incorporating coconut oil into their diets with good results. Many others, without any detectable neurological problems, are taking the oil as a preventative measure.

14 The Facts on Fats

FAT IS GOOD FOR YOU

Contrary to popular belief, fat is not some ugly beast that lurks in our food just to do us harm. It is a valuable, even an essential nutrient. Simply put, fat is good for you. It nourishes the body and can help protect you from disease.

All natural fats are good. However, good fats can become bad if they are adulterated by oxidation or chemically altered. Some fats are better for us than others. Some can be consumed in larger amounts than others. Some need to be eaten in balance with others. Some fats, those that are adulterated or man-made, should not be eaten at all. The problem is that most of us are confused as to which are which.

Advertising and marketing propaganda has greatly influenced and distorted our perception of dietary fats. We are told to reduce our fat intake to the bare minimum in order to lose excess weight and be healthy. In addition, some fats are portrayed as being good while others are depicted as being bad. Saturated fats get the brunt of the criticism and are blamed for contributing to just about every health problem experienced by mankind. Polyunsaturated vegetable oils, margarine, and shortening, on the other hand, are hailed as the "good" fats. The truth is that most saturated fats, and particularly coconut oil, are some of the healthiest you can eat. In contrast, many polyunsaturated fats are so far removed from their natural state as to become a serious health threat.

Natural fats which have undergone as little processing and adulteration as possible are the healthiest. People from all walks of life and throughout history have been eating natural fats without experiencing the health problems we commonly face today. These fats are not the troublemakers.

Fats are, in fact, vital nutrients that our bodies rely on to achieve and maintain good health. We need fat in our diet. Almost all foods in nature contain fat to one extent or another. An adequate amount of fat is necessary for proper digestion and nutrient absorption.

Fats slow down the movement of food through the stomach and digestive system. This allows more time for foods to bathe in stomach acids and digestive enzymes. As a consequence, more nutrients, especially minerals which are normally tightly bound to other compounds, are released from our foods and absorbed into the body.

Low-fat diets are actually detrimental because they prevent complete digestion of food and limit nutrient absorption, promoting mineral deficiencies. Calcium, for example, needs fat for proper absorption. For this reason, low-fat diets encourage osteoporosis. It is interesting that we often avoid fat as much as possible and eat low fat foods, including non-fat and low-fat milk, to get calcium—yet by eating reduced fat milks, the calcium is not effectively absorbed. This may be one of the reasons why people can drink loads of milk and take calcium supplements by the handful but still suffer from osteoporosis. Likewise, many vegetables are good sources of calcium. But in order to take advantage of that calcium, you need to eat them with butter and cream or other foods that contain fat.

Fat improves the availability and absorption of almost all vitamins and minerals and is essential in order to properly absorb fat-soluble nutrients. The fat soluble vitamins include vitamins A, D, E, and K. Other fat soluble nutrients include alpha-carotene, beta-carotene, lycopene, lutein, and other carotenoids. These nutrients are absolutely vital to good health.

Many of the fat-soluble vitamins function as antioxidants that protect you from free-radical damage. By reducing the amount of fat in your diet, you limit the amount of protective antioxidant nutrients available to protect you from destructive free-radical reactions. Low-fat diets speed the process of degeneration and aging. This may be one of the reasons why those people who stay on very low-fat diets for any length of time often look pale and sickly.

Carotenoids are fat-soluble nutrients found in fruits and vegetables. The best known is beta-carotene. All of the carotenoids are known for their antioxidant capability. Many studies have shown them and other fat-soluble antioxidants such as vitamins A and E to provide protection from degenerative disease and support immune system function.

Vegetables like broccoli and carrots have beta-carotene, but if you don't eat any oil with them you won't get the full benefit of the fat-soluble vitamins they contain. You can eat fruits and vegetables loaded with antioxidants and other nutrients, but if you don't include fat with them then you will only absorb a small portion of these vital nutrients. Taking vitamin tablets won't help much because they too need fat to facilitate proper absorption. Eating a low-fat diet, therefore, can actually be detrimental.

How much of an effect does fat have on nutrient absorption? Apparently a lot. In a study conducted at Ohio State University, researchers looked at absorption of three carotenoids (beta-carotene, lycopene, and lutein) in meals that had added fat. The researchers used avocado as the source of added fat.

Eleven test subjects were given a meal of fat-free salsa and bread. On another day the same meal was given, but this time avocado was added to the salsa, boosting the fat content of the meal to about 37 percent of calories. Blood levels of the test subjects showed that beta-carotene increased 2.6 times and lycopene 4.4 times. This showed that adding a little fat to the meal can more than double, triple, or quadruple nutrient absorption.

A second test involved eating a salad. The first salad included romaine lettuce, baby spinach, shredded carrots, and a non-fat dressing, resulting in a fat content of about 2 percent. After avocado was added, the fat content jumped to 42 percent. The higher fat salad increased blood levels of lutein 7 times and beta-carotene an incredible 18 times!

In a similar study, subjects were fed salads using dressings with a different fat content. Salad with non-fat dressing resulted in negligible carotenoid absorption. Low-fat dressing improved nutrient absorption some, but full-fat dressing showed a significant increase. The researchers were surprised not only by how adding fat improved nutrient absorption, but also how little is absorbed in the absence of fat.

So, if you want to get all the nutrients you can from a tomato, green beans, spinach, or any vegetable or low-fat food, you need to add a little fat. Eating vegetables without added fat is in effect the same as eating a nutritionally poor meal. Adding a good source of fat in the diet is important in order to gain the most nutrition from your foods.

Nathan Pritikin, a self-proclaimed nutritionist, became famous in the 1970s and 1980s as one of America's leading advocates for low-fat dieting as a means of achieving optimal health. He founded the Pritikin Longevity Center to promote his low-fat program. Pritikin was a fanatic about keeping fat out of the diet. He claimed there was enough fat in lettuce and other vegetables to meet our body's needs. His diet limited fat consumption to a mere 10 percent of total calories. People lost weight, but they also developed health problems as a result of fat deficiency. Charles T. McGee, MD, describes in his book *Heart Frauds* patients who tried the Pritikin low-fat diet. "Pritikin Program patients become deficient in essential fatty acids after they have been on the diet about two years. These people entered the office looking gaunt, with skin that was dry, droopy, pale, gray, and flaky. Fortunately this complication was seldom seen because most people find it difficult to keep fat intake down to the 10 percent level without cheating."

Pritikin claimed his low-fat way of eating would improve health, remove excess weight, and ward off degenerative disease. Unfortunately for Pritikin, it didn't work for him. He developed leukemia, went into deep depression, and committed suicide. Depression and suicide are well known side effects of low-fat dieting.[1-2] Even diets that allow 25 percent of calories as fat, over twice that recommended by Pritikin, can seriously affect mental health.[3] The diet he advocated to achieve optimal health and increase longevity and happiness was the thing that drove him out of his mind and to an early death.

Another low-fat advocate was Roy L. Walford, MD, a professor of medicine at UCLA medical school. Walford was considered one of the world's leading experts on calorie restriction and longevity. Since the 1930s researchers have observed that the lifespan of animals could be extended up to 50 percent by restricting the number of calories they ate. Walford believed human lifespan could be extended to 120 years on a calorie restricted diet. He wrote several books on the topic, including *The 120 Year Diet*, *Maximum Life Span*, and *The Anti-Aging Plan*. His plan was based on the concept of "calorie restriction with optimal nutrition" or what he termed "CRON." He claimed it would "retard the basic rate of aging in humans, greatly extending the period of youth and middle age; postpone the onset of such late-life disease as heart disease, diabetes, and cancer; and even lower the overall susceptibility to disease at any age."

Restricting the number of calories consumed was central to his program. Since fat contains more than twice as many calories as either carbohydrate or protein, fat was almost completely eliminated from his diet. Walford began eating this way when he was in his early 60s and fully expected to live to be a least 100. But things didn't work out the way he had planned. He developed amyotrophic lateral sclerosis (ALS) and died at the age of 79. The average lifespan for a white American male is 78 years.[4] So after 20 years of following a calorie restricted, low-fat diet, he added the sum total of only one year to his life and suffered with crippling neurodegenerative disease for his last few years of it. Instead of protecting him from degenerative disease, his low-fat diet was the thing that did him in.

Calorie restriction with optimal nutrition may very well extend lifespan and forestall aging, but the problem with Walford's diet was that he did not understand the importance of fat and how it is necessary in order to achieve optimal nutrition. Studies have shown that people eating low-fat diets have a higher rate of death due to degenerative disease than those with higher fat intake.[5] High-carbohydrate, low-fat diets are known to increase risk of ALS.[6]

One of the classic symptoms of neurodegenerative disease is chronic inflammation. Chronic inflammation is destructive, and ways to reduce neuroinflammation are actively being sought. While anti-inflammatory drugs have been suggested as a possible answer, for the most part they have proven to be ineffective. In fact, some accelerate the rate of neurodegeneration. Researchers continue to search for new drugs. The answer, however, is already available, and it doesn't require any drugs. Inflammation can be lowered through diet. In a study conducted at the University of Connecticut, investigators found that a low-carb, high-fat diet does an admirable job of lowering runaway inflammation. They showed that a high-fat diet (59 percent of calories as fat) greatly *reduces* inflammation and is much more effective than a low-fat diet (24 percent fat).[7]

The amount of fat people eat varies greatly around the world. Some people eat a lot while others relatively little. In many traditional diets fat historically accounted for 60 to 90 percent of their total caloric intake (and the vast majority was saturated fat). Some Pacific island communities consumed up to 60 percent of their calories as fat, 50 percent of it saturated, mostly from coconut.[8] Although these people ate large amounts of fat, diseases such as heart disease, diabetes, and Alzheimer's were completely unknown to them. Relatively isolated populations that still eat natural fats do not experience Alzheimer's or other degenerative diseases common in modern society.[9-10]

A QUICK COURSE IN FATS AND OILS

Fatty Acids and Triglycerides

The terms fat and oil are often used interchangeably. There is no real difference; however, fats are generally considered solid at room temperature while oils are liquid. Lard, for example, would be referred to as a fat, while liquid corn oil would be called an oil.

Fats and oils are composed of fat molecules known as fatty acids. Fatty acids are classified into three categories depending on their degree of saturation. There are saturated, monounsaturated, and polyunsaturated fatty acids. You hear these terms used all the time, but what makes a fat unsaturated? And what are saturated fats saturated with?

Fatty acids consist almost entirely of two elements—carbon (C) and hydrogen (H). The carbon atoms are hooked together like links in a long chain. Attached to each carbon atom are two hydrogen atoms. In a saturated fatty acid, each carbon atom is attached to a pair of hydrogen atoms (see illustration below). In other words, it is "saturated with" or holding as many hydrogen atoms as it possibly can. Hydrogen atoms are always attached in pairs. If one pair of hydrogen atoms is missing, you would have a monounsaturated fatty acid. "Mono" indicates one pair of hydrogen atoms is missing, while "unsaturated" indicates the fatty acid is not fully saturated with hydrogen atoms. If two, three, or more pairs of hydrogen atoms are missing, you have a polyunsaturated fatty acid ("poly" means "more than one").

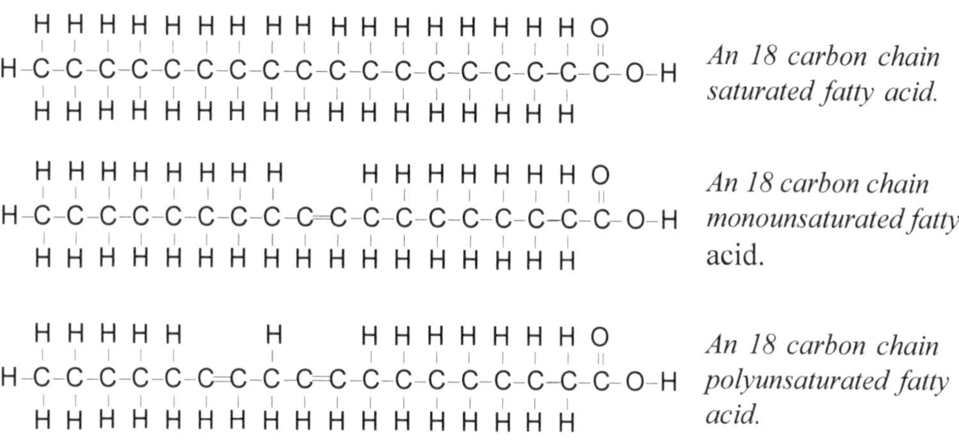

An 18 carbon chain saturated fatty acid.

An 18 carbon chain monounsaturated fatty acid.

An 18 carbon chain polyunsaturated fatty acid.

The fatty acids in the oil you pour on your salad for dinner and in the meat and vegetables you eat—in fact, even the fat in your own body—come in the form of *triglycerides*. A triglyceride is nothing more than three fatty acids joined together by a glycerol molecule. So you can have saturated triglycerides, monounsaturated triglycerides, or poly-unsaturated triglycerides.

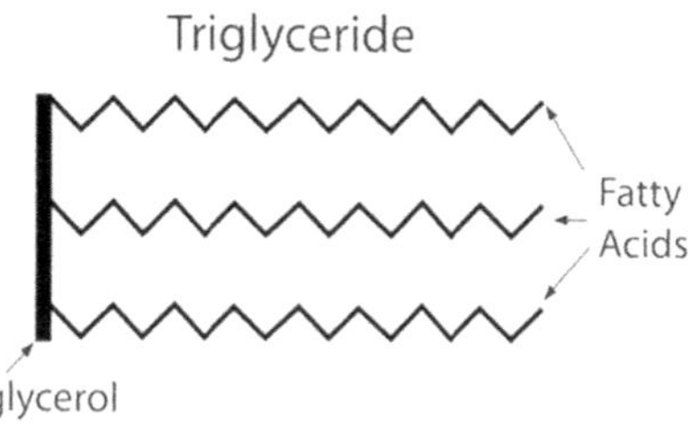

All vegetable oils and animal fats contain a mixture of saturated, monounsaturated, and polyunsaturated fatty acids. To say any particular oil is saturated or monounsaturated is a gross oversimplification. No oil is purely saturated or polyunsaturated. Olive oil is often called a "monounsaturated" oil because it is predominantly monounsaturated, but like all vegetable oils, it also contains some polyunsaturated and saturated fatty acids as well.

Generally, animal fats contain the highest amount of saturated fatty acids. Vegetable oils contain the highest amount of polyunsaturated fatty acids. Palm and coconut oils are exceptions; although they are vegetable oils, they contain a high amount of saturated fat.

Medium Chain Triglycerides

The different types of fatty acids can also be classified into three major categories depending on their size or, more precisely, the length of their carbon chains. There are long chain fatty acids (13 to 22 carbons), medium chain fatty acids (6 to 12 carbons), and short chain fatty acids (3 to 5 carbons). When a triglyceride is composed of three medium chain fatty acids, it is referred to as a medium chain triglyceride (MCT), and likewise with long chain triglycerides (LCT) and short chain triglycerides (SCT).

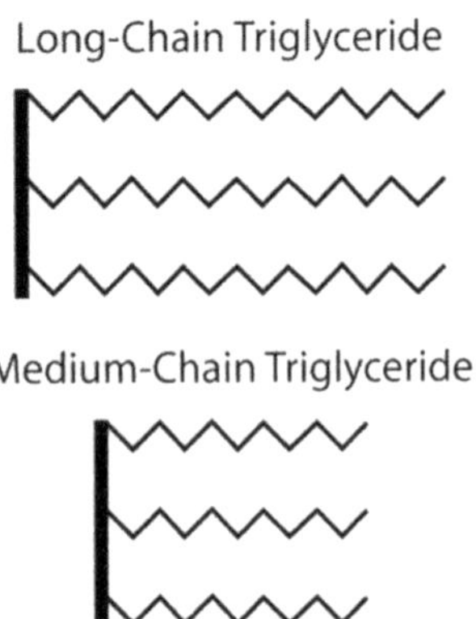

LCTs are by far the most plentiful in our diet, comprising 97 percent of the triglycerides we consume. MCTs make up most of the remaining 3 percent, and SCTs are very scarce. Fatty acids with chain lengths of 12 carbons or less are metabolized differently than those containing 14 or more. Consequently, many of the medium and short chain triglycerides are converted into ketone bodies, regardless of the amount of carbohydrate or glucose in the diet. LCTs are only converted into ketone bodies during severe glucose restriction, such as when fasting or eating a ketogenic diet.

Most fats and oils are composed of 100 percent LCTs. There are very few dietary sources of MCTs. By far the richest natural source of MCTs comes from coconut oil, which consists of 63 percent medium triglycerides. The next largest source of MCTs comes from palm kernel oil, which consists of 53 percent. Butter is a distant third, containing only 12 percent medium and short chain fatty acids. Milk from all species of mammals contains MCTs. Human milk contains more than cow, goat, and other animal milks. Ketones produced from MCTs are essential for brain development in infants, supplying 25 percent of the brain's energy needs. Since the human brain is larger in proportion to the rest of the body in comparison to animals, the need for MCTs in humans is much greater.

POLYUNSATURATED FATS

The Essential Fatty Acids

Polyunsaturated fats are found most abundantly in plants. Vegetables oils such as soybean oil, safflower oil, sunflower oil, cottonseed oil, corn oil, and flaxseed oil are composed predominantly of polyunsaturated fatty acids and, therefore, are commonly referred to as polyunsaturated oils.

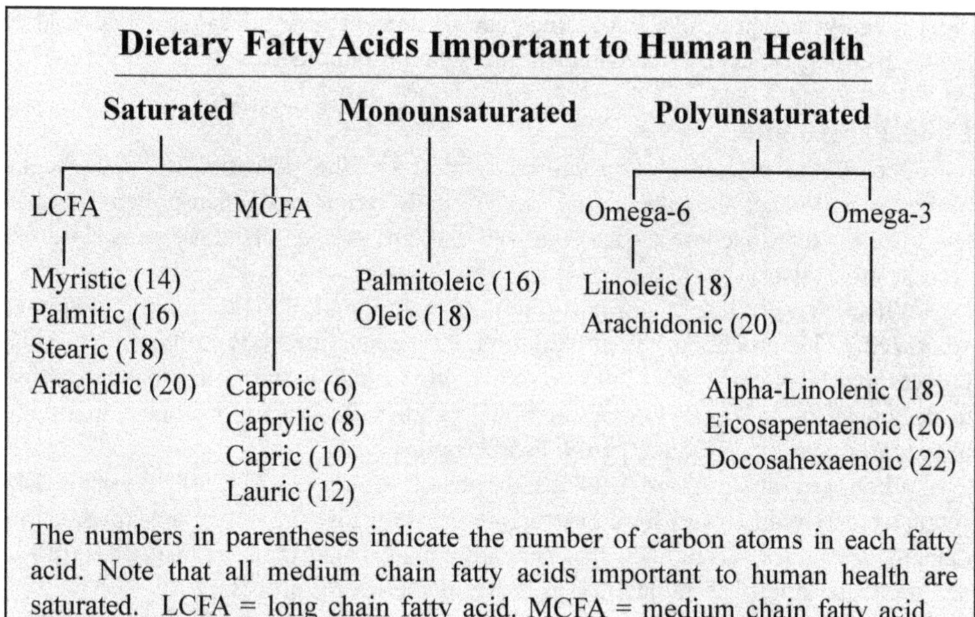

The numbers in parentheses indicate the number of carbon atoms in each fatty acid. Note that all medium chain fatty acids important to human health are saturated. LCFA = long chain fatty acid. MCFA = medium chain fatty acid.

Some fatty acids are classified as being essential. This means our bodies cannot make them from other nutrients, so we must have them in our diet in order to achieve and maintain good health. Our bodies can manufacture saturated and monounsaturated fats from other foods. However, we do not have the ability to manufacture polyunsaturated fats. Therefore, it is *essential* that they be included in our diet.

When we talk about saturated, monounsaturated, or polyunsaturated fats, we are not referring to just three types of fatty acids, but three families of fatty acids. There are many different types of saturated fatty acids as well as many different monounsaturated and polyunsaturated fatty acids. Two families of polyunsaturated fatty acids are important to human health: omega-6 and omega-3 polyunsaturated fatty acids. There are several omega-6 and omega-3 fatty acids. Two are considered essential because the body can use these two to make all of the rest—linoleic acid and alpha-linolenic acid. These are the essential fatty acids (EFAs) nutritionists often talk about. Linoleic acid belongs to the omega-6 family. Alpha-linolenic acid belongs to the omega-3 family.

Theoretically, if you eat an adequate source of linoleic acid, the body can make all the other omega-6 fatty acids it needs. Likewise, if you have an adequate source of alpha-linolenic acid, it can make all the other omega-3 fatty acids.

Nutritional studies indicate that we need about 3 percent of our total calories to come from EFAs. In a typical 2000 calorie diet, that is equivalent to about 7 grams, which isn't very much. A teaspoon holds 5 grams. So 1½ teaspoons or ½ tablespoon of EFAs will supply minimum daily needs.

Since these fatty acids are considered "essential," people often get the impression that they possess special health properties and that the more they eat the better. But this is not necessarily the case. While we must have some in our diet, too much can be detrimental. Researchers have found that the consumption of polyunsaturated oil, most notably omega-6 oils, exceeding just 10 percent of total calories can lead to blood disorders, cancer, liver damage, and vitamin deficiencies.[11]

Lipid Peroxidation

One of the reasons polyunsaturated fats have the potential to cause health problems is because they are highly vulnerable to oxidation. When polyunsaturated fats oxidize, they become toxic. Oxidized fats are rancid fats. Free radicals are a product of oxidation.

When oxygen reacts normally with a compound, the compound becomes "oxidized." This process is called oxidation. Polyunsaturated fats readily oxidize in a process that biochemists call lipid peroxidation. "Lipid" is the term biochemists use to designate fat or oil, and "peroxidation" signifies an oxidation process involving unsaturated fats that produce peroxide free radicals.

When polyunsaturated oils are exposed to heat, light, or oxygen, they spontaneously oxidize and form destructive free radicals. Once they are formed, free radicals can attack unsaturated fats and proteins, causing them to become oxidized and generate more free radicals. It is a self-perpetuating process.

Liquid vegetable oils can be deceiving because they look and taste harmless even after they become rancid. The oil may not smell bad and may look as fresh as the day you bought it, yet be teaming with free radical terrorists.

When oil is extracted from seeds, the oxidation process is set in motion. The more the oil is exposed to heat, light, and oxygen, the more oxidized it becomes. By the time the oil is processed and bottled, it has already become oxidized to some extent. As it sits in the warehouse, the back of a truck, the grocery store, and your kitchen cabinet, it is continuing to oxidize. When you buy vegetable oil from the store, it has already gone rancid to some degree. In one study, various oils obtained off the shelf from local stores were tested for oxidation of the polyunsaturated fatty acids.[12] The researchers found that oxidation was already present in every sample tested. When you use these oils in cooking, oxidation is greatly accelerated. This is why you should never cook foods using any polyunsaturated oil.

Oxidation occurs inside our bodies as well. Our only defense against free radicals is antioxidants. Antioxidants stop the chain reactions which create new free radicals. If we consume too much processed vegetable oil, the free radicals they create deplete antioxidant nutrients such as vitamins A, C, and E as well as zinc and selenium and can actually promote nutrient deficiencies.

Polyunsaturated fats are found in all of our cells to one degree or another. A polyunsaturated fatty acid in a cell membrane attacked by a free radical will oxidize and become a free radical itself, then attack a neighboring polyunsaturated molecule, likely in the same cell. The destructive chain reaction continues until the cell is severely crippled or utterly destroyed. Random free-radical reactions occurring throughout the body day after day, year after year take their toll.

Several studies have shown a relationship between processed vegetable oil consumption and damage to the central nervous system. In one study, for example, the effect of dietary oils on the mental ability of rats was determined by analyzing the animal's maze-learning abilities. Different oils were added to the rats' food. The study was initiated after rats had aged considerably, allowing enough time for the effects of the oils to become measurable. Rats were tested on the number of maze errors they made. The animals that performed the best and retained their mental capacities the longest were the ones fed saturated fats. The ones given polyunsaturated oils lost their mental abilities the most quickly.[13]

Age-related macular degeneration is the most common cause of blindness in the US, Canada, Australia, and most other industrialized countries. The incidence of this condition has skyrocketed over the past 30 years. Several studies have shown that the primary culprit in causing this rise in macular degeneration is the increased consumption of unsaturated vegetable oils.[14-16]

In contrast, saturated fats are very resistant to oxidation. They do not form destructive free radicals. In fact, they act more like protective antioxidants because they prevent oxidation and the formation of free radicals. A diet high in protective saturated fats can help prevent lipid peroxidation.

Polyunsaturated fatty acids are very easily oxidized. Saturated fatty acids are very resistant to oxidization. Monounsaturated fatty acids are in between. They are more stable than polyunsaturated fatty acids but less stable than saturated fatty acids.

Replacing polyunsaturated fats with saturated and monounsaturated fats in the diet can help reduce the risks associated with free radicals. Also, eating a diet rich in antioxidant nutrients such as vitamin E and beta-carotene will help protect the polyunsaturated fatty acids in your body from oxidation.

Heat Damaged Vegetable Oils

Most cooks recommend polyunsaturated vegetable oils in cooking and food preparation as a "healthy" alternative to saturated fats. Ironically, these unsaturated vegetable oils, when used in cooking, form a variety of toxic compounds that are far more damaging to health than any saturated fat could be. Polyunsaturated vegetable oils are the least suitable for cooking.[17]

When vegetable oils are heated, these unstable polyunsaturated fatty acids are easily transformed into harmful compounds, including a particularly insidious compound known as 4-hydroxy-trans-2-nonenal (4-HNE). When you cook with polyunsaturated oils, your food is littered with these toxic substances.

Even heating these oils at low temperatures causes damage to the delicate chemical structure of polyunsaturated fatty acids. Cooking foods at high temperatures accelerates oxidation and harmful chemical reactions. Numerous studies, in some cases published as early as the 1930s, have reported the toxic effects of consuming heated vegetable oils.[12]

Over the past 20 years, an increasing number of studies have found links between 4-HNE and increased risk for heart disease, stroke, Parkinson's disease, Alzheimer's disease, Huntington's disease, liver problems, osteoarthritis, and cancer. Every time you use unsaturated vegetable oils for cooking or baking, you are creating 4-HNE.

One of the conditions linked to 4-HNE in heated vegetable oils is heart disease. This may come as a surprise to most people because polyunsaturated vegetable oils are supposed to be heart friendly, yet recent studies show a clear link between

4-HNE and heart disease.[18-20] Studies also show that 4-HNE levels are high in the diseased regions of the brain in Alzheimer's patients.[21-22]

Studies show that diets containing heat-treated liquid vegetable oils produce more atherosclerosis than those containing unheated vegetable oil.[23] Any unsaturated vegetable oil can become toxic when heated. And even a small amount, especially if eaten frequently over time, will affect your health. Oxidized oils have been found to induce damage to blood vessel walls and cause numerous organ lesions in animals.

The oils that are most vulnerable to the damage caused by heating are the ones that contain the highest amount of polyunsaturated fatty acids. Monounsaturated fatty acids are chemically more stable and can withstand higher temperatures, yet they too can oxidize and form toxic byproducts if heated to high temperatures. Saturated fatty acids are very heat stable and can withstand relatively high temperatures without oxidation. Therefore, saturated fats are the safest to use for day-to-day cooking and baking.

We need some polyunsaturated fats in our diet, but if all commercial polyunsaturated vegetable oils are rancid to some degree before we even purchase them, and if they become more harmful to health when used in cooking, how are we going to get our daily requirement of essential fatty acids? The answer is simple. You can get your EFA requirement just as your ancestors did—from foods! You do not need to eat processed vegetable oils to satisfy your daily EFA requirements. You can get all your EFAs from foods. This is by far the best way to get them because while they are still packaged in their original cellular containers, they are shielded from the damaging effects of oxygen and protected by naturally occurring antioxidants to keep them fresh.

Omega-6 essential polyunsaturated fatty acids are found in almost all plant and animal foods—meat, eggs, nuts, grains, legumes, and vegetables. Omega-6 fatty acids are so abundant in the diet that a deficiency isn't likely to happen. Less common are the omega-3 polyunsaturated fatty acids found in seeds, leafy green vegetables, seaweed, eggs, fish, and shellfish. You can get all the omega-3 fatty acids you need by making sure you include some fish, eggs, and leafy greens as a part of your weekly menu. Grass-fed beef and game meats also supply omega-3 fatty acids. Cattle that graze on grass, which is rich in omega-3s, incorporate these fats into their own tissues. Grain-fed beef, however, is a poor source of omega-3 fatty acids.

Hydrogenated Vegetable Oils

Many packaged foods are made using hydrogenated or partially hydrogenated vegetable oil. These are among the most health-damaging fats you can possibly eat—just as bad, if not worse, than oxidized polyunsaturated fats.

Hydrogenated oils are made by bombarding liquid vegetable oil with hydrogen atoms in the presence of a metal catalyst. In the process, polyunsaturated vegetable oils become saturated with hydrogen. This makes the liquid oil transform into a more hardened or solid fat. In the process of hydrogenation, however, a new type of fatty acid known as a *trans fatty acid* is created. Trans fatty acids are artificial man-made fats. This toxic fatty acid is foreign to our bodies and can create all sorts of trouble.

"These are probably the most toxic fats ever known," says Walter Willett, MD, professor of epidemiology and nutrition at Harvard School of Public Health.[24] Studies show that trans fatty acids can contribute to atherosclerosis and heart disease. Trans fatty acids increase blood LDL (bad cholesterol) and lower the HDL (good cholesterol), both regarded to be undesirable changes.[25] Researchers now believe it has a greater influence on the risk of cardiovascular disease than any other dietary fat.[26]

Trans fatty acids affect more than just our cardiovascular health. They have been linked with a variety of adverse health effects, which include cancer, multiple sclerosis, diverticulitis, diabetes, and other degenerative conditions.[27] Trans fatty acids disrupt brain communication. Studies show that the trans fatty acids we eat get incorporated into brain cell membranes, including the myelin sheath that insulates neurons. Trans fatty acids alter the electrical activity of brain cells, causing cellular degeneration and diminished mental performance.[28]

Under pressure from many health organizations and the public, the United States Institute of Medicine spent three years reviewing all the published studies on trans fatty acids. After the study was completed, the Institute of Medicine issued a statement declaring that no level of trans fatty acid consumption was safe. What surprised everyone was that the Institute of Medicine didn't give a recommendation as to what percentage of trans fats were safe to consume, as is often done with food additives, but flatly stated that *no level* of trans fats is safe. If you see a packaged food that contains hydrogenated oil, margarine, or shortening, don't touch it. If you eat out, ask the restaurant manager what type of oil they use to cook their food. If they say "vegetable oil," it almost definitely is hydrogenated vegetable oil: avoid it. The reason you can safely count on it being hydrogenated vegetable oil is because regular vegetable oil breaks down too quickly and becomes rancid. Restaurants like to reuse their oils as long as possible before they have to be tossed out. Ordinary vegetable oils have too short a life span.

Many of the foods you buy in the store and in restaurants are prepared with or cooked in hydrogenated oil. Fried foods sold in grocery stores and restaurants are usually cooked in hydrogenated oil because it makes foods crispy and is more resistant to spoilage than ordinary vegetable oils. Many frozen processed foods are cooked or prepared in hydrogenated oils. Hydrogenated oils are used in making French fries, biscuits, cookies, crackers, chips, frozen pies, pizzas, peanut butter, cake frosting, and ice cream, especially soft serve ice cream.

SATURATED FAT

Saturated Fat Is a Vital Nutrient

Probably no food component in history has been as misunderstood and maligned as saturated fat. It is labeled the cause of nearly every health problem of modern civilization. If it really is as dangerous as they say, it's truly a miracle how our ancestors survived for thousands of years eating a diet dominated by saturated fat. Animal fats, butter, and palm and coconut oils were the most common fats used throughout history. These fats are easy to produce using the simplest of tools.

Vegetable oils from seeds such as soybeans, cottonseed, safflower seeds, and such are very difficult to extract. Consequently, polyunsaturated vegetable oils were not used much until after the invention of hydraulic oil presses in the 19th century. Interestingly enough, when people ate primarily saturated fats, the so-called diseases of modern civilization—heart disease, diabetes, and the like—were uncommon. As we've replaced saturated fats with unsaturated oils, these diseases have come upon us like a plague. From a historical point of view it is easy to see that saturated fats don't cause these diseases.

The truth of the matter is that saturated fat is a vital nutrient. Yes, saturated fat is a nutrient, *not* a poison. It is necessary in order to obtain and maintain good health. Saturated fat serves as an important source of energy for the body and aids in the absorption of vitamins and minerals. As a food ingredient, fat helps us feel full and provides taste, consistency, and stability. Saturated fat is necessary for proper growth, repair, and maintenance of body tissues. It is essential for good lung function. It is the preferred source of energy for the heart muscle and also helps protect the unsaturated fats in your body against the destructive action of free radicals.

We hear a lot about the importance of the essential fatty acids. Because they are called "essential," we get the mistaken belief that they are the most important fats. However, the reason they are "essential" is because they are the *least* important of the fats. Believe it or not, saturated fat is far more important to your health than the EFAs! Let me explain why.

Saturated fat is so necessary to your health that our bodies have been programmed to make it out of other nutrients. Getting an adequate amount of saturated fat is so important that it is not left to chance. The consequences of a saturated fat deficiency are so serious that the body is capable of manufacturing its own.

The EFAs (polyunsaturated fats), on the other hand, are far less important to our health, so the body has not developed a means of manufacturing its own. It relies totally on what is in the diet.

The foods that we eat provide the building blocks for our cells and tissues. This is true for the fats we consume as well. The fat in our bodies consists of 45 percent saturated, 50 percent monounsaturated, and only 5 percent polyunsaturated fat. That's right. Only 5 percent of the fat in your body is polyunsaturated. Consequently, the body's need for polyunsaturated fat or EFAs is very small. Your body needs nearly 10 times as much saturated fat, as well as monounsaturated fat, as it does EFA. So which is more essential?

While the body can manufacture saturated and monounsaturated fats, it cannot make enough on its own for optimal health. We still need them in our diet to avoid nutritional deficiencies.[29-30]

Saturated Fat Does Not Promote Heart Disease

Reducing dietary saturated fat has generally been thought to improve cardiovascular health and protect against heart attacks and strokes. This assumption is based on the belief that dietary saturated fat increases blood cholesterol, thus promoting cardiovascular disease. You learned in Chapter 12 that blood cholesterol has little to do with heart disease; therefore, even if saturated fat did raise total cholesterol, it would not increase heart disease risk. There has been debate on this issue in the medical community for decades. A recent meta-analysis study published in the *American Journal of Clinical Nutrition* now has conclusively proven that saturated fats are not harmful and do not cause heart disease.[31]

Over the years, many studies have sought to prove the lipid hypothesis of heart disease—that diets high in saturated fat and cholesterol promote heart disease. Results have been mixed. Some seemed to support it, while others did not. However, the majority of the medical community, along with the pharmaceutical industry (which profits greatly from the saturated fat-heart disease idea) supports the theory. Those studies that support the theory receive national press and are used as justification to establish government policies on health, while those that do not support the theory are generally ignored.

The evidence in favor of the lipid hypothesis is no greater than the evidence that contradicts it. In fact, there is a substantial amount of evidence that challenges the hypothesis. The number of studies for or against is not a major issue; some of the studies have used relatively few participants, while others have used much larger numbers. Obviously, the results of a study involving 50,000 test subjects carries more weight than one involving only 1,000. One large study using 50,000 participants produces more reliable results than 10 small studies with a total combined number of 10,000 participants. So the total number of studies is not as important as the number of people *in* the studies. If *all* the subjects in these many different studies were combined and evaluated equally, what would the final outcome be? Would it prove the lipid hypothesis or disprove it?

Researchers at the Children's Hospital Oakland Research Institute in California and Harvard School of Public Health got together to find out. They analyzed all the previous studies with data for dietary saturated fat intakes and risk of cardiovascular disease. The studies also had to be of high quality and reliable. Twenty-one studies were identified that fit their criteria. This meta-analysis study included data on nearly 350,000 subjects. With such a large subject database, the results would be far more reliable than a study consisting of only 10,000 or even 100,000 subjects. The focus of the researchers was to determine if there was sufficient evidence linking saturated fat consumption to cardiovascular disease. Their results said "no." Intake of saturated fat was not associated with an increased risk of cardiovascular disease. Those people who ate the greatest amount of saturated fat were no more likely to suffer a heart attack or stroke than those who ate the least. It didn't matter how much saturated fat one ate, the incidence of heart disease was not affected.[31] This study demonstrates that the combined data from all available studies in the medical literature disprove the lipid hypothesis.

This new study is not likely to change policies and recommendations about eating saturated fat any time soon. Doctors have been warning us about the dangers of eating saturated fat for so many years that it is thoroughly ingrained into their minds, and they will continue to give this advice despite facts to the contrary. In other words, many health professionals will continue to ignore these studies and try to convince you to accept their opinions based on nothing more than a longstanding prejudice against saturated fat. The bottom line here is that you do not need to fear eating saturated fat or cholesterol even when you hear criticism about it in the media or from your own doctor.

A Word of Caution

In the world of scientific investigation there is often a difference of opinion. Consequently, studies are frequently published that contradict one another. We see this in the newspaper all the time. The media is constantly reporting new studies that show results contrary to previous studies.

The outcome of many studies is influenced by personal bias of the investigators or by the corporation funding the study. This is plainly evident in the investigation of fats and oils. Numerous researchers and their funding institutions (pharmaceutical, supplement, and weight loss industries, as well as others) have a bias against fat and especially saturated fat. Their studies often reflect this bias and perpetuate common myths. One of these myths is that saturated fat and cholesterol promote heart disease.

There have been a number of animal studies published that implicate saturated fat as a contributing factor in various health concerns, including heart disease and dementia. When one of these studies is published, news reporters and anti-fat proponents immediately jump on it, writing blaring articles about the dangers of eating saturated fat and cholesterol, reinforcing the fat-heart disease myth.

What most people do not understand, and for that matter neither do the reporters or anti-fat proponents, is that these studies are scientifically meaningless. The studies are purposely designed to give these results.

In many of these studies, the researchers combine relatively high amounts of saturated fat with cholesterol and mix it in the rats' food. After a period of time, these rats are compared to a group of rats that were fed normal rat chow. What they find is that within weeks the fat/cholesterol fed rats start developing arterial lesions that are commonly associated with heart disease. Clogged arteries, in turn, increase risk of stroke and dementia. Such studies appear to suggest that saturated fat is the cause of these problems.

However, that is not the case. When people eat the most heart-damaging foods around, they do not develop clogged arteries in just a few weeks like the animals in these experiments. Atherosclerosis is a lifelong process that takes decades to develop. This should tell you that something is wrong with the diet that is fed to the rats and that it does not match what happens in real life.

What is wrong in these studies is the cholesterol. The cholesterol used in these studies comes in powder form. The cholesterol powder is dissolved in fat and then added to the rat chow. The problem here is that powdered cholesterol is not ordinary cholesterol. It is not the same as the cholesterol in most of your foods or in your body. When the cholesterol is "dried," it becomes fully oxidized. Oxidized cholesterol is highly toxic, just like oxidized polyunsaturated fats are. Oxidized cholesterol damages artery walls promoting atherosclerosis. Only oxidized cholesterol is found in clogged arteries; normal cholesterol is not.

It is the oxidized cholesterol that is used in these studies that causes the damage to the rats' arteries. When oxidized cholesterol is added to *any* type of fat, be it saturated or unsaturated, it causes arterial lesions. If the investigators combined oxidized cholesterol with soybean oil or corn oil the outcome would be the same: the rats would all develop lesions. However, the conclusions the authors of these types of studies come to is that it is the saturated fat that is the culprit.

In other studies, saturated fat is combined with high amounts of sugar and then added to the rat chow. When the rats develop insulin resistance or some other problem they blame it on the saturated fat and conveniently ignore the added sugar!

A little common sense will tell you these studies are deceptive. Ketogenic diets that consist of 90 percent fat, mostly saturated fat, have been used successfully for nearly a century without causing heart disease, stroke, or dementia. In fact, contrary to the rat studies, they improve memory. Likewise, many populations around the world who eat traditional diets consisting of 60-90 percent fat, again mostly saturated fat, do not experience increased rates of heart disease or Alzheimer's. In fact, they are remarkably free of these diseases.

In contrast, the rats in these studies are given only about 20 percent fat, nothing near the 90 percent of the ketogenic diet, yet in a few weeks they were developing atherosclerotic lesions and memory impairment. Obviously, something is wrong with the fat they fed the rats, and that something is the oxidized cholesterol.

So when you see studies reported in the news or when people tell you of some study that shows that high-fat diets or saturated fat promotes heart disease or Alzheimer's, don't believe it!

Now that you are aware of the trouble oxidized cholesterol causes, you might be wondering if there are sources of this type of cholesterol in our diet. The answer is yes! Cholesterol is not found in plants, so you don't have to worry about getting any from plant-based foods. Cholesterol comes only in animal foods like meat, dairy and eggs. When animal products are dehydrated or powdered, the cholesterol in them becomes oxidized. Examples of these types of products include powdered whole milk, dried grated cheese, and powdered eggs and butter. Right now you may be saying to yourself, "Well, I don't eat powdered foods." Well, think again. Powdered products are used in the ingredients of many processed foods sold at your local grocery store, the most obvious being prepared cake, pancake, and muffin mixes. If the ingredient label lists eggs, milk or butter, you know for sure it means *powdered* eggs, milk or butter, otherwise the product wouldn't be in a *dry* mix. Sometimes the label will specify if an ingredient is powdered, but not always. Even products such as frozen pizza, TV dinners, cookies, bread, and the like could include powdered ingredients. This is a good reason to make your own meals from fresh ingredients rather than rely on prepared packaged foods.

Although vegetable oils do not contain cholesterol, if they are oxidized they become toxic. If an oil is powdered or dehydrated, it is oxidized and should never be eaten. This includes powdered shortening, fish oil, coconut oil, and MCT oil. Powdered oils are often found in dietary supplements and protein shake mixes.

15 The Ultimate Brain Food

COCONUT OIL: THE ULTIMATE BRAIN FOOD

If any food could be labeled as "Brain Food," it would have to be coconut oil. The MCTs in coconut oil are converted into ketones, which act as high-potency fuel for the brain. This superfuel bypasses the glucose metabolic pathway to overcome defects in glucose metabolism. In doing so, it boosts energy output, normalizes brain function, stops erratic signal transmission that leads to seizures, improves cognition and memory, improves motor function, and supplies building blocks for the repair, maintenance, and growth of new brain tissue. Ketones reduce the brain's need for oxygen, protecting it from injury caused by physical trauma or lack of blood and oxygen supply due to stroke, asphyxiation, or other causes. Ketones have proven useful in stopping the progression of neurodegenerative diseases and even reversing the symptoms.

Coconut MCTs are also converted into MCFAs (medium chain fatty acids), which provide additional brain support. Unlike long chain fatty acids, MCFAs can pass through the blood-brain barrier. They provide the brain with a third source of energy. Although not as potent as ketones, MCFAs still provide more energy than glucose and are preferred over glucose by brain cells as a fuel. The energy-producing, antioxidant, anti-inflammatory, antimicrobial, and antitoxic properties of MCFAs protect the brain from a variety of insults.

Insulin resistance is the primary characteristic of type 2 diabetes and is believed to be an underlying problem of Alzheimer's disease. It also increases the risk of Parkinson's disease and various forms of dementia. Studies have shown that when insulin is delivered directly to the brain, Alzheimer's patients experience marked cognitive improvement. Coconut oil is proving to be useful in the treatment of insulin resistance and associated conditions by improving insulin secretion and insulin sensitivity.[1] Thus, coconut oil can help reverse brain insulin resistance and improve cognitive function.

When added to foods, coconut oil slows down the digestion of carbohydrate, allowing glucose to be released into the bloodstream at a steady, even pace and moderating blood sugar levels. All of this improves insulin and blood sugar control, which is important for both the body and the brain.

MCTs are absolutely *essential* for the growth and development of the fetal and newborn brain. From what researchers have been discovering in recent years, they are also of great value in maintaining healthy brain function and protecting against neurodegenerative disease.

In this chapter you will learn how coconut oil can protect against infections and toxins that promote neurodegeneration.

A NATURAL DEFENSE AGAINST INFECTION

In the womb, unborn infants rely on ketones as an important source of energy and as an essential source of raw materials for the building of brain tissue. After birth, ketones are still necessary for a period of time to satisfy these same needs. Infants get their nourishment from mother's milk. While ketones are not supplied in the milk, their precursors MCTs are. As milk is digested, MCTs are broken down into individual MCFAs. Some of these fatty acids are converted into ketones while others are released into the bloodstream as free fatty acids.

When starving or on a calorie restricted diet or even between meals when glucose levels are low, body fat is broken down into fatty acids and used to power our cells. The fatty acids that come from stored body fat are almost entirely long chain fatty acids (LCFAs) and cannot cross over the blood-brain barrier. If the brain had access to LCFAs, it would use them for energy production, just as other cells in the body do. Since the brain does not have access to LCFAs, it must rely on ketones, which easily cross the blood-brain barrier. MCFAs are also allowed to pass through the blood-brain barrier and, therefore, provide a third source of energy for the brain.

The fact that MCFAs can enter the brain is very important, particularly for those with neurodegenerative disease. Besides supplying energy and building blocks much like ketones, MCFAs do something ketones cannot do. MCFAs can protect the brain from infection. These unique fatty acids possess powerful antimicrobial properties capable of killing disease-causing bacteria, viruses, and fungi.[2] This apparently is another reason why nature puts MCTs in mother's milk. In fact, MCFAs in mother's milk serves as the infant's primary defense against infection for the first few months of its life, while the immune system is still developing.[3]

Other than breast milk, there are very few good dietary sources of MCTs. By far, the richest natural source of MCTs is coconut. There are more MCTs in coconut oil than there are in mother's milk, a lot more. For this reason, coconut oil can have a pronounced impact on our health, just as mother's milk does on newborn infants. The MCTs in coconut oil are identical to those found in mother's milk and possess the same antimicrobial potential. Food manufacturers have been putting coconut oil, or MCTs derived from coconut oil, into baby formula for years in order to give the formula the same qualities as natural breast milk.[4]

MCFAs derived from coconut oil have been studied extensively as potential antimicrobial agents that can be used in foods, cosmetics, and drugs. Studies show that these MCFAs are effective in killing bacteria that cause health problems such as gastric ulcers, sinus infections, bladder infections, gum disease and cavities, pneumonia, gonorrhea, and many other illnesses.[5-10] They kill fungi and yeasts that cause ringworm, athlete's foot, jock itch, and candidiasis.[11-13] They kill viruses that cause influenza, measles, herpes, mononucleosis, and hepatitis C.[14-18] They are so potent that they can even kill HIV—the AIDS virus.[19-21] There are numerous published studies and even entire books describing the antimicrobial effects of MCFAs derived from coconut oil.[22]

Because of the published studies that have shown MCFAs to be effective in killing the AIDS virus, many HIV-infected individuals have added coconut in one form or another to their treatment programs with success. For example, Tony V. was diagnosed with full-blown AIDS but was able to overcome the disease using coconut oil therapy. AIDS attacks the immune system of its victims, thus increasing their vulnerability to other infections. In fact, AIDS patients usually die from secondary infections rather than from the AIDS virus itself. Tony was in terrible shape. His immune system was so weakened that he was riddled with secondary infections. He had lost a substantial amount of weight, suffered with chronic pneumonia, struggled with chronic fatigue, experienced repeated bouts of nausea and diarrhea, had oral candidiasis, and was covered from head to foot with skin infections. His skin was an angry red, cracking, flaking, and weeping. His skin was so bad that the hair on his head was falling out in clumps. He wore a wig to hide the bald spots and oozing sores. He was so far gone that his doctors told him he had only a matter of months to live.

Unable to work because of his illness, he had little money and could not afford to continue to buy medication. He asked the government for help. He was referred to a doctor who had published studies on the therapeutic effects of coconut oil. He told Tony to consume 6 tablespoons of coconut oil daily, along with rubbing more oil on the lesions all over his body. Tony began doing as he was directed. To the surprise of his other doctors, nine months later Tony was not only alive, but thriving. The coconut oil healed him from all of his secondary infections and brought the HIV under control. He regained his lost weight, his hair grew back, and his skin was clear and healthy with no sign of infection.[23] While Tony may never be completely free of the HIV virus, coconut oil has given him a better life.

Studies by Gilda Erguiza, MD, and colleagues have shown that coconut oil added to standard antibiotic therapy improves recovery from community-acquired pneumonia. Community-acquired pneumonia is an infection of the lungs that is contracted outside a hospital setting. It is a serious infection in children. In a presentation delivered to the American College of Chest Physicians in Philadelphia, Dr. Erguiza described her findings.[24] The study included 40 children between the ages of three months to five years, all suffering from pneumonia and treated intravenously with the antibiotic ampicillin. Half of the group was also given a daily dose of coconut oil at 2 ml per kilogram of body weight. The oil was given for three days in a row. The researchers found that the respiratory rate normalized in 32.6 hours for the coconut oil group versus 48.2 hours for the control group. After three days, patients in the control group were more likely than those in the coconut oil group to still have wheezing in the lungs—60 percent of the controls still had wheezing compared to only 25 percent of the coconut oil group. Those in the coconut oil group also recovered from their fevers quicker, had normal oxygen saturation faster, and had shorter hospital stays.

The fact that coconut oil can be used to fight infection has important implications to those with neurodegenerative disease. In at least 90 percent of Alzheimer's cases examined, the presence of infection has been found in the brain. Many cases of Parkinson's and other neurodegenerative diseases also appear to be associated with infection. Unlike most drugs, including antibiotics, MCFAs can cross over the blood-brain barrier and actively kill an infection. All of the major microorganisms associated with neurodegeneration, including Treponema spirochetes, herpes virus, *Chlamydia pneumonia*, *Helicobacter pylori*, and cytomegalovirus, are killed by MCFAs. In addition, MCFAs also kill many other microorganisms such as candida, streptococcus, and staphylococcus which all cause systemic infections that can trigger neuroinflammation.

Although MCFAs are deadly to many disease-causing microorganisms, they are completely harmless to us. They are so safe that nature puts them into mother's milk to nourish newborn infants.

As safe and as effective as they are, MCFAs do not kill all microorganisms. Consequently, some disease-causing organisms are unaffected. Rhinovirus, which causes the common cold, and hepatitis A virus are two such organisms. The fact the MCFAs do not kill all microorganisms is actually a good thing. Our digestive tract is filled with many helpful organisms that aid in digestion and nutrient absorption. MCFAs do not kill these friendly gut bacteria—they kill the bad guys but leave the good guys alone.

MCFAs are used in a variety of medications and dietary supplements. Caprylic acid, one of the MCFAs in coconut oil, is a popular ingredient in some anti-candida formulations. Monolaurin, another coconut oil-derived supplement, is used as a general-purpose antibiotic. Fractionated coconut oil, also known as MCT oil, is a common ingredient in many health and fitness products. Coconut oil has even been put into gel capsules as a dietary supplement. Of course, you can also find pure coconut oil in just about any health food store.

About 85 percent of the fatty acids in coconut oil exhibit antimicrobial activity. The most important germ-fighting fatty acids in coconut oil are lauric acid, myristic acid, caprylic acid, and capric acid. All are saturated fats and all except myristic acid are MCFAs. These fatty acids are generally absent from other oils.

While each of these fatty acids demonstrate antimicrobial properties, lauric acid has the greatest overall antibacterial, antiviral, and antifungal effect. It is also the most abundant fatty acid in coconut oil, constituting about 50 percent of the oil. Each of these fatty acids, however, exert a different effect on various microorganisms. For example, one may be more effective at killing *Chlamydia pneumonia* than another, but less effective against herpes. All of them work together synergistically to provide the widest and strongest germ-killing potential.

WHAT PEOPLE ARE SAYING ABOUT COCONUT OIL

Thousands of people are currently using coconut oil as a home-remedy against infections with good success. Some people prefer to use *virgin* coconut oil over ordinary coconut oil. The term "virgin" indicates that the oil has undergone minimal processing so it retains all of its natural nutrients and flavor. Both forms of coconut oil have been used successfully.

"I've had chronic bladder infections for twenty years," says Cindy D. "I've been to numerous doctors with no positive results and most of the time I was worse. After the last doctor I swore I would not go to another doctor unless I was dying and had no choice. I began to research natural remedies. I tried so many things it would be hard to list. They helped to some extent but didn't cure my infections. I found your website and tried coconut oil. In one month's time I have not had one bladder infection. I'm taking one tablespoon 3 times a day with meals. I've put the oil on cuts and healed so quickly I couldn't believe it. My husband eats popcorn every night and I started using coconut oil instead of canola oil. He loves the flavor of the popcorn."

Mike says, "I wanted to thank you for enlightening me to the benefits of coconut oil. I am 29 years old and have been suffering with ulcerative colitis for 14 years. My father had ulcerative colitis that went untreated and led to cancer and his death at the age of 46, so I have always been aware of the seriousness. I never experienced coconut oil until my wife found your cookbooks! I visited your website and ordered your *Coconut Cures* book and was blown away page after page. In addition to colitis, I have several other medical problems that were treated with coconut oil so how can I not give it a shot.

"I built up to a maintenance level of 1-2 tablespoons in my coffee every morning and started feeling better after about one month. Nine months later I had my yearly colonoscopy check up (required for colitis patients of any age) and my doctor was shocked! Not only has the disease reversed itself, none of the biopsies revealed any indication of colitis and I essentially have a normal person's colon!! I told him about coconut oil and, of course, my doctor thought that the medication was cause for improvement but said to definitely keep doing whatever I'm doing. If only my father had this knowledge when my father was young, he could have seen his kids grow up."

"I am not scratching for the first time in a month," says Elizabeth. "What a relief. I first noticed it as persistent itchiness at the top of my thigh. After a week or so, a small rash appeared. It quickly spread across my hip. Then the rash appeared on my other hip. Before long, I was itchy on the back of my knees, the inside of my elbows, and the back of my hands, as well as across both hips. I went to a conventional doctor who couldn't diagnose the source but prescribed antihistamines and a prednisone 'burst.' After a week on prednisone, the rash was as itchy as ever, and my skin was even more red and swollen. I tried every topical remedy I could think of with little relief. I saw a naturopathic doctor who was also unable to diagnose my problem but suggested treating it through a process of elimination, trying an antifungal first, and going to an antibacterial if the antifungal didn't work. After several days on the antifungal with no relief—in fact, the rash was now spreading to my back, my belly, and my forearms—it flashed through the back of my mind that I had once read that coconut oil had anti-fungal, anti-bacterial, and anti-virus properties. Feeling fairly desperate—and with nothing to lose—I pulled my bottle of virgin coconut oil out of the kitchen cupboard and applied it topically to all my itchy places. The results were miraculous. Almost instantly, the itching stopped. Within hours, my skin began to soothe, and the redness faded. This absence of itching is such a wonderful feeling that I'm truly grateful. I am now a coconut oil convert."

"There has been a nasty stomach virus going around the New York City area," says Vince. "I was hit with it on a Sunday mid-afternoon. I had two bowel 'episodes' which made me know I had the virus, just like my brother and our mother and father. Later that day I took about two tablespoons of liquid virgin coconut oil and I also took some cider vinegar with water. For dinner, I had a sweet potato drenched in coconut oil. I never had another episode. My friends and family had been telling me about how long the virus stayed with them—some for seven days or more. Mine only lasted for an afternoon. That evening I was back to normal. I'm glad I've been finding out about all the incredible things coconut and coconut oil can do for you."

Holistic minded medical doctors, nurses, and nutritionists are also using coconut oil and recommending it to their patients. Dr. Eliza Perez Francisco, MD, says, "In my clinical practice at St. Luke's Medical Center, I use virgin coconut oil for the elderly in relation to physiologic changes that occur with aging. Virgin coconut oil can address sensory losses, tooth and gum problems, changes in the intestinal tract, changes in the immune system, changes in body composition, and changes that come with menopause and andropause...A combination of old age and malnutrition makes older people vulnerable to pneumonia, UTI, and bedsores. Virgin coconut oil can help fight infection in the early stages. Take the case of a 76-year-old who developed painful herpes zoster on his trunk. The antibiotic cream given to him only lasted for one application because the area affected was so wide. But when virgin coconut oil was applied all over the skin for a week, the patient reported relief from itch and the lesions dried up."

Dr. S. Kumar, MD, states, "I am a primary care practitioner or general practitioner with priority in nutritional medicine as the healing component. I have read Dr. Fife's, Dr. Dayrit's, and Prof Mary G. Enig's books and am using only virgin coconut oil (VCO) for cooking and also orally when down with the flu, etc. I strongly advise my patients to consume more VCO when sick and advocate to all ages from newborns to the old and sick, including those with diabetic, hypertensive, heart, and skin ailments and even those stricken with cancer. Over the last two years I've seen patients get better. It is difficult sometimes for some patients initially to accept VCO. They think I am going 'nuts'! The truth is being revealed and allopathic medicine has to admit all this while they have been wrong and it is still not too late to rectify this mistake. I still get criticisms from many but I believe in due time the critics will be silenced."

Most doctors are still unaware of the incredible effects coconut oil can have on neurodegenerative disease. "I currently care for my 85-year-old father who has a multitude of problems, including dementia, Parkinson's symptoms, and lymphatic cancer," says Donna. "When I told the doctor that he had been shaking, shuffling gait, flat-faced affect, stooped over walking and it had cleared up with virgin coconut oil, he just looked at me and said that it could not have been Parkinson's because it does not reverse like that…What can I say?"

"My husband, who suffers from dementia, has had fever blisters almost constantly for many years," says Grace. "Since starting coconut oil four months ago he has had only one tiny outbreak which lasted only a few days. I don't know if the herpes was affecting his brain but I do know that he doesn't have outbreaks anymore and his memory has improved and he is much more social now."

"I can tell you from personal experience that it definitely works," says Loretta. "Almost immediately my husband became more alert and that vacant look he used to have is gone. His conversational skills have returned. In testing at the rehab center last fall, when my husband drew the clock as part of the testing, he started hesitantly with the 1 and then continued around to the top stopping at number 15! After two months using coconut oil, he drew the circle, with all the numbers in the right place—a remarkable improvement!" It is impossible to say how much of her husband's improvement was due to the ketones and how much of it may have resulted from MCFAs clearing out a possible infection, but what is apparent is that coconut oil is definitely helping.

"I grew up in Puerto Rico, where coconut was widely available and consumed for a myriad of remedies," says Carlos Diaz. "I remember my mother using the coconut milk to feed us in lieu of regular milk. I come from a big family and none of my brothers and sisters had any serious health problems when they were young. This is amazing, when you consider we had no running water at that time, and access to healthcare was very scarce. Coconut oil was used as a remedy for any stomach problem (i.e., constipation, diarrhea, ulcers, etc). It was also used as a purging agent and as an ointment to prevent wound or insect bite infections…It's interesting that when a Puerto Rican wants to say he is in superb good health, he says 'estoy como coco' which literally means 'I'm as good as a coconut.'"

ORAL INFECTIONS

The headlines in the newspaper could have read "Man Dies of Toothache." As unlikely as this may sound, it is true. Boyd was a healthy 54-year old. His only complaint was the sudden appearance of a toothache. The dentist identified the problem as an abscess—an infection near the base of the tooth. The tooth was salvageable, so it was not extracted, and the infection was scraped out of the gum tissue and drained.

That evening Boyd experienced shaking chills and fever. He took an aspirin and felt better the next day. Fourteen days later he developed a severe headache with involuntary twitching of the muscles on the left side of his face and neck. He was taken to the hospital. A CAT scan revealed a mass in the frontal lobe of his brain, which was diagnosed as a brain abscess. He was given massive doses of antibiotics and underwent surgery to drain the infection.

Boyd seemed to improve immediately after the surgery. Six days later, however, he became noticeably disoriented and developed swelling on his head. A CAT scan revealed the recurrence of the brain abscess. He was given more antibiotics and underwent a second surgery to drain the pus and remove infected tissue including part of his skull.

After surgery, he began to improve but two more times the infection came roaring back and he underwent two more surgeries and the complete removal of the frontal lobe of his brain. After the last surgery and in spite of massive doses of antibiotics, his condition deteriorated. After struggling for more than a month in the hospital, he died.

Samples taken from each of the surgeries revealed the infection was caused by three species of bacteria, the origin of which were traced back to his abscessed tooth. Bacteria from his infected gums spread to the bloodstream and localized in his brain. Cause of death was listed as a brain abscess, but the real culprit was the infected tooth.

Because of the close proximity of the mouth to the brain, oral bacteria can have a pronounced effect on neurological function and mental health. Whenever there is an injury, infection, or inflammation in gum tissue, bacteria can seep into the bloodstream. Major dental infections, such as a tooth abscess, can cause massive amounts of bacteria to enter the bloodstream, leading to a brain abscess or some other secondary infection elsewhere in the body.

Minor oral infections, which often go unnoticed and may remain active for years, can also affect our brains. These infections slowly release bacteria into the bloodstream or infect facial nerves and travel up into the brain. If the immune system is working properly, no secondary infection occurs. However, the continual stream of bacteria into surrounding tissues causes chronic inflammation. Near the jaw it causes bone to disintegrate, eventually leading to bone and tooth loss. Chronic inflammation in nerve and brain tissue can lead to neurological degeneration. There may be no symptoms immediately noticeable, but over time as inflammation damages nerve tissue, mental or physical function declines. Most viruses and bacteria found in the brains of Alzheimer's and Parkinson's disease patients originate in the mouth.

Over 90 percent of the population has some degree of tooth decay or gum disease. Having a bright white smile and no obvious problems is no guarantee that you are free of infection. Regardless of how clean your mouth appears, you could have an active infection right now and be completely unaware of it. More brushing, flossing, or mouthwash will not stop it. Antibiotics will not stop it.

But there is something that will work. Believe it or not, a spoonful of coconut oil can clean your teeth more thoroughly than brushing, flossing, or gargling with antiseptic mouthwash. The oil is not used in brushing the teeth, although it can be. It is used in an entirely different way. The method is called oil pulling.

Oil pulling is a modified version of *oil gargling*, which comes from Ayurvedic medicine and dates back thousands of years. Various oils have been used for oil gargling but for oil pulling, coconut oil works best.

The process of oil pulling is very simple. You put a spoonful of coconut oil into your mouth and swish it around (do not gargle) for a period of 15 to 20 minutes. The coconut oil is "worked" in the mouth by pushing, pulling, and sucking it through the teeth. As you work the oil, it sucks up bacteria, toxins, pus, and mucous. Don't swallow it! When you are finished pulling, spit it into the trash. You do not want to discard it in the sink or down the toilet because over time the oil may build up and clog the pipes. After spitting it out, rinse your mouth with water. Although 20 minutes sounds like a long time, if you busy yourself with other things such as dressing, preparing breakfast, reading the paper, or such, the time goes by quickly.

Oil pulling is best done first thing in the morning before eating breakfast. After eating, brush your teeth as you normally would. Oil pulling can be done one to three times a day on an empty stomach. Just before meals are good times.

Coconut oil acts like a cleanser. When you put it in your mouth and work it around your teeth and gums it "pulls" out bacteria and other debris. It acts much like the motor oil you put in your car engine. The motor oil picks up dirt and grime. When you drain the oil, it pulls out the dirt and grime with it, leaving the engine relatively clean. Consequently, the engine runs more smoothly and lasts longer. Likewise, when we expel harmful substances from our mouths, our teeth and gums work better and last longer.

A study published in the *Journal of Oral Health and Community Dentistry* demonstrates the effectiveness of oil pulling compared to other forms of oral hygiene.[25] The subjects in the study had mild to moderate gum disease and plaque accumulation, typical of the population as a whole. They were instructed to continue their normal home oral hygiene practices, along with oil pulling. Oil pulling was performed once each morning for a period of 45 days. Plaque levels and the severity of gum disease were assessed periodically during the study. The subjects were instructed to suck and pull the oil through their teeth for 8-10 minutes daily.

At the end of the 45 days no adverse reactions to the teeth or soft tissues in the mouth were found, indicating that the procedure caused no physical harm. Most people would have assumed this, but the study gave confirmation. Plaque formation was significantly reduced, with most of the reduction coming during the latter half of the study, indicating that the longer you do the treatment the better the results. Gingivitis (gum disease) was also significantly reduced in all subjects, decreasing by more than 50 percent. The researchers rated the changes as "highly" significant.

Mouthwashes have shown to reduce plaque by 20-26 percent and gingivitis by about 13 percent. Tooth brushing reduces plaque by 11-27 percent and gingivitis by 8-23 percent.[26] Oil pulling beats them both. Data from this study shows that oil pulling reduced plaque by 18-30 percent and gingivitis by an amazing 52-60 percent. The reduction in plaque using oil pulling is only slightly better than antiseptic mouthwashes and brushing, but reduction in gingivitis is two to seven times better. So, oil pulling significantly out-performs brushing and mouthwash as a means of oral cleansing. If the subjects had oil pulled for 15-20 minutes daily, as is normally recommended, and done it over a longer period of time, the results would have undoubtedly been even better.

While oil pulling can significantly reduce plaque and gingivitis, it shouldn't be used in place of tooth brushing, but can be an effective supplemental aid in a daily oral hygiene regimen.

Oil pulling isn't only good at preventing oral infections, but can actively fight them as well. The oil pulls the infection out of the tissues, allowing the body to heal itself. Inflammation is quieted, gums stop bleeding, loose teeth tighten, and pain and sensitivity vanish. Teeth become whiter and gums become pinker and healthier-looking. Infection no longer drains into the bloodstream. To learn more about oil pulling and how it works to fight infection and improve mental and physical health, see the book *Oil Pulling Therapy* by Bruce Fife.

PROTECTION AGAINST ENVIRONMENTAL TOXINS

As seen in previous chapters, environmental toxins can have a profound effect on the initiation and progression of neurodegenerative disease. Everyone is exposed to chemical toxins to some degree. According to a study by the US Centers for Disease Control and Prevention (CDC), Americans carry in their bodies dozens of pesticides and toxic compounds used in consumer products, many of which are linked to potential health problems. These chemicals include pyrethroids that are ingredients of virtually every household pesticide and phthalates found in nail polish and other beauty products as well as in soft plastics.

The study looked for 148 toxic compounds in the urine and blood of about 2,400 people. The discovery of more than 100 chemicals in human bodies is of great concern because we don't know what effect they can have on the body. Evidence suggests that the rise in Alzheimer's, cancer, and other chronic diseases over the past several decades may be due, in part, to the accumulation of these chemicals in our bodies.

However, removing pesticides, drain cleaners, plastic bottles, and other items isn't going to happen anytime soon. The best solution to the problem is to remove the toxins from our bodies. Certain foods have detoxifying effects that can absorb or neutralize environmental chemicals that collect in our bodies. Simply adding these detoxifying foods to the diet can help eliminate many of the toxins we are exposed to each day. Coconut oil is of particular interest because it has been shown to be highly effective in nullifying the toxic effects of a variety of chemicals.

An interesting case report published in the journal *Human and Experimental Toxicology* revealed the effectiveness of coconut oil in neutralizing aluminum phosphide, a poison used in rodent control.[27] The article described an incident in which a 28-year-old man ingested a lethal amount of the chemical in an attempt to commit suicide. There is no known antidote for aluminum phosphide poisoning. Doctors had little hope of saving him. He was given the standard treatment for acute poisoning as well as the oral administration of coconut oil. To the surprise of the medical staff, the patient survived. As a result of the success of this case, the authors of the report recommend that coconut oil be added to the treatment protocol of all cases of acute aluminum phosphide poisoning.

Using coconut oil to help nullify the effects of a poison is not as strange as it may sound. Researchers have known for some time about the detoxifying properties of coconut oil. Numerous animal studies have shown that coconut oil blocks the deleterious action of a number of chemical toxins. While the exact mechanisms involved are not fully understood, part of the reason for coconut oil's protective effects can be attributed to its antioxidant, anti-inflammatory, and immune-boosting properties, as well as its ability to improve oxygen circulation throughout the body. For these reasons, MCTs from coconut oil are being investigated as a means to aid cancer patients and to block the detrimental side effects of chemotherapy drugs.[28-29]

Studies show that coconut oil or MCTs can protect animals from a variety of carcinogenic chemicals.[30-32] Dr. C. Lim-Sylianco and colleagues demonstrated coconut oil's antimutagenic effects against six potent mutacarcinogens—benzpyrene, azaserine, dimethylhydrazine, dimethylnitrosamine, methylmethanesulfonate, and tetracycline. Administration of coconut oil either in bolus form or as part of the diet protected the animals from the toxic effect of all six mutagens. Fertility tests were also performed and coconut oil was shown to protect fertilized female mice against the sterilizing and abortifacient effects of the carcinogens. Dr. Lim-Sylianco reported that coconut oil was "strongly protective" against all six chemicals.[33-34]

Aflatoxin is a very potent carcinogen that comes from a fungus that often infests grains, especially corn. In Asia and Africa, aflatoxin is a serious problem. Corn has been found to be the most aflatoxin contaminated food eaten in the Philippines. In certain areas of that country corn consumption is high. A correlation exists between the incidence of liver cancer caused by aflatoxin and the amount of corn consumed. Those people who eat the most corn also have the highest rates of liver cancer. Coconut oil consumption appears to protect the liver from the cancer-causing effect of aflatoxin. The population of Bicol, in the Philippines, has an unusually high intake of aflatoxin infested corn, yet they have a low incidence of liver cancer. The reason for the low cancer rate is believed to be due to the high coconut consumption in the area.[35]

Studies have shown that the harmful effects of exotoxins and endotoxins—the poisons produced by bacteria that cause illness—can also be neutralized or reduced by the use of coconut oil and its monoglycerides. Monoglycerides of coconut oil are individual MCFAs that are attached to a glycerol molecule. They function much like MCFAs and possess the same antimicrobial and antitoxic properties. Monoglycerides are commonly used in the food and cosmetic industry to inhibit the production of exotoxins produced by streptococci and staphylococci.[36-37]

Both monoglycerides and MCFAs mitigate the effects of these poisons inside the body. For example, in one study guinea pigs were separated into two groups. One group was given a mixture of MCTs and fish oil in their diet. The other group received safflower oil. After 6 weeks on these diets the animals were injected with an endotoxin. The group fed safflower oil developed severe metabolic and respiratory shock. The group that received MCTs showed only mild symptoms.[38]

In another study, the protective effect of coconut oil was tested on E. coli endotoxin shock in rats.[39] A total of 180 rats were used in the study. The animals were separated into three equal groups. The first group was given coconut oil at 5 percent of daily calories in their diet, the second group 20 percent, and the third received no coconut oil and served as the control. After one month on the diet the mice were given a dose of E. coli endotoxin via oral tube. The number of survivors was monitored at intervals of up to 96 hours. The results showed that rats in the control group had only a 48 percent survival rate. Those given coconut oil at 5 percent

Toxins Mitigated by Coconut Oil/MCFAs

Coconut oil or MCFAs are known to temper or block the toxic effects of many chemicals including the following:

Aflatoxin
Aluminum phosphide
Azaserine
Azoxymethane
Azo dyes
Benzpyrene
Dimethylbenzanthracene
Dimethylhydrazine
Dimethynitrosamine
E. coli endotoxin
Ethanol
Glutamic acid/MSG
Methylmethanesulfonate
N-nitrosomethylurea
Streptococci endotoxin/exotoxin
Staphylococci endotoxin/exotoxin
Tetracycline

and 20 percent of total calories had survival rates of 77 percent and 72 percent, respectively. Both coconut oil fed groups had about the same level of survival. This indicated that even a small amount of coconut oil (5 percent of calories) offered the same amount of protection against E coli endotoxin as a larger amount (20 percent of calories). In humans consuming a typical 2,000-calorie diet, 5 percent of calories would equate to about 1 tablespoon of coconut oil.

Glutamic acid, a potential neurotoxin that affects the function of the brain and nerves, is tempered by monoglycerides from coconut oil.[40] Glutamic acid is the primary component of monosodium glutamate (MSG), a common food additive. In animals, glutamic acid causes brain lesions and neuroendocrine disorders. It can do the same in humans. Some of the symptoms associated with it include seizures, stroke, and heart irregularities, among others.

Many environmental toxins can adversely affect the brain. The antitoxic effects of MCFAs provide another reason for adding coconut oil into the diet.

Looking at all that coconut oil can do, it can definitely be called the ultimate brain food. The benefits of coconut oil and MCFAs don't stop there. They provide a degree of protection against a number of adverse health conditions that can afflict the entire body, including cancer, diabetes, liver disease, kidney disease, heart disease, colitis, and a number of infectious diseases. A more complete description of the incredible health benefits of coconut oil can be found in the book *Coconut Cures* by Bruce Fife.

COCONUT OIL AND DIABETES

Since diabetes is a strong risk factor for neurodegeneration, it is important to get blood sugar under control. Coconut oil works wonders for alleviating symptoms associated with diabetes and insulin resistance. Studies show that MCFAs improve insulin secretion and insulin sensitivity. When added to meals, dietary fat and particularly coconut oil slows down the absorption of sugar into the bloodstream, thus moderating blood sugar levels. Taken with meals, coconut oil can be very effective in keeping blood sugar under control. Even when taken after or between meals it can lower high blood sugar.

Blood sugar levels vary throughout the day depending on frequency of eating and the types of foods consumed. In non-diabetics daily blood sugar levels should stay below 140 mg/dl even after eating. Those with early diabetes have readings over 140 mg/dl; values over 200 mg/dl indicate full-blown diabetes. Coconut oil can have a dramatic effect on reducing elevated blood sugar. For example, Michele's non-fasting blood sugar was 290 mg/dl, definitely in the diabetic range. She was instructed to take two tablespoons of coconut oil. She did and almost immediately her blood sugar levels fell by 130 mg/dl, down to a much safer 160 mg/dl. This is a common occurrence among diabetics using coconut oil. She now uses coconut oil on a daily basis to help control her blood sugar.

This effect reduces the need for insulin injections. Some people have discovered that taking coconut oil even eliminates their need for additional insulin. "Virgin coconut oil has a substantial effect on blood sugar levels," says Ed. "My wife and daughter (both have type 2 diabetes) measure their blood sugar levels at least three times a day. When they eat the wrong foods and their blood sugar levels get to 80-100 points above normal, they don't take extra medication, they take 2-3 tablespoons of the coconut oil directly from the bottle. Within a half hour their blood sugar levels will come back to normal."

"I was diagnosed as type 2 diabetic in July of 2001 and immediately put on the Amaryl RX," says Sharon. "I have been looking for a way to reverse this condition since diagnosed. I have found a world of info out there on various supplements and diet. BUT not from my doctor who just said 'Welcome to the club' and told me to take my meds. (I was crying and he seemed happy!)... Bottom line is this. I have been able to slowly remove myself from the RX and now control my blood sugar by diet, supplements and with coconut oil! Cool, huh? I do still check my blood sugar levels once or twice daily and they are as good, and usually *better* than when I was on the Amaryl RX! And I have been off the RX since the end of March of 2003."

Coconut oil does more than just balance blood sugar, it can actually reverse damage caused by insulin resistance. Diabetic neuropathy is a condition in which nerves throughout the body degenerate. The effects are often evident as pain or numbness in the feet and legs. Other symptoms include digestive problems, muscle weakness and cramps, loss of bladder control, dizziness, speech impairment, vision changes, and loss of sense of warm or cold. Approximately 50 percent of people with diabetes will eventually develop nerve damage.

Neuropathy is often accompanied by poor blood circulation, which retards healing. Poor circulation to the extremities is a common cause of diabetic foot ulcers that can lead to gangrene and amputation. Because of poor circulation, relatively minor cuts or injuries on the feet or legs of a diabetic can persist for months and become gangrenous. If the limb is numb, the injury and accompanying infection and decay can be painless.

Coconut oil can reverse these conditions. Many diabetics have experienced the reawaking of nearly dead limbs when they start adding coconut oil into their diets.

"I did have a minor scrape on my lower right leg that has been trying to heal for a couple of months," says Edward K. "My wife called it an ugly wound. Six years ago my feet started to get numb, starting with the large toe and, over the years, the feet would become more and more numb. I began taking around 3 to 4 tablespoons per day of coconut oil. Within 10 days the injury on my leg healed up totally. I am so happy because now I feel the feeling coming back. The numbness is leaving. I have more feeling now." Edward was at serious risk of having his wound become infected and perhaps eventually undergoing surgery or amputation. In just 10 days coconut oil improved his circulation, allowing the cut to completely heal, and brought life back into legs and feeling to feet that had been numb for six years. Edward's story isn't unusual. Many diabetics experience the same response when they start taking coconut oil regularly.

Coconut oil improves circulation and reverses nerve damage in the extremities. It is reasonable to assume that it does the same in the brain. Every diabetic and anyone with any degree of insulin resistance should be using coconut oil on a regular basis.

Adding Coconut Oil into Your Life

As you have learned about the many benefits of coconut oil, it should be obvious that this extraordinary brain food plays a central role in the fight against Alzheimer's and other neurodegenerative disorders. Therefore, understanding how to incorporate it into your daily life is important. The simplest way to do this is to prepare your foods with it. Coconut oil is very heat stable, so it is excellent for use in the kitchen. You can use it for any baking or frying purpose. In recipes that call for margarine, butter, shortening, or vegetable oil, use coconut oil instead. Use the same amount or more to make sure you get the recommended amount in your diet (see Chapter 19 for more details on the recommended daily dose).

Not all foods are prepared using oil, but you can still incorporate the oil into the diet. You can add coconut oil to foods that aren't normally prepared with oil. For example, add a spoonful of coconut oil to hot beverages, hot cereals, soups, sauces, and casseroles, or use it as a topping on cooked vegetables.

Although I recommend that you consume coconut oil with foods, you don't have to prepare your food with it or add it to the food. You can take it by the spoonful like a dietary supplement. Many people prefer to get their daily dose of coconut oil this way. If you use a good quality coconut oil, it tastes good. Many people don't like the thought of putting a spoonful of oil, any oil, into their mouths. It may take some people a little time to get used to it.

There are two primary types of coconut oil you will find sold in stores. One is called *virgin* coconut oil; the other is refined, bleached, and deodorized (RBD) coconut oil. Virgin coconut oil is made from fresh coconuts with very minimal processing. The oil basically comes straight from the coconut. Since it has gone through little processing, it retains a delicate coconut taste and aroma. It is delicious.

RBD coconut oil is made from copra (air dried coconut) and has gone through more extensive processing. During the processing all the flavor and aroma has been removed. For people who don't like the taste of coconut in their foods, this is a good option. RBD oil is processed using mechanical means and high temperatures. Chemicals are not generally used. When you go to the store, you can tell the difference between virgin and RBD coconut oils by the label. All virgin coconut oils will state that they are "virgin." RBD oils will not have this statement. They also do not say "RBD." Sometimes they will be advertised as "Expeller Pressed," which means that the initial pressing of the oil from the coconut meat was done mechanically, without the use of heat. However, heat is usually used at some later stage in the refining process.

Many people prefer the virgin coconut oil because it has undergone less processing and retains more of the nutrients and the flavor that nature put into it. This is why it maintains its coconut flavor. Because more care is taken to produce virgin coconut oil, it is more expensive than RBD oil.

Most brands of RBD oil are generally tasteless and odorless and differ little from each other. The quality of the different brands of virgin coconut oil, however, can vary greatly. There are many different processing methods used to produce virgin coconut oil. Some are better than others. Plus, the care taken also affects the quality. Some companies produce excellent quality coconut oil that tastes so good you can easily eat it off the spoon. Other brands have a strong flavor and may be nearly unpalatable. You generally cannot tell the difference just by looking at the jar. You have to taste it. If the oil has a mild coconut flavor with a mild coconut smell and tastes good to you, then that is a brand you should use. If the flavor is overpowering or smells smoky, you might want to try another brand.

Coconut oil is available at all health food stores, many grocery stores, as well as on the Internet. There are many different brands to choose from. Generally the more expensive brands are the best quality, but not always. The cheaper brands of virgin coconut oil are almost always of inferior quality. All brands, however, have basically the same culinary and therapeutic effects and are useful.

If you purchase coconut oil from the store, it may have the appearance of shortening, being firm and snow white in color. When you take it home and put it on your kitchen shelf, after a few days it may transform into a colorless liquid. Don't be alarmed. This is natural. One of the distinctive characteristics of coconut oil is its high melting point. At temperatures of 76 degrees F (24 C) and above the oil is liquid like any other vegetable oil. At temperatures below this, it solidifies. It is much like butter. If stored in the refrigerator, a stick of butter is solid, but let it sit on the countertop on a hot day and it melts into a puddle. A jar of coconut oil may be liquid or solid depending on the temperature where it is stored. You can use it in either form.

Coconut oil is very stable, so it does not need to be refrigerated. You can store it on a cupboard shelf. Shelf life for a good quality coconut oil is 1 to 3 years. Hopefully, you will use it long before then.

MCT Oil

Most of the health benefits associated with coconut oil come from its medium chain triglycerides. If MCTs are good, then it might be reasoned that a source that contains more than coconut oil may be even better. Coconut oil is the richest "natural" source of MCTs, but there is another source that contains more: MCT oil. Coconut oil consists of 63 percent MCTs, while MCT oil is 100 percent. MCT oil, which is sometimes referred to as fractionated coconut oil, is produced from coconut oil. The 10 fatty acids that make up coconut oil are separated out and two of the medium chain fatty acids (caprylic and capric acids) are recombined to form MCT oil.

The advantage of MCT oil is that it provides more MCTs per unit volume than coconut oil. It is tasteless and, being liquid at room temperature, can be used in cooking or as a salad dressing. The disadvantage of MCT oil is that it is more likely to cause nausea and diarrhea than coconut oil. So there is a limited amount that can be used without experiencing this side effect. It also contains no lauric acid—the most important of the medium chain fatty acids.

In contrast, about 50 percent of coconut oil consists of lauric acid. Lauric acid possesses the most potent antimicrobial power. When combined with the other fatty acids in the oil, its antimicrobial potential is enhanced. Consequently, coconut oil has a far greater germ-fighting ability than MCT oil.

The MCFAs in MCT oil are quickly converted into ketones. Blood ketone levels peak 1½ hours after consumption and are gone after 3 hours. The conversion of lauric acid into ketones is slower. Ketone levels peak at 3 hours after consumption of coconut oil, but remain in the blood for about 8 hours. MCT oil may give a quicker and higher peak in ketosis, but fizzles out much sooner. This is important because a brain suffering from neurodegeneration needs a *constant* supply of ketones. Without them, brain cells struggle and die.

MCT oil would need to be administered every 2 hours or so day and night to maintain blood ketone levels. During sleep, brain function remains fully active and needs energy just as it does when awake. The patient would need to be awakened constantly throughout the night to receive doses of MCT oil. This amount of MCT oil is unrealistic because of the undesirable digestive disturbances it would cause.

Coconut oil only needs to be taken three or four times a day and can last throughout the night. Some people who had been using coconut oil in treating Alzheimer's and switched to MCT oil have reported a decline in patients' progress. The conclusion is that MCT oil is not a suitable substitute for coconut oil in the treatment of neurodegeneration. It can, however, be added to coconut oil, which may produce a quicker rise in ketosis, but it really isn't needed. Coconut oil lasts longer, has fewer side effects, and is more effective in treating chronic infections.

16 Malnutrition and Neurodegeneration

SUGAR AND STARCHES

Sugar, Sugar Everywhere

Throughout human history, sugar has never been a very significant part of the diet. Two hundred years ago people ate, on average, only about 15 pounds (6.8 kg) of sugar a year. During the latter half of the 1800s, as sugar refining technology improved and more became available, sugar consumption dramatically increased. By 1900 annual sugar consumption in the United States had risen to 85 pounds (38.5 kg). Today we consume an average of about 160 pounds (72.6 kg) of sugar per year. This is over ten times the amount consumed in 1815.

On average, we consume about 200 grams (nearly half a pound) of sugar every day. Total carbohydrate consumption from all foods (fruits, vegetables, grains, beverages, etc.) for an averaged sized adult amounts to about 300 grams a day. If 200 grams of that is in the form of sugar, then two-thirds of our total daily carbohydrate intake comes from empty calories with no nutritional value whatsoever, calories that drain nutrients from the body without replacing them, calories that cause the body to go into metabolic shock, leading to insulin resistance and poor health.

Just because you don't add sugar to your foods or eat candy doesn't mean you are not consuming massive amounts of the sweet poison. Sugar is found as an ingredient in thousands of products from bread to nuts to soda and fruit drinks. Today sugars come in a variety of forms: sucrose (white table sugar), fructose, high fructose corn syrup, dextrose—the list goes on and on. Ingredient labels list the contents, starting with the most predominant one and followed in order to the least at the end. Sugar is often listed multiple times. In many packaged products, although sugar may not be listed first, if you combined all the many forms of sugar under the name "sugar," it would be the first ingredient on the list.

We get additional sugar that comes naturally in foods. Fruits and especially fruit juices are loaded with sugar. If you include these sources, our total daily sugar intake is even higher than 200 grams.

As sugar has increased in the diet over the years, other, more nutritious foods have been displaced. Despite the variety of foods available to us nowadays, the nutritional value of these foods is so poor that we can eat and eat and even overeat, and yet still be malnourished. We can easily get way too many calories without the nutrients needed for optimal health. Our foods, in effect, are slowly killing us.

Sugar Doesn't Make Memories Sweeter

One of the major benefits of cutting down on sugar consumption is better memory. Excess sugar consumption can keep you from remembering what day it is, where you live, or the name of your spouse. Compelling evidence suggests that the overconsumption of sugary foods and drinks can lead to Alzheimer's. Read that again: it's possible that sugar will cause Alzheimer's disease.

Sugar has become a major component of the modern human diet. Studies show that excess consumption of sweet foods, particularly sugar-sweetened beverages, play an important role in the epidemic of obesity and diabetes.[1] Diabetes is strongly associated with an increased risk of Alzheimer's disease, and evidence suggests it may also be a contributing factor in Parkinson's and other neurodegenerative diseases. Evidence is now emerging that shows a relationship between high sugar consumption and mental deterioration, learning difficulties, and memory loss.[2]

Researchers at the University of Alabama in Birmingham have shown that mice fed diets high in sugar develop the same amyloid plaque deposits and memory defects that characterize Alzheimer's disease. Over 25 weeks, one group of mice received a diet consisting of mouse chow and regular water. The other group ate the same chow, but drank a sugar water solution. The sugar-fed mice gained about 17 percent more weight over the course of the study. They also were more likely to develop insulin resistance, a hallmark of diabetes. These mice also performed worse on tests designed to measure learning and memory retention. The brains of the sugar-fed mice also had substantially more plaque deposits, a common feature of Alzheimer's.[3]

The amount of sugar water consumed by the mice was equivalent to a human drinking five 12-ounce cans of regular soda a day. Five cans of soda contain about 210 grams of sugar. While most people don't drink five cans of soda every day, they do get sugar from other sources—fruit juice, candy, donuts, pancakes, coffee, pastry, ice cream, and even everyday foods like spaghetti, catsup, barbeque sauce, bread, and fruit—that can easily surpass 210 grams. On average, every man, woman, and child consumes about this much every day. Of course an infant or a child will consume less, and some people eat almost no sugar at all, so those adults who do eat sugar are consuming well over 210 grams daily. It is interesting that the memory defects and plaque deposits in the sugar-fed mice occurred after only 25 weeks. What happens in our brains after years of eating a high-sugar diet?

As you recall from Chapter 4, high levels of blood sugar promote the formation of brain-destroying AGEs. Sugar in the blood tends to glycate or "stick" to proteins and fats, causing permanent damage to tissues and generating destructive free radicals. The accumulation of AGEs in the body is correlated with the process of aging. The more you accumulate, the more quickly you and your brain age. AGE accumulation is associated with neurodegenerative disease. Like excessive oxidation, it is one of the characteristics of neurodegeneration. AGEs develop in the body whenever sugar or starch is consumed, regardless of the amount. The more sugar and starch consumed, however, the more AGEs are created.

The overconsumption of sugar leads to chronically high blood sugar levels associated with insulin resistance. You don't have to be a diabetic to have insulin resistance. Anyone who has fasting blood sugar levels over 90 mg/dl (5.0 mmol/l) has some degree of insulin resistance. That includes most people who eat the typical American or western-type diet high in sugar and refined grains.

Some of the damaged glycated proteins and fats can stick around for life, contributing to sagging skin, cataracts, and hardened blood vessels. But we are not completely defenseless against AGEs; the white blood cells of our immune system can remove some of these little troublemakers. They do this by eating them in a process biologists call *phagocytosis.* AGEs are engulfed by the white blood cells, broken down or digested and made harmless. The same process is used on invading bacteria.

The ability of white blood cells to phagocytize toxic particles and bacteria, however, is strongly influenced by sugar consumption. Sugar depresses the white blood cells' ability to phagocytize these harmful substances. Studies have shown that after a single dose of sugar, phagocytosis drops by nearly 50 percent and remains depressed for at least five hours.[4] If you eat a sugary meal, your immune system will be severely depressed and remain that way at least until your next meal. So if you eat pancakes or sugary breakfast cereal in the morning, drink a sugary soda with your lunch, and end your dinner with a bowl of ice cream, your immune system will be severely depressed all day long. You will be less able to remove AGEs and more susceptible to infection and inflammation, all of which can adversely affect the brain.

Because sugar depresses immune function, it increases risks of any type of infection, including oral infections which can spread to the brain, reduces the body's ability to neutralize and dispose of environmental toxins, and increases risk of cancer. Cancer cells feed on sugar. The more sugar you give them, the better they grow.[5]

Sugar comes in a variety of forms. Sucrose, commonly known as white table sugar, is the most common. Others include brown sugar, honey, corn syrup, maple syrup, sucanat (unrefined dehydrated sugarcane juice), molasses, date sugar, fruit juice concentrate, barley malt, agave nectar, and brown rice syrup. In addition to these sugars, you may find others included on ingredient labels such as dextrin, dextrose, fructose, high fructose corn syrup, glucose, and maltodextrin. So-called "natural" sugars such as fruit juice concentrate or agave nectar are no better than refined sucrose. The end results are the same. Whether you eat table sugar, honey, or molasses makes little difference. Sugar by any other name is still sugar.

Starch Is Just a Form of Sugar

Refined sugar isn't the only problem. Starch can be nearly as bad. Starch is the carbohydrate found in grains, tubers, beans, and other starchy vegetables. Starch is sugar. It is composed of pure glucose. The only difference is that in starch, the glucose molecules are all linked together in a long chain but, once we eat it, however, digestive enzymes break the links into individual sugar molecules. Like any other source of sugar, starch causes blood sugar levels to rise rapidly, increases AGE formation, depresses immune function, and has all the other detrimental effects associated with sugar. Eating a slice of white bread is essentially equivalent to eating

3 teaspoons of sugar. White bread begins to turn into sugar in our mouths as soon as we start chewing. Saliva contains digestive enzymes that immediately begin to transform the starch into sugar.

People who do not eat many sweets or use sugar may think they are immune to sugar's detrimental effects. Yet, if they eat white bread, white rice, white potatoes, and products made with white flour they are getting just as much sugar as anyone else and maybe even more. White bread can cause insulin resistance and diabetes, reduce resistance against cancer, and set the stage for Alzheimer's or Parkinson's disease.

White flour is made by refining whole wheat flour. During the refining process many nutrients are removed, along with most of the fiber. Manufacturers add back a few of the nutrients but not the fiber. Fiber plays an essential role in the digestion of starch. Fiber slows down the release of glucose into the bloodstream. This is very important because it slows down sugar absorption, making it more manageable.

Starch in and of itself is not necessarily bad. After all, the glucose in starch is used as a source of fuel for our cells. The problem is the overconsumption of starch or the disproportion of starch in the diet in comparison to fat, protein, and fiber. A moderate amount of starch and even sugar can be handled as long as adequate amounts of fat, protein, and fiber are also consumed.

A typical diet consisting of 2,000 calories per day includes about 300 grams of carbohydrate on average. Out of this total, 200 grams comes from added sugars, 15 grams comes from fiber, and most of the remaining 85 grams comes in the form of starch. The number of calories in 285 grams of sugar and starch amounts to 1,140—that is almost *60 percent* of the total daily calories consumed! It's no wonder diabetes, Alzheimer's, and other degenerative diseases are on the rise.

Artificial Sweeteners

If real sugar wasn't bad enough, we can now "enjoy" artificial sugar—aspartame, saccharin, and such. These man-made products have the sweetness of sugar yet fewer calories. Like sugar, these crystalline powders are addictive, but they are even more detrimental to health. Yes, they contain fewer calories than sugar, but like any drug, they have undesirable side effects that range from headaches to death.

Artificial sweeteners look like sugar, taste like sugar, and can be used to sweeten foods just like sugar but without the calories or the carbohydrates of sugar. For someone who is trying to cut down on carbohydrate consumption, artificial sweeteners sound like an ideal solution. However, artificial sweeteners have a dark side much more sinister than sugar.

Sugar, even as refined as it is, is still a product the body recognizes and can process, even though the processing causes the body a great deal of stress and drains nutrients. Artificial sweeteners, on the other hand, are strange new creatures the human body has never seen before and isn't programmed to handle safely or efficiently. This creates problems. While the materials that scientists use to make artificial sweeteners may come from "natural" sources, they are combined in such a way as to form unique chemicals that are harmful causing all types of mischief.

One of the most widely used artificial sweeteners is aspartame. Aspartame is sold under the brand names AminoSweet, NutraSweet, Equal, Spoonful, and Equal-Measure. Discovered in 1965, it was approved for use as a food additive in the US in the early 1980s. The US Food and Drug Administration allowed its use even under the heavy criticism by several scientists who warned of its dangers. Despite objections, approval was granted based on research funded by aspartame's manufacturer (Monsanto and its subsidiary, The NutraSweet Company).

Since its approval, aspartame has accounted for over 75 percent of the adverse reactions to food additives reported to the FDA. At least 90 different symptoms have been documented as being caused by aspartame. Some of these include headaches/migraines, dizziness, seizures, nausea, numbness, muscle spasms, rashes, depression, fatigue, irritability, tachycardia, insomnia, vision problems, hearing loss, heart palpitations, breathing difficulties, anxiety attacks, slurred speech, loss of taste, tinnitus, vertigo, memory loss, joint pain, and, believe it or not, weight gain. In addition, aspartame has triggered or worsened brain tumors, multiple sclerosis, epilepsy, chronic fatigue syndrome, Parkinson's disease, Alzheimer's disease, birth defects, fibromyalgia, and diabetes. Would any sane person knowingly eat a substance that caused or even contributed to these types of problems?

Aspartame is a relative newcomer compared to saccharin. Discovered in 1879, saccharin was the first of the artificial sweeteners. In 1937 cyclamate came on the scene. This was followed by aspartame in the 1960s and more recently acesulfame K and sucralose. These artificial sweeteners are many times sweeter than sugar. Saccharin has a sweetening power 300 times that of table sugar. Cyclamate is about 30 times as sweet as sugar and aspartame is 200 times sweeter. Gram for gram, these sweeteners contain about the same number of calories as sugar, but since they are so much sweeter, only a fraction of the amount is needed for the same effect.

Saccharin and cyclamate have fallen in stature since the late 1960s when it was discovered that they caused tumorous growths in laboratory animals. Cyclamate was banned in the US in 1970, although it has remained in limited use in the United Kingdom and Canada. In Canada it is only allowed as a tabletop sweetener on the advice of a physician and as an additive in medicines.

In 1977, a ban was also proposed for saccharin. Since it was the only remaining artificial sweetener in use at the time many people opposed the ban, claiming the action was unfair to diabetics and the overweight. In response to the public outcry the ban was put on hold. Instead of the ban, products containing saccharin are required to carry a warning which reads "Use of this product may be hazardous to your health. This product contains saccharin, which has been determined to cause cancer in laboratory animals." Saccharin, however, is banned completely in Canada.

Acesulfame K is of the same general chemical family as saccharin. It has the same potential drawbacks as saccharin in regards to cancer. Like saccharin, it also stimulates insulin secretion which makes it less desirable for diabetes.

The newest kid on the block is sucralose, better known by the trade name Splenda. It is 600 times sweeter than sugar. This chemical sweetener is so alien to our bodies that the digestive system doesn't know what to do with it. It travels through the digestive tract without being absorbed. Thus it provides no calories and does not affect insulin or blood sugar levels and, therefore, is considered safe for diabetics. Sound too good to be true? Judging from the number of complaints filed with the FDA, it is.

If you're not convinced that artificial sweeteners are harmful, I recommend that you read *Excitotoxins: The Taste That Kills* Dr. Russell L. Blaylock, MD. This book provides details on the medical research documenting the dangers of aspartame and other food additives.

SUBCLINICAL MALNUTRITION

Most of the foods we eat nowadays are nutrient deficient. Processing and refining remove and destroy many nutrients. Sugar, for example, has a total of zero vitamins and minerals but contains fattening calories. White flour, likewise, has been stripped of its vitamin- and mineral-rich bran and germ, leaving almost pure starch. When you eat products made with white flour, you are eating primarily sugar, which is essentially void of any nutritional value. White rice is the same; the vitamin-rich bran is removed, leaving the white starchy portion behind. Potatoes are almost all starch. The skins contain most of the nutrients, but how many people eat the skins with their potatoes?

Most of the foods we typically eat are made from sugar, white flour, white rice, and skinless potatoes. These foods supply roughly 60 percent of the daily calories of most people. Another 20 to 30 percent comes from fats and oils. The most popular oils are margarine, shortening, and processed vegetable oils like soybean and corn oils. Oils are often hidden in our foods. All packaged, convenience, and restaurant foods contain loads of fats, including a high percentage of hydrogenated fats. Like sugar, processed oils contain no vitamins and minerals, only calories.

For the most part our typical diet consists of foods which are mostly empty calories—starch, sugar, and processed oils. Few of us eat fruits and vegetables. When we do, it's generally as condiments—pickles and lettuce on a sandwich, tomato sauce on a pizza. Our food is loaded with calories, but nutritionally deficient. We consume lots of calories but few nutrients. The consequence is that you can eat and eat and eat even to the point of becoming overweight yet still be malnourished.

The US Department of Agriculture states that most of us don't get enough (100 percent RDA) of at least 10 essential nutrients. Only 12 percent of the population obtains 100 percent of seven essential nutrients. Less than 10 percent of us get the recommended daily servings of fruit and vegetables. Forty percent of us eat no fruit and 20 percent no vegetables. And most of the vegetables we do get are fried potatoes cooked in hydrogenated vegetable oil.

It's bad enough that most of the foods we eat are nutritionally poor, but the problem is compounded even further by the fact that these same foods also destroy the nutrients we get from other foods. Sugar, for example, has no nutrients, yet it still uses up nutrients when it is metabolized. Eating sugary and starchy foods can drain the body of chromium, a mineral vital to potentiating insulin. Without insulin, you develop blood sugar problems like a diabetic. The more processed our food is, the more nutrients we need in order to metabolize it. Polyunsaturated oils, another source of empty calories, eat up vitamins E and A and deplete zinc reserves; other food additives, including iron, burn up vitamins A, C, and E. A diet loaded with white flour products, sugar, and processed vegetable oil quickly depletes nutrient reserves, pushing us further toward malnutrition.

Advanced stages of malnutrition can exhibit themselves by a number of characteristic diseases such as scurvy (vitamin C deficiency), beriberi (thiamin deficiency), and pellagra (niacin deficiency). Such conditions depress immunity, leave the body vulnerable to infections, slow down healing, disrupt normal growth and development, and promote tissue and organ degeneration.

According to the World Health Organization, 70–80 percent of people in developed nations die from lifestyle- or diet-caused diseases. The majority of cancers are caused by what we put into our bodies. Heart disease, stroke, and atherosclerosis, the biggest killers in industrialized nations, are dietary diseases. Diabetes is a diet-related disease. And for the most part, so are Alzheimer's and Parkinson's disease. Numerous studies have shown that vitamins, minerals, and other nutrients in foods protect us from these diseases.

When we think of malnutrition, we usually think of emaciated drought victims in Africa or starving people in India. In more affluent countries, the problem is more insidious. Symptoms of malnutrition are not as evident. People don't look malnourished, and methods of diagnosing deficiency diseases require malnutrition to be in an advanced stage before they can be detected.

When a variety of foods are available, few people develop obvious symptoms of malnutrition, even when their diets are nutritionally poor. Instead, they suffer from subclinical malnutrition. Subclinical malnutrition is a condition where a person consumes just enough essential nutrients to prevent full-blown symptoms of severe malnutrition, but the body is still nutrient deficient and prone to slow, premature degeneration. This condition can go on unnoticed indefinitely. In Western countries the problem of subclinical malnutrition is epidemic. Our foods are sadly depleted of nutrients. We eat, and even overeat, but may still be malnourished because our foods do not contain all the essential nutrients our bodies need to function optimally. As a result, the immune system is chronically depressed, the body cannot fight off infections well, and tissues and cells starving for nutrients slowly degenerate.

A diet that is loaded with sugar and refined carbohydrates, as is typical in our society today, is nutrient deficient. The best way to improve the diet is to reduce the total amount of carbohydrate consumed. Replace refined carbohydrates with more fat, protein, and complex carbohydrates (those accompanied by fiber). Although vegetables are considered carbohydrate-rich foods, most non-starchy vegetables, such as zucchini, tomatoes, and broccoli, are low in carbohydrate because they are around 90 percent water. These are also good sources of fiber, vitamins, minerals, antioxidants, and other phytonutrients.

NUTRIENT DEFICIENCIES AND NEURODEGENERATION

The brain, like the rest of the body, needs good nutrition to develop and function properly. A deficiency in just one nutrient can have serious consequences.

Folate, one of the B vitamins, has long been known to be important for fetal brain and spinal cord development. Babies born to folate-deficient mothers often have a severe spinal cord deformity called spina bifida. Folate is important for adult brain and nerve function as well, and a lack of this vitamin has been associated with neurodegenerative disease. In one study involving 575 people over age 50, investigators found that those getting 400 micrograms or more of folate per day, the recommended daily allowance of this vitamin, had a 55 percent lower risk of developing Alzheimer's than people getting less than that amount.[6]

One of the characteristics of Alzheimer's disease is the loss of brain mass due to shrinkage. Our brains normally shrink a little with age, but in Alzheimer's the rate of shrinkage is accelerated. Deficiencies in folate and other B vitamins such as vitamins B_6 and B_{12} appear to accelerate brain aging and shrinkage. Researchers at the University of Oxford found that giving large doses of these vitamins to elderly people with cognitive impairment (but not yet diagnosed with Alzheimer's) reduced the rate of brain shrinkage by nearly half, thus delaying or completely avoiding the onset of dementia.[7]

Folate deficiency can influence Parkinson's disease as well. In one study, lab mice were given the drug MPTP to induce Parkinson's disease. The mice were split into two groups, one of which was fed a folate-deficient diet. In mice that were fed adequate amounts of folate, dopamine-producing nerve cells were able to repair damaged DNA and counteract the adverse effects of the drug. However, the dopamine cells in folate-deficient mice could not repair the damage. As a result, these cells died.[8]

Folate does not cure Alzheimer's or Parkinson's disease, but a deficiency appears to significantly increase susceptibility. Getting adequate folate is important in reducing risk. Good dietary sources of folate include spinach, bok choy, broccoli, chicken, and fish. A diet that includes ample amounts of vegetables and fresh meat supplies the needed folate.

The mineral magnesium has been identified as a cofactor in over 300 enzymatic reactions involving energy metabolism and protein and DNA synthesis. Magnesium deficiency can cause muscle weakness, tremors, seizures, and disturbances to the heart and circulatory system. Evidence suggests it may also increase risk of Alzheimer's, Parkinson's, MS, and glaucoma. The majority of adults in the United States (68 percent) do not consume even the minimum RDA of magnesium, which many health professionals consider to be too low in the first place. To make matters worse, some common foods pull what little magnesium we do eat out of our bodies. Blood levels of magnesium are decreased by excess consumption of alcohol, caffeine, and phosphoric acid (used in sodas). Good dietary sources are spinach, beet greens, beets, asparagus, sesame seeds, sunflower seeds, and shrimp.

There are dozens of trace minerals that support brain health. The mineral lithium has long been known to be an effective therapy for bipolar disorder (formerly known as manic depression). Lithium stimulates the release of proteins that protect brain cells from harm, improve their survival, and promote neuronal growth and repair. For instance, after four weeks of lithium supplementation, three-dimensional magnetic resonance imaging showed grey matter volume increased in patients with bipolar disorder.[9] Animal studies show that lithium can decrease areas of cell death after a stroke by 56 percent. By promoting brain cell regeneration, lithium can function as an anti-aging nutrient for the brain.

Lithium has also shown to block the destructive effects of neurotoxins such as MSG, caffeine, and anti-convulsant drugs.[10] Certain toxic metals, such as aluminum, are chelated by lithium and removed from the body.[11] Food sources of lithium include eggs, dairy, whole grains, and vegetables.

Another important trace mineral is zinc. As many as one-fourth of older women have zinc intakes that are less than half of the daily recommended allowance. A study in England showed that people with senile dementia had much lower levels of zinc than those without dementia.[12] Good sources of zinc are shellfish, fish, meat, milk, whole wheat, and leafy green vegetables.

The highest concentrations of vitamin C in the body are found in the brain and in neuroendocrine tissues such as the adrenals.[13] Vitamin C acts as a protective antioxidant, participates as a cofactor in several enzyme reactions, and functions as a neuromodulator of several neurotransmitters including glutamate, dopamine, and choline. Vitamin C is depleted by excessive oxidative stress, injury, and infection—important issues involving neurodegeneration. Dietary sources include dark leafy green vegetables, broccoli, cauliflower, peppers, tomatoes, citrus fruits, mangos, and papayas.

One group of researchers studied the relationship between nutrition status and cognitive functioning in 260 healthy, independent-living men and women over 60 years of age.[14] The researchers evaluated nutrient intakes by way of diet records and nutrition status by way of biochemical tests. Participants in the study were given two tests of cognitive function. One was a test of short-term memory and the other a test of problem-solving ability. Participants with low blood concentrations of vitamin C or vitamin B_{12} scored worse than better-nourished participants on both tests. Those with low blood concentrations of riboflavin or folic acid scored worse on the problem-solving test. The researchers concluded that subclinical malnutrition may play a role in the depression of cognitive function detectable in some elderly individuals.

Memory impairment due to vitamin B_{12} deficiency can precede the blood symptoms of deficiency by years. Evidence that vitamin B_{12} deficiency accounts for some cognitive deficits in older people comes from a study that revealed abnormal short-term memory in more than two-thirds of clients with pernicious anemia.[15] Treatment with vitamin B_{12} restored memory within one month in three-fourths of the clients. Good sources of vitamin B_{12} include meat, fish, poultry, dairy, and eggs. Vegetables, fruits, and grains don't supply this important vitamin. Consequently, vitamin B_{12} deficiency is a serious problem among strict vegetarians.

One of the hallmark features of neurodegenerative disease is runaway oxidative stress and free-radical destruction. The brain is particularly vulnerable to lipid peroxidation of polyunsaturated fatty acids because of its relatively high concentration of these fats.[16] Chronic oxidative stress severely depletes protective antioxidants. The only way to boost brain antioxidant levels is by eating foods rich in antioxidant nutrients. The major dietary antioxidants include vitamins A, C, D, E, and K, the minerals zinc and selenium, alpha-lipoic acid, CoQ10, and flavonoids such as beta-carotene, alpha-carotene, lutein, and lycopene. Blood levels of many of these antioxidants are lower in Alzheimer's patients in comparison to normal individuals, suggesting a dietary inadequacy in many important antioxidant nutrients.[17-18]

Studies show that those people who regularly eat vegetables and fruits are less likely to develop age-related mental decline and neurodegenerative disease than those who eat little.[19-20]

Eating vegetables appears to retard the aging process. Researchers at Rush Institute for Healthy Aging analyzed the eating habits and cognitive function of nearly 2,000 people over the age of 65. Those who consumed the most servings of vegetables each day had about 40 percent slowing in age-related mental decline. The greatest benefits were seen in people who consumed three or more servings of vegetables daily. Interestingly, fruit intake did not seem to protect against mental decline.

The slower mental decline was "equivalent to about five years of younger age," according to the researchers. Leafy green vegetables, which are rich in antioxidants and folate, were the most protective.[21]

Blood tests that measure antioxidant levels show that people of any age who have high levels of beta-carotene, lycopene, and vitamin E, score higher on cognitive tests in comparison to those with low antioxidant levels.[22] High blood levels of antioxidants were associated with a high daily intake of vegetables and fruits.

Taking a multiple vitamin and mineral supplement may help make up for some of the missing nutrients in the diet, but it is not a solution in itself. Studies have repeatedly shown that dietary supplements do not afford the same degree of protection obtained from eating whole foods.[23] Apparently, there are benefits associated with whole foods that go beyond their basic vitamin and mineral content.

Please note that pizza, donuts, white bread, soda, and other packaged processed foods were not listed above as good sources for any of the vitamins and minerals essential for good health. Good nutrition only comes from fresh, whole foods.

17 Brain Boosters

EAT YOUR VEGETABLES

Remember your mother telling you to "Eat your vegetables?" She knew that vegetables were important for good health. It's almost instinctive. Science has confirmed it. Study after study shows that a diet rich in vegetables and fruits wards off disease and promotes good health. Please note that vegetables are mentioned here before fruits because they are far more important to your health. Eating plenty of vegetables and fruits can help protect against heart disease and stroke, control blood pressure, prevent some types of cancer, avoid painful digestive ailments, guard against cataract and macular degeneration, and protect the brain against neurodegeneration.

You may have heard the advice to get five ½ cup servings of vegetables and fruits every day; the latest dietary guidelines actually recommend that we should get at least five to 13 servings (2½ to 6½ cups) a day. The amount depends on your total caloric requirements.[1] An average sized adult needs about 2,000 calories a day to maintain weight and health, this translates into nine servings, or 4½ cups per day.

What counts as a cup of vegetables and fruits? For most fresh or cooked vegetables and fruits, 1 cup is simply what you would put in a measuring cup. There are three main exceptions to this rule: lettuce, dried fruit, and potatoes. You need 2 cups of lettuce and other raw leafy greens to get the equivalent of 1 cup of vegetables. For dried fruit, you only need to eat ½ cup to get the equivalent of 1 cup of fruit. Potatoes are not counted as vegetables, since they are mostly starch and should be used sparingly.

Technically, vegetable and fruit juices would count as part of the daily serving requirement. However, juices are very high in sugar and devoid of fiber that would ordinarily moderate sugar absorption. The sugar content of pure fruit juice is the same as an equal amount of cola—about 10 teaspoons per 12-ounce serving. While the juice may include some vitamins and minerals, it is really little more than just flavored sugar water.

Insulin resistance is one of the major risk factors for neurodegeneration. Studies have shown that adding just one more serving of vitamin-rich leafy green vegetables or three servings of whole fruit a day can significantly decrease the risk of developing insulin resistance and, consequently, diabetes. With an additional ½ cup serving of vegetables, risk decreases by almost 10 percent. Adding 1½ cups

(3 servings) of fruit reduces risk about the same. Interestingly, risk decreases only with *whole* fruit. Fruit juices actually *increase* the risk; adding just one serving of fruit juice per day leads to an 18 percent increase in the risk of diabetes. The high sugar content of the juice and lack of fiber apparently cancel out the positive effects of the vitamins and minerals.[2] So, vegetable and fruit juices do not count as part of the daily requirement.

The average American gets a total of just three servings of vegetables and fruits a day. If people are not eating vegetables and fruits, what are they eating? Most likely lots of processed, packaged foods loaded with sugar and refined carbohydrates that have been stripped of their nutrients.

The recommendation is to get *at least* five to 13 thirteen servings of vegetables and fruits in the diet. That is a minimum. If you could get more, that would be even better. These servings are not to be added on top of everything you already eat but should replace less healthy foods like potatoes, white bread, and pasta in the diet. This would surely improve the nutrient content and reduce the amount of empty carbohydrate eaten. You are not adding more calories, you are replacing empty calories with more nutritious calories.

Studies have consistently shown that diets rich in vegetables, fruits, and whole grains protect against degenerative disease. Reducing carbohydrate consumption by replacing it with vegetables as well as fat and protein improves health and protects against disease.[3]

WHOLE FOODS

Why are vegetables, fruits, and whole grains so good for us? The answer is because they contain the basic vitamins and minerals, along with a myriad of phytonutrients that nourish our bodies, protect us from disease, and keep us healthy. Phytonutrients are chemicals produced in plants that have vitamin-like characteristics. One of these is beta-carotene. Beta-carotene acts as an antioxidant and helps protect us from cancer and heart disease. It can also be converted into vitamin A, if the body needs it. Beta-carotene gives carrots, squash, and other vegetables their characteristic yellow and orange colors. Lycopene is another phytonutrient that has gained recognition lately for its ability to lower the risk of prostate cancer. It produces the red pigment in tomatoes, watermelon, and pink grapefruit. There are over 20,000 phytonutrients that have been identified in plant foods.

In the past, individual vitamins and minerals were thought to be adequate in curing health problems. We now know that while a single nutrient may be helpful, a variety of nutrients working together provides the greatest benefit. Nutrients work together in concert, like all the different instruments in a philharmonic orchestra together produce music. All of the instruments are needed to create the best sound. Likewise, a wide variety of nutrients is needed in the proper proportion, like that found in whole foods, to provide the health benefits scientists see in nutritional studies.

This is why it is better to eat food containing hundreds of phytonutrients than to take a vitamin tablet which only has a dozen or so. This is why it is better to eat bread made from whole wheat flour than white flour which has had some 20 nutrients removed in the refining process. This is why fresh vegetables and fruits are superior to processed, packaged foods containing refined carbohydrates.

Most people will admit that they need to add more vegetables into their diets. But some people just don't care for vegetables. They were raised on white bread and pasta and other junk foods and never developed a taste for vegetables. Too often, vegetables are served more or less plain—maybe with a squeeze of lemon and a dash of salt—but without butter or any other type of sauce in order to avoid adding fat into the diet. Adding sources of fat such as butter, cheese, cream, nuts, seeds, meat drippings, crumbled bacon, pieces of ham, and rich creamy sauces greatly improve both the nutritional value of the vegetables and their taste. When served this way, even the staunchest vegetable haters will love to eat their veggies. As you begin to add more vegetables into your diet, you will develop a greater liking for them, especially when they are prepared this way.

GOOD QUALITY MEATS ARE IMPORTANT

As good as vegetables and other plant-based foods are, they don't provide all the nutrients necessary for optimal nutrition. Meat, fish, eggs, and dairy are the best sources of vitamins A, B_6, and B_{12}. In fact, it is impossible to get adequate amounts of these vitamins from plant sources alone. Meats and dairy supply fats which are required for the proper absorption and utilization of fat soluble vitamins. They also supply high quality protein needed for maintenance and growth of organs and tissues, including the brain.

Phosphatidylcholine, is a fatty substance that makes up a major constituent of cell membranes and also plays a role in membrane-mediated cell signaling. Phosphatidylcholine is a source of choline, one the B vitamins important to human health—particularly brain health. Phosphatidylcholine levels in the brain membranes decline with age, which may contribute to memory loss. Choline is one of the few substances able to penetrate the blood-brain barrier. It goes directly into the brain, where it is used to produce the neurotransmitter acetylcholine, which is important in memory function. A number of studies have shown a positive effect of phosphatidylcholine on preventing dementia and improving cognitive function. Evidence suggests it may also help to slow the deterioration of the myelin, which is depleted in multiple sclerosis sufferers. For these reasons, it is gaining recognition as a valuable dietary supplement to support brain health. Egg yolk is the richest natural source of phosphatidylcholine. Eating one or two eggs a day provides a good source of this important substance.

A similar substance that also plays an important role in cell membrane function is phosphatidylserine. This substance enables the brain cells to metabolize glucose and to release and bind with neurotransmitters. Phosphatidylserine modulates the fluidity of the cell membranes—essential to the brain cells' ability to send and receive chemical communication, which is important to learning, memory, and other cognitive functions.. It restores the brains' supply of acetylcholine. It also stimulates the brain to produce dopamine.

Dietary sources of phosphatidylserine come from meat and fish. Plants are very poor sources. The typical North American diet supplies about 130 mg of phosphatidylserine a day. Diets with optimal meat and fish consumption provide 180 mg, while low-fat diets supply only 100 mg and vegetarian diets less than 50 mg. Many people, especially older people, can benefit by adding more good quality meat into their diets.

BASK YOURSELF IN VITAMIN D

Vitamin D has long been known to be important for proper bone development; a lack of the vitamin can lead to osteomalacia, or rickets as it is known in children, and to osteoporosis in adults. Vitamin D also plays a protective role in many types of cancer, bacterial and viral infections (including dental cavities and periodontal disease), arthritis, inflammatory bowel disease, diabetes, cardiovascular disease, macular degeneration, hypertension, and depression. Now studies are showing the vitamin to be important for brain function as well. Researchers began studying the possible link between neurodegeneration and vitamin D after Alzheimer's and multiple sclerosis patients reported symptoms improving with large doses of vitamin D.

According to researchers at Cambridge University, low blood levels of vitamin D is associated with an increased risk of dementia. Scientists measured blood levels of the vitamin in 1,766 people over 65 and assessed their mental function. Those with the lowest levels of vitamin D were 2.3 times as likely to be cognitively impaired.[4]

Researchers at Emory University School of Medicine in Atlanta, Georgia have found a similar connection. The study involved 99 healthy adults who served as controls along with 97 Alzheimer's patients and 100 Parkinson's patients. Thirty-six percent of the healthy subjects had low vitamin D levels compared to 41 percent of those with Alzheimer's and 55 percent of those with Parkinson's. Ten percent of the healthy subjects had *severe* vitamin D deficiency, while 16 percent of the Alzheimer's patients and 23 percent of the Parkinson's patients were severely deficient.[5] A number of other studies have shown similar results.[6-7]

An interesting correlation exists between vitamin D deficiency due to a lack of sunlight and multiple sclerosis. The incidence of MS is nearly zero in equatorial regions, where solar radiation is greatest, and increases dramatically with latitude in both hemispheres, where UV radiation is weakest. This suggests that sunlight may help protect against MS. Studies show that MS prevalence is highest where environmental supplies of vitamin D are the lowest.[8] This explains two peculiar geographic anomalies, one in Switzerland with high MS rates at low altitudes and low MS rates at high altitudes, and one in Norway with a high MS prevalence inland and a lower MS prevalence along the coast. Ultraviolet light intensity is higher at high altitudes, resulting in a greater vitamin D production rate, thereby accounting for low MS rates at higher altitudes. On the Norwegian coast, fish is consumed at high rates; fish oils are rich in vitamin D.

Vitamin D deficiency affects most MS patients, as demonstrated by their low bone mass and high fracture rates. The clearest evidence linking vitamin D deficiency to MS comes from experiments with experimentally induced encephalomyelitis

(EAE)—an animal model of MS. Treatment with vitamin D completely inhibits EAE induction and progression.[9]

Vitamin D deficiency is not the cause of Alzheimer's, Parkinson's, or MS but can increase the risk. Neurons in the brain contain vitamin D receptors, suggesting that the vitamin may play a role in brain development and protection. Vitamin D acts as a molecular switch, activating more than 200 genes. This may be one of the reasons why it can have such great influence on health.

Defense against infections and the speed at which the body can overcome infection are directly related to vitamin D levels. Activation of white blood cells to fight infection requires vitamin D. Without adequate vitamin D, the immune system is sluggish. Infections can be more frequent, last longer, and even linger indefinitely when the immune system is crippled by a lack of vitamin D. This holds true for infections in the brain as well. Inflammation from infection anywhere in the body can ignite inflammation in the brain. Therefore, vitamin D deficiency can have a significant effect on brain health.

Vitamin D is known as the sunshine vitamin because it is produced by exposure to sunlight. The ultraviolet (UV) rays from the sun penetrate the skin and initiate chemical reactions that convert cholesterol into vitamin D. It is estimated that 85 percent of the population in North America has sub-optimal levels of vitamin D. Vitamin D deficiency is the result of too little sun exposure. The best way to remedy that is to get out into the sun more often.

Exposing your skin to direct sunlight, without sunscreen, is the most effective and the most natural way to get vitamin D. You don't want to use sunscreen because it blocks the UV rays that trigger vitamin synthesis. Contrary to overcautious recommendations to avoid the sun at all costs, we actually need some sun exposure to produce vitamin D. For a light skinned person, about 15 minutes a day is usually adequate. More time is needed if the sun is not directly overhead, as in the early morning or late in the afternoon, or if it is cloudy, because the sun's intensity is decreased. A dark-skinned person may need two or three times this amount of exposure to produce the same amount of vitamin D.

You should expose as much skin as possible; just your face and arms is not enough. For maximum benefit, stay in the sun just until your skin begins to turn a slight shade of pink. If you have any reservations about getting burned, you can apply a thin coat of coconut oil over all your exposed skin. The oil protects the skin from damage without interfering with vitamin D synthesis. Coconut oil will allow you to stay under the sun longer without fear of burning. Other oils do not have this protective characteristic and are not recommended. With coconut oil you will be able to stay under the sun at least twice as long before the pink coloration develops, generating twice as much vitamin D.

In latitudes greater than 35 degrees (all states north of Alabama and all of Europe), sun exposure is greatly reduced in the winter. It is impossible to get enough sun exposure to produce sufficient amounts of vitamin D. Virtually everyone at a latitude greater than 35 has a chronic vitamin D deficiency during the winter no matter how much sun they get. In this case, you need to get your vitamin D another way. One option is to use a safe tanning bed. Another option is to eat foods that contain vitamin D. Foods, even those with the highest vitamin D levels, are generally insufficient, but the highest sources are found in milk, fish, eggs, Shitake mushrooms, and liver. Lard from pigs that have had ample exposure to sunlight is a modest source of vitamin D. Pigs get vitamin D just as humans do, from the sun. Pigs lack a thick covering of hair, so skin exposure to the sun produces the vitamin, which is stored in the animal's fat. The best dietary source of vitamin D, however, is cod liver oil. A spoonful a day will supply your minimum daily requirement.

One more source is from dietary supplements. If you take a supplement, make sure it contains vitamin D_3 (cholecalciferol), which is human vitamin D. Do not use the synthetic and inferior vitamin D_2. The recommended dietary allowance (RDA) for vitamin D is 15 micrograms (600 IU) per day. Based on the latest research, however, 2,000-5,000 IU per day appears to provide the best overall health benefit.[10]

The synthesis of cholesterol into vitamin D from sunlight is much more productive than that obtained from dietary sources. For example, full body summer sun exposure for 30 minutes may produce about 20,000 IU of vitamin D, which is the amount provided by consuming 200 glasses of milk (100 IU/8 oz glass) or taking 50 standard multivitamins (400 IU/tablet). The best way to build up vitamin D reserves is to get out into the sun.

NATURAL INFLAMMATION FIGHTERS

A common feature in all neurodegenerative disease is chronic inflammation. Inflammation promotes much of the destructive action that takes place in the brain. Logically then, calming the inflammation should relieve much of the stress and ease symptoms. Some success has been achieved with this approach. Administering MPTP to mice to induce Parkinson's, along with rosiglitazone, an insulin-sensitizing drug that moderates inflammatory responses, investigators were able to completely prevent motor and olfactory dysfunctions. Anti-inflammatory drugs, however, carry the risk of adverse side effects, some of which may promote neurodegeneration.

An alternative to drugs are natural anti-inflammatory phytonutrients found in vegetables, fruits, herbs, and spices. Eating foods rich in these substances can help fight destructive free radicals and douse inflammation associated with neurodegeneration. Unlike drugs, these compounds are constituents of everyday foods that nourish the body without causing unwanted side effects.

Luteolin, a plant flavonoid found in a number of vegetables and fruits in particularly celery and bell peppers, has been shown to exert potent anti-inflammatory effects within the central nervous system.[11]

Many anti-inflammatory compounds are found only in certain plants. Some of the herbs and spices we use every day contain these unique compounds. One of these is thymol, the oil from the herb thyme. Another is gingerol, from ginger root. Gingerol is chemically very similar to capsaicin, the spicy ingredient that gives chili peppers their bite.

One of the most potent natural anti-inflammatory compounds is curcumin—the pigment that gives the spice turmeric its distinctive yellow color. Turmeric is a popular spice used in Asian cooking for making curries. The yellow color of curry powder comes from turmeric. Because of curcumin's potent antioxidant and anti-inflammatory action, investigators are actively studying its effect on neurodegenerative disease.

A fungal neurotoxin known as 3-nitropropionic acid causes motor and cognitive defects resembling Huntington's disease. When rats are given curcumin a few days before and during the administration of this neurotoxin, it protects their brains from much of the destructive action of the toxin.

Researchers have reported that when mice genetically bred to develop the equivalent of Alzheimer's disease are fed foods spiced with turmeric, brain inflammation is greatly reduced and they develop only half the amyloid plaque as those not eating the spice.[12]

If curcumin provides protection against neurodegeneration, Alzheimer's might be expected to be less common among those people who consume a lot of curry. This idea was the basis for a study conducted in Singapore. In this study over 1,000 residents over the age of 60 who had not been diagnosed with any form of dementia, took a diet survey and were evaluated using the Mini Mental State Examination for Alzheimer's. Participants who reported consuming curry "often" had a 49 percent lower risk of cognitive problems compared with those who "never or rarely" ate curry. Those who ate curry "occasionally" had a 38 percent lower risk of cognitive impairment.[13]

Researchers from the University of Pittsburgh performed a similar study. Curry dishes are immensely popular throughout India. The researchers gathered data on the incidence of Alzheimer's in a community near New Delhi where curries are commonly eaten and compared it with a population that rarely eats curry near Pittsburgh, Pennsylvania. The incidence rate of those 65 years of age and older in the US population was 17.5 per 1,000 people. In contrast, the incidence rate of the Indian population was only 4.7 per 1,000 people. The rate in the Indian population is among the lowest in the world and only a fourth of that reported in the United States.[14] The extraordinary low incidence of Alzheimer's may be due to the consumption of turmeric in curry, but curries are frequently made using coconut milk, which is rich in medium chain triglycerides, so the study results could be due to the coconut, the turmeric, or both.

There are hundreds of phytochemicals that possess anti-inflammatory and antioxidant properties, most of which have not yet been studied in any significant detail. Eating a variety of plant foods can provide a great deal of protection against neurodegenerative disease.

Plant foods aren't the only sources of anti-inflammatory compounds. Fish, and more specifically fish oil, may also help ease runaway inflammation. Fish oil is a rich source of omega-3 fatty acids. These fatty acids are converted by the body into hormone-like substances known as prostaglandins that have potent anti-inflammatory properties. The best source of fish oil is from eating fresh fish. Another source is cod liver oil. The advantage of cod liver oil over fish oil supplements is that it has a higher antioxidant content and is the best dietary source of vitamin D.

Studies do suggest that eating fish can reduce the risks of Parkinson's and Alzheimer's.[15] One study showed that eating at least one serving of fish per week lowered the risk of developing Alzheimer's disease by 60 percent, compared to those who rarely or never eat fish.[16]

Some people have expressed concern about eating fish or even cod liver oil due to possible contamination by mercury and other pollutants. This is a legitimate concern. Toxic levels of mercury can accumulate in fish as a result of biomagnification. The higher up on the food chain the fish is, the greater the risk of contamination (see Chapter 9 for a list of the safest fish to eat). For this reason, some people prefer to get their omega-3s from krill oil. Krill are tiny shrimp-like crustaceans that live in the arctic oceans and feed on microscopic plankton. They are near the bottom of the food chain, so mercury contamination is not an issue. Krill oil also contains a number of antioxidants, including vitamins E, A, and D and a super antioxidant called astaxanthin. It has 48 times more antioxidant potency than ordinary fish oil. You can find krill oil at your health food store or online.

Fish oils contain two important omega-3 fatty acids: docosahexaenoic acid (DHA) and eicosapentaenoic acid (EPA). Both can be converted into anti-inflammatory prostaglandins and help reduce runaway inflammation. DHA is the more important of the two because it is also used as a structural component for some brain tissues.

While studies show that eating fish can benefit those with Alzheimer's, fish oil supplementation has proven to be a disappointment. While some studies have indicated a possible benefit to using fish oil dietary supplements in treating Alzheimer's, others have shown no benefit.

One of the concerns about fish oil supplements is quality. Fish oil is highly vulnerable to oxidation. If not processed, handled, or stored properly it can easily become oxidized (rancid) and be totally useless and even harmful. Many of the fish oil supplements on the market are partially rancid before they are even purchased from the store and others go rancid quickly after opening. Fish oil should always be stored in the refrigerator and be used within a few weeks after purchase, regardless of the expiration date. Rancid oils can promote inflammation. This may be the reason why fish oil supplementation has been ineffectual in treating Alzheimer's. Krill oil is preferred to other fish oils because it has a much higher antioxidant content protecting it from oxidation.

Another popular source of omega-3 fatty acids is flaxseed oil. Some people prefer flaxseed oil because it comes from a plant source. The omega-3 fatty acid in flaxseed, as well as other plant sources, is called alpha-linolenic acid (ALA). Unlike DHA, ALA is not needed in brain tissue or converted directly into prostaglandins. However, the body, through a long series of chemical steps, can convert ALA into EPA. The process is not very efficient and only about 10 percent of the ALA ends up as EPA. Little if any is converted into DHA. Even with a very high consumption of ALA, DHA levels in the brain do not change.[17] Therefore, it is essential that you get your omega-3s from fish or other animal sources (i.e., eggs, grass-fed beef), rather than rely on flaxseed or other plant sources.

A DAILY DOSE OF ANTIOXIDANTS FROM A COOKING OIL

In recent years there has been a wealth of exciting research on a relatively little known class of nutrients called tocotrienols. Tocotrienols are super-potent forms of vitamin E, possessing up to 60 times the antioxidant power of ordinary vitamin E. Their effects on health are far beyond that of regular vitamin E. Research shows that tocotrienols reduce high blood pressure, dissolve arterial plaque, extend lives of stroke and heart disease patients, possess powerful anticancer properties, and protect the brain from degenerative conditions such as Alzheimer's and Parkinson's disease.

Ordinary vitamin E can be found in many foods. Tocotrienols, on the other hand, are not as common. They can be found in small amounts in some nuts, seeds, and grains. By far the most abundant source of these super antioxidants comes from palm oil. Palm oil is one of the richest natural sources of vitamin E in general, and by far the richest source of tocotrienols.

Because tocotrienols are powerful antioxidants, they are being investigated in the treatment of heart disease. Heart disease is characterized by atherosclerosis—build-up of plaque in the arteries. A number of studies have demonstrated the ability of antioxidants to prevent fat and cholesterol oxidation and, thereby, arrest the development of atherosclerosis. Although ordinary vitamin E is a potent antioxidant, it has only shown modest benefit in this respect. Palm tocotrienols, however, have shown to be very effective in stopping and even reversing atherosclerosis, and therefore, protecting against heart attacks and strokes.

Studies show that tocotrienols can actively remove plaque build-up in arteries and reverse the progression of atherosclerosis. This has been demonstrated in both animal and human studies. In one study, for instance, 50 subjects were divided into two equal groups. All the participants had been diagnosed with atherosclerosis and had suffered at least one stroke. At the beginning of the study the degree of blockage of their carotid arteries—the artery that feeds the brain—ranged from 15 to 79 percent. Without any other changes to their diets or medications, half of the subjects began taking a daily palm oil supplement containing tocotrienols. The other half received placebos and served as the controls. The degree of atherosclerosis was monitored using ultrasound scans over an 18 month period. In the group receiving tocotrienols, atherosclerosis was halted in 23 of the 25 subjects. In seven of these subjects, atherosclerosis regressed. In comparison, none of those in the control group showed any improvement; in fact, in 10 of them, the condition worsened.[18] This study demonstrated that tocotrienols not only stop the progression of atherosclerosis but can reverse it as well.

Tocotrienols also help protect against heart disease and stroke by maintaining proper blood pressure. This powerful antioxidant inhibits platelets from sticking to one another, thereby "thinning" the blood. It also reduces inflammation and assists in keeping blood vessels properly dilated so that circulation remains normal and blood pressure stays under control.

In one study, researchers induced inflammation in the arteries of test animals. Inflammation causes swelling, narrowing artery passageways and restricting blood flow to vital organs such as the heart. Half of the animals received tocotrienols in their diet while the other half served as the control. In the control group artery passageways were severely constricted and 42 percent of the animals died. However, those that received the tocotrienols showed far less inflammation and constriction, resulting in a 100 percent survival rate.

Tocotrienols strengthen the heart so that it can better withstand stress. Researchers can purposely induce heart attacks in lab animals by cutting off blood flow to the heart. This causes severe injury and death. However, if the animals are fed tocotrienol-rich palm oil beforehand, survival rate is greatly increased, injury is minimized, and recovery time is reduced.[19]

While tocotrienols appear to be powerful aids in preventing heart disease, they have gained more notice in the fight against cancer. Antioxidants have long been known to offer protection against various forms of cancer. Tocotrienols, being highly potent antioxidants, have demonstrated remarkable anticancer properties far superior to most other antioxidants, including their more common vitamin E cousins.

Studies show tocotrienols inhibit the growth of skin, stomach, pancreas, liver, lung, colon, prostate, breast and other cancers. Most of the research to date has been done with breast cancer, where tocotrienols show great promise. Initial research has been so impressive that cancer researchers have called tocotrienols the most powerful natural anticancer substances known to science.[20] That's quite a bold statement, but it illustrates the potential of tocotrienols in cancer prevention and treatment.

The antioxidant power of palm oil has also shown to be of benefit in protecting against neurological degeneration. Two of the most significant factors that affect brain function are oxidative stress and poor circulation. Oxidative stress generates free radicals that damage brain and nerve tissue. Poor circulation affects the brain by restricting oxygen and glucose. Researchers have found correlations between oxidative stress and reduced blood flow to the brain to senile dementia, Alzheimer's disease, Parkinson's disease, Huntington's disease, and even schizophrenia. All of these conditions involve brain cell death. Tocotrienols aid the brain by reducing oxidative stress and improving blood flow.

Researchers can mimic much of the destruction seen in the above neurological disorders by feeding test animals glutamate—an amino acid that in large amounts kills brain cells. The primary action of cell death is caused by free radicals. Ordinary vitamin E is not strong enough to prevent glutamate-induced cell death, but palm tocotrienols can quench the destructive action of glutamate. In laboratory studies tocotrienol-treated neurons maintain healthy growth and motility even in the presences of excess glutamate.[21]

Research is showing that tocotrienols can be of help with a number of common health problems including osteoporosis, asthma, cataracts, macular degeneration, arthritis, and liver disease as well as stunting the processes that promote premature aging.

Palm oil comes from the fruit of the oil palm. Palm fruit is about the size of a small plum. The oil is extracted from the fruit or pulp surrounding the seed. Palm fruit is a dark red color and produces an orange-red colored oil. This crude or virgin oil is called *red palm oil*. Red palm oil has undergone minimal processing, and retains most of the naturally occurring fat soluble vitamins and other nutrients. The red color comes from the rich abundance of beta-carotene and other carotenes in the fruit.

Red palm oil is a virtual powerhouse of nutrition. It contains far more nutrients than any other dietary oil. Besides being the richest natural source of tocotrienols, it is also the richest dietary source of beta-carotene, a precursor to vitamin A. It has 15 times more beta-carotene than carrots and 300 times more than tomatoes. In addition, it contains lycopene, alpha-carotene, and at least 20 other carotenes along with vitamin E, vitamin K, CoQ10, squalene, phytosterols, flavonoids, phenolic acids, and glycolipids. There are four tocotrienols—palm oil contains all of them. The combination of vitamin E, tocotrienols, carotenes, and other antioxidants makes red palm oil a natural super-antioxidant supplement. In fact, it is currently being encapsulated and sold as a vitamin supplement. The oil is also available in bottles, like other vegetable oils, for kitchen use.

One tablespoon supplies more than enough to meet daily requirements of vitamins E and A. The best way to take red palm oil is to incorporate it into daily food preparation and use it like you would any other cooking oil. It is very heat tolerant and makes an excellent cooking oil.

Because of its distinctive orange-red color, red palm oil is easy to spot on store shelves. At room temperature it is semisolid, somewhat like soft butter. If refrigerated, it will harden. On the countertop on a warm day, it will liquefy. Red palm oil doesn't need to be refrigerated; it is very resistant to oxidation. You can use the oil when it is hard or soft. Nutritionally, there is no difference.

Red palm oil has a distinctive flavor and aroma. In cultures where palm oil is produced, it is an important ingredient in food preparation and gives the food much of its characteristic flavor. The oil has a pleasant, somewhat savory taste that enhances the natural flavor of meats and vegetables. The flavor complements soups, sauces, sautéed vegetables, eggs, and meats. In recipes that call for vegetable oil, butter, or margarine, you can usually replace them with red palm oil.

Please note that red palm oil is not the same as coconut oil. Besides the obvious difference in color, red palm oil does not contain any MCTs. Therefore, it does not produce the ketones needed by the brain. The benefit of red palm oil is its excellent cooking properties and its rich vitamin and antioxidant content.

Palm fruit produces two types of oil; one from the fleshy fruit and the other from the seed or kernel. Red palm oil comes from the soft fruit. *Palm kernel oil* is extracted from the seed. The two are not alike. Palm kernel oil is almost identical to coconut oil, containing about 53 percent MCTs, and like coconut oil, is colorless.

Red palm oil is available at most good health food stores and online. To learn more about the health benefits of tocotrienols and palm oil, I recommend the book *The Palm Oil Miracle* by Bruce Fife.

THE ANTI-AGING DIET

The ketogenic diet was developed as a means to mimic the metabolic and therapeutic effects of fasting. Another approach to simulate the therapeutic effects of fasting is through calorie restriction. The calorie restricted diet, or so-called CR diet, limits daily calorie consumption to about 50-90 percent of normal intake. The CR diet has often been referred to as an "anti-aging diet" because it slows down the aging process and extends life span. The basis for the CR diet first emerged in the 1930s when scientists learned that underfed rodents lived up to 40 percent longer than their well-fed counterparts. Over the years these results have been duplicated in fruit flies, worms, fish, and other lab animals.

Most of the recent studies use a naturally long-lived strain of mice. In one typical study, for example, half of the mice were kept on a normal diet and half on a diet restricted in calories but adequate in everything else (this is referred to as "calorie restriction with adequate nutrition"). The maximum life span of the mice on the normal diet was 41 months. However, for the calorie-restricted mice, maximum life span was pushed out to 56 months. In humans that would be the equivalent of extending life to 150 years!

These added years are not sickly years, but mostly youthful, disease-free years. Animals on a CR diet experience far less age-related disease. For example, one published report showed that breast cancer incidence fell from 40 percent in fully fed animals to only 2 percent in CR animals; lung cancer fell from 60 percent to 30 percent; liver cancer fell from 64 percent to 0 percent; leukemia fell from 65 percent to 10 percent; kidney disease fell from 100 percent to 36 percent; and cardiovascular disease fell from 63 percent to 17 percent.[22] Other conditions that are delayed or avoided by CR include arthritis, diabetes, atherosclerosis, Alzheimer's, Parkinson's, Huntington's, and virtually all age-related degenerative diseases.[23-24]

Exactly how CR extends life and mitigates disease is not fully understood. But it is known to increase DNA repair, decrease oxidative damage, increase the body's own antioxidant defense system, lower blood pressure, lower inflammation, improve glucose metabolism and insulin sensitivity, delay age-related immunological decline, and is associated with less glycation, all of which undoubtedly play a part in the improved health and longevity.

All of these factors come into play in protecting the brain from trauma and disease. In addition, CR increases brain-derived neurotrophic factor (BDNF), which increases the resistance of neurons in the brain to dysfunction and degeneration and supports repair and regrowth. Calorie restriction also diminishes or negates the detrimental effects of various neurotoxins, including the Parkinson's-causing MPTP.[25-26]

Even a small restriction in calorie consumption has been shown to be beneficial. Just 10 percent restriction shows a very measurable beneficial effect. The effect increases with 20, 30, and even 50 percent restriction. There is, of course, a lower limit. Much below 50 percent leads to starvation, and the death rate begins to increase.

In animal studies, 40-50 percent calorie restriction has produced the greatest extension in life span. In humans, restricting calories this much is too difficult to maintain. A 25 percent restriction is more doable. A normal 2,000 calorie diet would be reduced to 1,500 calories. Even still, it takes a great deal of willpower to maintain this level of restriction for life. At this level, human studies have reported improvement in various measures of health status, just as those seen in animal studies. A change in maximum life span has not yet been determined because the studies have not gone on long enough.

Since the total amount of food is decreased, what is eaten must be nutrient dense, so there are no empty calories (i.e., junk foods). Eating empty calories on a restricted diet will lead to malnutrition. This is why semi-starved populations in certain parts of the world don't live longer—they are calorie restricted *and* malnourished. Even calorie restriction proponents who load up on dietary supplements to assure complete nutrition yet neglect to get adequate amounts of fat, suffer from deficiency diseases; as was the case of the most famous CR proponent of all, Dr. Roy Walford, who after 20 years of calorie restriction died unexpectedly early from the brain wasting disease ALS.

Although CR has shown to improve many aspects of health, it is not without some problems. Even if nutrient intake is adequate, the reduction in calories stunts growth and retards development. Body mass is reduced; this includes less body fat but also results in loss of muscle. The lack of dietary fat and calories seriously affects hormone production, causing loss of libido, menstrual irregularities, and reduced bone density, which increases risk of osteoporosis later in life. Fewer calories also shift the body into a survival mode where metabolism slows down and body temperature declines, causing an increased sensitivity to cold and temperature changes. The most noticeable symptom, and the one that makes CR difficult to endure, is constant gnawing hunger.

In recent years a large number of human studies have demonstrated that low-carb diets produce the same metabolic benefits seen in CR.[27-32] Combining an ample amount of fat with a low-carbohydrate diet appears to enhance these benefits. All of the metabolic improvements associated with CR can be duplicated with a low-carb, high-fat diet without any calorie restriction.[33]

Aging is associated with elevated levels of glucose, insulin, and triglycerides. People who live over a century in relatively good health have lower blood glucose, insulin, leptin (a hormone involved in regulating body weight and metabolism), free T3 (a thyroid hormone), and serum triglycerides than those who do not live to be over one hundred years old. Researchers at Duke University and the University of Arizona have postulated that the fundamental mechanism by which calorie restriction improves life span is by an alternation in these metabolic parameters. Using a high-fat, adequate protein, low-carbohydrate diet, the researchers were able to duplicate the metabolic effects of calorie restriction completely independent of caloric intake. The diet is based on the premise that by shifting much of the body's dependence of energy from glucose to fat, many of the same physiologic changes that are seen in calorie-restricted animals will also be seen in individuals following this type of diet.[34]

In their research, patients were told to eat when they were hungry. Calories were not explicitly restricted; calorie intake was determined solely by appetite. Protein intake was limited to approximately 1.0 grams/kg lean body mass per day. As a result, most patients were instructed to eat from 50-80 grams of protein per day. Only non-starchy, fibrous vegetables were allowed. Though not explicitly stated, the general dietary intake as percent of daily caloric intake for most participants ended up to be approximately 20 percent carbohydrate, 20 percent protein, and 60 percent fat. By comparison, a typical American diet ordinarily consists of 50-60 percent carbohydrate, 10-20 percent protein, and 25-35 percent fat. Essentially, fat replaces much of the carbohydrate. As a consequence, health improves dramatically.

The study lasted for three months. During this time patients lost on average 7 pounds (3 kg) of excess body weight, even though they were not dieting and ate as much as they wanted. They showed a significant reduction in blood pressure, an average drop of over 10 mmHg. Blood levels of leptin, insulin, fasting glucose, and free T3 significantly decreased. Insulin sensitivity improved. In addition, despite the increased intake of fat, they experienced a significant decrease in triglyceride levels. Their triglyceride/HDL ratios decreased on average from 5.1 to 2.6. This is very significant. The triglyceride/HDL ratio is considered one of the most accurate indicators of heart disease risk.[35] A ratio of 4.0 or greater indicates high risk. The patients' beginning average of 5.1 was much too high. By the end of the study the average ratio dropped to a much safer 2.6. A ratio of 2.0 is considered ideal. So, within just three months' time on a high-fat, low-carb diet, they went from being at very high risk of heart disease to low risk as well as lowering their risk of diabetes and a multitude of other health problems, thus avoiding or delaying diseases that would otherwise shorten their lives.

Longevity studies using calorie restriction examine the same metabolic parameters measured in this study. This and other studies have demonstrated that high-fat, low-carbohydrate diets produce the same physiological effects as CR, but without all the drawbacks like constant hunger and disturbed hormone balance.

The low-carb, adequate protein, high-fat diet is a mild ketogenic diet, which makes it more advantageous then CR diets. In fact, studies show the low-carb, high-fat diet produces better results on metabolic parameters than calorie restriction. One study did a direct comparison of the two diets. Investigators compared a low-carb, high-fat ketogenic diet to a calorie restricted diet over a 24-week period in patients with obesity and type 2 diabetes. The low-carb diet was restricted to 20 grams or less of carbohydrate a day, with no explicit limitation on total calorie intake. The CR diet was 500 calories/day lower than normal intake, or about a 25 percent reduction. Both diets led to improvements in metabolic parameters.

Metabolic measurements included fasting glucose, blood triglyceride levels, HDL (good) cholesterol levels, VLDL (bad) cholesterol levels, total cholesterol/HDL cholesterol ratio, triglyceride/HDL cholesterol ratio, blood pressure, waist circumference, body weight, and body mass index. In every case, the measurements of the low-carb group exceeded those of the CR group. It is interesting that the low-carb group consumed more calories than the CR group, yet lost more weight and more inches around the waist. This is apparently a result of superior metabolic control and improved insulin sensitivity in the low-carb group. In diabetic patients taking insulin, the effects were often dramatic. For example, participants taking 40 to 90 units of insulin before the study were able to eliminate their insulin use while also improving glycemic control. Over 95 percent of the participants in the low-carb group were able to reduce or completely eliminate their medications (insulin, metformin, pioglitazone, glimiperide) by the end of the study. The results of this study are in agreement with a number of other studies that have evaluated the metabolic effects of low-carb, high-fat diets.[36-40]

The reason why calorie restriction protects against degenerative disease and prolongs life is not due to the reduction in calories, but to the reduction in carbohydrate. A low-carb diet, which does not restrict calories, produces better changes in metabolic parameters without the adverse side effects associated with calorie restriction. The true anti-aging diet, therefore, is one that supplies enough protein to meet the body's needs and in which fat replaces much of the carbohydrate so as to maintain adequate calorie consumption. Basically, this is a low-carb diet with no restriction on fat consumption. This type of diet has proven to improve insulin sensitivity and glucose metabolism, reduce inflammation, glycation, and free-radical generation, and therefore protect the brain from degenerative disease.[41]

EXERCISE SHARPENS THE MIND

"If exercise could be packaged in pill form, it would immediately become the number one anti-aging medicine, as well as the world's most prescribed pill," says Dr. Robert Butler of the International Longevity Center at Manhattan's Mt. Sinai Hospital. Exercise tones the muscles, strengthens the bones, improves circulation, increases energy, and sharpens the mind.

Just as exercise can bulk up the muscles, it can also bulk up the brain—literally! Regular exercise stimulates brain growth and repair, like it does with the muscles. Whether it is lifting weights or running on a treadmill, exercise tones the brain, slowing down the aging process.

As neurons age and die the brain shrinks and cognitive ability declines. Most people would assume that brain shrinkage begins when we reach middle age or later. But actually, shrinkage begins as early as your 30s and normally progresses at a rate of about 0.5 to 1 percent a year. The rate of shrinkage can increase substantially as a result of trauma, toxic exposure, infection, etc.

According to a study by Dr. Arthur Kramer and colleagues at the University of Illinois-Urbana, the rate at which the brain ages (i.e., shrinks) can dramatically slow down with just three hours of aerobic exercise a week. Kramer divided up a group of 59 adults, aged 60-79, into two groups and followed them for six months. One group participated in 1 hour of aerobics three times a week at a level of 60-70 percent of their maximum heart rate, which is pretty moderate. The other group spent 1 hour three times a week doing stretching and toning exercises. Three-dimensional MRI scans of the participants' brains were taken at the beginning and at the end of the study period. This allowed the researchers to visually compare the before and after pictures of the participants' brains. Kramer found that after only six months, the participants who exercised aerobically had the brain volumes of people three years younger. Exercise not only prevented brain shrinkage, but *stimulated neuron growth.* The exercisers were able to regain lost brain mass. Most of the growth occurred in the frontal lobe of the brain, which is involved in memory and reasoning. There was no improvement in the brains of those who did only the toning and stretching exercises.[42]

Why such remarkable improvement? Exercise improves brain health, in part by improving circulation. More blood, carrying oxygen and nutrients, is brought in to feed and nourish the brain. Exercise reduces insulin resistance and improves glucose metabolism allowing the brain to function better. In addition, exercise stimulates the activation of special neuroprotective proteins such as brain derived neurotrophic factors (BDNF) and insulin-like growth factor 1 (IGF-1), both of which defend the brain against oxidative stress and promote neuronal growth and repair.

Exercise not only slows down the normal aging process but protects against neurodegenerative diseases such as Alzheimer's and Parkinson's. Dr. E.B. Larson and colleagues at the Center for Health Studies in Seattle, Washington, found that persons

65 years of age or older who exercised three or more times a week experienced a much lower rate of Alzheimer's disease than those who exercised less or not at all.[43]

In another study, brisk walking improved memory in older people who were at high risk of developing Alzheimer's. The study involved 138 men aged 50 years or older who reported memory problems but did not yet meet the criteria for dementia. The participants were divided into two groups, one of which began a 24-week exercise program of walking for 50 minutes three days per week. The other group continued at their normal activity level. After 24 weeks, participants in the exercise group scored better on memory assessments and cognitive tests and lower on dementia ratings. Those in the control group, on the other hand, showed a decline, as would be expected as part of the normal process of aging and continued brain shrinkage. The positive effects of the exercise were still evident 18 months later.[44] The researchers stated that the effects of exercise were at least as good, and actually better, than those seen with drugs approved to aid mental function in Alzheimer's disease.

Even in Alzheimer's patients, where brain shrinkage is severe, exercise improves brain volume. The area of the brain most involved in storing and retrieving memory—the hippocampus—is protected from shrinkage.[45]

Researchers at St Jude Children's Research Hospital, in Memphis, Tennessee demonstrated that exercise increases the brain's capacity for self-repair. They showed that neurotoxic drugs that damage certain areas of the brain and induce Parkinson's disease were rendered completely harmless by regular exercise.[46]

Studies such as those described above suggest that exercise can not only slow down normal aging but potentially provide protection against a variety of neurodegenerative conditions. In essence, exercise acts as an antidote against neurodegeneration.

Many studies have shown a clear benefit with aerobic exercise—exercise that involves continuous vigorous movement such as jogging, swimming laps, or hiking. But weight lifting—a nonaerobic exercise—can also be beneficial.

Researchers at the University of British Columbia, Canada found that older women who did 1-2 hours of strength training exercises each week had improved cognitive function a year later.[47]

The researchers randomly assigned 155 women ages 65 to 75 either to strength training with dumbbells and weight machines once or twice a week, or to a comparison group doing balance and toning. The strength training classes were fairly intense. All major muscles from the shoulders and arms to the lower legs and feet were covered, so the participants received a hearty workout. The balance and toning classes consisted of a more leisurely regimen of stretching, range of motion exercises, exercises to strengthen the pelvic floor muscles, balance exercises, and relaxation techniques.

A year later, the women who did strength training improved their performance on tests of so-called executive function by 10.9 percent to 12.6 percent, while those assigned to balance and toning exercises experienced a slight deterioration of 0.5 percent. The improvements in the strength training group included an enhanced ability to make decisions, resolve conflicts, and focus on subjects without being distracted by competing stimuli.

How strength training compares with aerobic exercise has yet to be determined, but it appears that an exercise program that combines aerobic exercise with some strength training may give the greatest brain boost.

As noted in a few of the above studies, light exercise consisting of only toning and stretching exercises are of little value. Apparently, for exercise to have any real benefit it must be vigorous enough to increase heart rate, stimulate circulation, and activate neuroprotective proteins in the brain. Fortunately, you don't need to run a marathon every day to accomplish this. Moderate exercise is adequate. Significant effects can be achieved with just 1-3 hours of exercise per week.

In one study it was learned that burning as few as 209 more calories per week resulted in a 27 percent reduced risk of vascular dementia.[48] Walking at a moderate pace (3 miles or 4.8 kilometers per hour) can easily burn off 209 calories in a single hour. This study showed that adding even one hour per *week* of exercise was beneficial to the brain.

In another study, participants over the age of 55 filled out a questionnaire that categorized them into one of three levels of physical activity: none, moderate, or high. Moderate activity was defined as exercising fewer than three times a week. High activity was defined as three or more times a week. The type of exercise included walking, hiking, biking, swimming, and similar activities.

At the end of 2 years, the researchers found that 13.9 percent of the non-exercisers had developed cognitive impairment. However, in the moderate and high activity groups only 6.7 and 5.1 percent respectively developed cognitive impairment.[49] The researchers were amazed by the magnitude of the findings. "Physical activity *cut in half* the odds of developing incident cognitive impairment. We were also surprised that moderate physical activity had nearly the same effect as high physical activity," says Thorleif Etgen, MD, the lead author of the study. "The take-home message is: keep on moving," said Etgen.

Exercise doesn't have to be strenuous or of long duration. Walking is adequate if it is done at a moderate pace. A bare minimum is 30 minutes three times a week; 60 minutes three times a week is better and 5-6 days a week is best. But be careful not to overdo it. Pushing yourself too hard can lead to injury.

> Exercise has proven to be more effective than any of the drugs currently used to treat Alzheimer's disease.

18 Low-Carb Therapy

KETONE THERAPY

Ketone therapy in the form of the ketogenic diet has been used successfully for 90 years to treat epilepsy. Recent research has shown that ketone therapy can also be of benefit in treating Alzheimer's, Parkinson's, Huntington's, MS, and a number of other neurological disorders.

Neurodegenerative disorders involve a disruption of the brain's ability to metabolize glucose and produce energy. Ketones have been the key to bypass this defect, maintain energy levels, and normalize brain function. Ketone therapy, whether through a ketogenic diet or the administration of MCTs or ketone-producing medications, strives to provide the brain with the fuel it needs to achieve and maintain normal, healthy function.

With this in mind, some investigators have assumed that the higher the blood ketone levels are, the better. Research is being done to develop drugs that can increase ketone levels 10 times higher than what is possible from eating coconut or MCT oils. While some level of ketosis is necessary in order to supply the brain with the energy it needs, high blood ketone levels have not been shown to be any more effective than much lower levels. The idea that "more is better" isn't necessarily true when it comes to ketones. This is apparently the case with seizure control in epileptics. Measures of seizure protection and seizure incidence with ketones levels do not correlate.[1]

We always have measurable concentrations of ketones in our blood and urine regardless of our diet. The concentration of beta-hydroxybutyrate (BHB), the primary ketone, is typically around 0.1 mmol/l (millimoles per liter). During starvation or prolonged fasting, BHB levels increase to 2-7 mmol/l, which is also the same level achieved on the classic ketogenic diet. Therapeutic levels of ketosis that are effective in treating Alzheimer's disease can be achieved with blood levels of BHB less than 0.5 mmol/l.[2] This level can easily be achieved by consuming a 2 tablespoon dose of coconut oil. Blood levels of ketones at about this level have shown to be just as effective as those which are many times higher and typically associated with the ketogenic diet.[3] High ketone levels are not necessary.

You can think of it like filling the gas tank of your car. The tank can be filled to the top with fuel, but the engine can only burn a little at a time. The amount of gas in the tank has no effect on the rate at which the engine can burn the fuel. As long as enough gas is available to keep the engine continually running, it doesn't matter how full the tank is. The same is true with ketones. Pumping the body with more ketones than it needs will have no additional benefit. Excess ketones are not stored, like fuel is in the gas tank, or like glucose (which is stored as glycogen or fat). Ketones have a short life span in the blood. If they are not used within a few minutes, they are flushed out of the body in the urine. So a large influx of ketones into the bloodstream will end up being removed from the body and do absolutely no good.

Even when blood ketones are high, the addition of carbohydrate into the diet can initiate seizures. It is apparent that blood glucose levels also have an influence on brain function. Ketone therapy alone is not the complete answer. Controlling blood glucose levels is also vitally important.

While excessive ketone levels are not necessary, therapeutic levels should be maintained constantly throughout the day and night. Medications or supplements that boost ketone levels only last a few hours and need to be retaken often. During the day this is not a big problem, but at night it can be. At night, ketosis tapers off, and by morning, it is gone. Ketone therapy prevents the brain from dying during the day, but when ketones run out, the brain is starved and death and degeneration continue.

It is kind of like being able to breathe for 16 hours of the day and then being denied oxygen for 8 hours at night. As long as you have oxygen you are alive and well, but take away your oxygen and you begin to suffocate and die. You need oxygen 24 hours a day, not just 16. The same is true for the brain. It needs energy, ketones, 24 hours a day.

Ketone therapy that lasts only a few hours a day may slow down the progression of the disease and may even produce some improvement, but unless ketones are present day and night, the brain will gradually degenerate.

Coconut oil is better than current ketone medications or MCT oil because it produces ketones over a much longer period of time, up to eight hours. Taken just before bedtime, coconut oil keeps ketone levels elevated through the night. One drawback to this is that coconut oil also stimulates metabolism, so after eating it, a person may have so much energy that he or she may find it difficult to fall asleep.

The solution to this problem is to combine ketone therapy with a low-carb, ketogenic diet. The diet will allow the body to produce ketones continually, 24 hours a day. Even a mild ketogenic diet, when combined with the coconut oil, can maintain ketosis at a therapeutic level. Coconut oil is consumed only at mealtime, so it doesn't interfere with sleep. The brain is never denied the energy it needs. Healing continues night and day.

THE LOW-CARBOHYDRATE DIET

Insulin resistance appears to be a common problem in all forms of neurodegeneration. All the major forms of neurodegeneration improve when blood sugar is brought under control. Therefore, blood sugar control is vital in the treatment of Alzheimer's and related conditions.

The overconsumption of carbohydrate-rich foods is at the heart of the problem. Carbohydrates raise blood glucose levels. Insulin is pumped into the bloodstream to shuttle glucose from the bloodstream into the cells. When carbohydrate consumption is high, so is blood glucose—and insulin. Cells exposed to high insulin levels for extended periods of time become desensitized to the action of insulin. That is to say, they become insulin resistant. Glucose is not able to effectively get into the cells and remains elevated in the blood for extended periods of time. More insulin is then released to clear the glucose out of the blood, so insulin levels rise. As insulin levels rise, cells become more insulin resistant. This sets into motion a vicious cycle of increasing degrees of insulin resistance.

Insulin resistance affects the brain's ability to utilize glucose, which may progress to brain insulin resistance, starving the brain of energy and promoting brain cell degeneration. For this reason, Alzheimer's disease has been labeled type 3 diabetes. Simply feeding the brain ketones doesn't solve this problem. Ketone therapy is only a partial solution that provides temporary relief without addressing the underlying problem—insulin resistance.

The only way to compensate for insulin resistance is to control blood glucose levels. This is accomplished by restricting the amount of carbohydrate consumed. Prior to the discovery of insulin in the 1920s, a low-carb diet consisting of 75 percent fat, 17 percent protein, and 8 percent carbohydrate was used successfully in the treatment of diabetes. The problem with this diet, as well as the classic ketogenic diet (90 percent fat, 8 percent protein, and 2 percent carbohydrate), is that it is too difficult for most people to adhere to for any length of time. Fortunately, such a strict diet isn't necessary in order to limit carbohydrate consumption or boost ketone levels. The Atkins or low-carbohydrate diet has shown to provide a similar degree of protection while allowing a much greater variety of foods and even a higher, yet still restricted, intake of carbohydrate.

The diet proposed in this book is a modified form of the Atkins diet combined with the ketone-producing, brain-protecting power of MCTs from coconut oil. This dietary program produces enough ketones to supply the brain with the fuel it needs to function properly. In addition, it enhances insulin sensitivity, normalizes metabolic parameters, neutralizes neurotoxins, calms inflammation, stops runaway oxidative stress and destructive glycation, and subdues harmful microorganisms. In other words, it removes the underlying factors that lead to neurodegeneration and provides the energy and the building materials needed for brain revitalization.

Ketone therapy alone is not enough. Controlling blood sugar through a low-carbohydrate dietary plan is also necessary—indeed essential for optimal improvement.

This program consists of three dietary plans based on the patient's degree of insulin resistance as determined by fasting blood glucose levels.

Low-Carb 25 Gram Diet

If fasting blood glucose is 126 mg/dl (7 mmol/l) or greater, carbohydrate consumption is limited to a maximum of 25 grams per day. No single meal should exceed half of the day's total carbohydrate allowance (12.5 grams).

Low-Carb 50 Gram Diet
If fasting blood glucose is 101-125 mg/dl (5.6-6.9 mmol/l), carbohydrate consumption is limited to a maximum of 50 grams per day. No single meal should exceed half of the day's total carbohydrate allowance (25 grams).

Low-Carb 100 Gram Diet
If fasting blood glucose is 91-100 mg/dl (5.0-5.5 mmol/l), carbohydrate consumption is limited to a maximum of 100 grams per day. No single meal should exceed half of the day's total carbohydrate allowance (50 grams).

If after following the dietary guidelines in this book for a period of time, your fasting blood glucose has dropped to a lower category, you can move to the next level and increase your carbohydrate intake. For example, if you started the program at the Low-Carb 25 Gram Diet level and your fasting blood sugar is now consistently under 126 mg/dl, then you can move into the Low-Carb 50 Gram diet. But if your fasting blood sugar goes above 126 mg/dl while at this level, you need to go back to the Low-Carb 25 Gram diet regimen. Likewise, if your fasting blood glucose is consistently below 101 mg/dl, you can go to the Low-Carb 100 Gram diet.

If fasting blood sugar levels are below 91 mg/dl (5.0 mmol/l), blood sugar and insulin control is normal and apparently working properly. Neurodegenerative disorders are very unlikely at this stage. However, disregard for carbohydrate consumption, especially refined carbohydrates and particularly sweets, can eventually lead to problems later in life. For someone who has normal fasting blood glucose levels, the Low-Carb 100 Gram Diet or even a more indulgent 150 gram diet would help to forestall or even avoid the consequences of insulin resistance and neurodegeneration. However, if one of your parents or even a spouse suffers from insulin resistance, your risk of developing insulin resistance is increased.

This book is written just as much for the person who is concerned about his or her future mental health as it is for those who are already experiencing a measurable decline. Taking care of your brain starting now, before symptoms surface, is your best insurance that you will remain mentally fit long into old age.

BASIC GUIDELINES FOR THE LOW-CARB DIET

All three of the above low-carb diets are ketogenic when combined with coconut oil. Obviously, the lower the carbohydrate intake, the greater the ketogenic effect and the better the blood sugar control. Therefore, those who have the greatest problem with insulin resistance and blood sugar control need a more carbohydrate restricted diet. The Low-Carb 25 Gram Diet is the most ketogenic of the three and is low enough in carbohydrate that it can even be used for seizure control.

The low-carb diet accomplishes many things. In addition to the benefits mentioned above, this diet will condition your body to burn fat in place of sugar; change destructive eating patterns; stop uncontrollable food cravings; break addictions to sugar, soda, caffeine, white bread, alcohol, and other junk foods; allow you to enjoy eating full-fat and full-flavored foods without guilt; let you experience how delicious whole, natural foods taste; change your mental frame of mind about foods; stabilize blood sugar; allow your body a chance to heal; relinquish your dependence on drugs; and enjoy life to a greater extent.

Depending on your fasting blood sugar readings, you will follow the 25, 50, or 100 gram diet. These are the maximum amounts of carbohydrate you are allowed for the entire day. You do not need to count calories, measure the amount of fat or protein consumed, or limit what you eat, except for the carbohydrate. Eat until you are satisfied, but not stuffed. Overeating reduces the effectiveness of the diet. As much as 58 percent of the protein you eat can be converted into glucose, so you do not want to over-consume high-protein foods either. Since fat produces very little glucose, you can eat as much as you desire.

A person can live on any of these, including the 25 gram diet, indefinitely. It is not lacking in nutrients. It provides all the nutrients needed for good health. Consider the fact that the Eskimo traditionally lived, and even thrived, on a diet consisting totally of meat and fat. Carbohydrate from plant foods constituted less than 1 percent of their total calories. They were healthy without diabetes, Alzheimer's, Parkinson's, cancer, or any other degenerative disease common in our high-carb society today. This new diet allows many more plant foods, greater variety, and more nutrients then the traditional Eskimo diet. It is probably a far healthier diet than you have ever eaten before.

You do need to calculate every gram of carbohydrate you eat. This is important. As you gain experience you will be able to prepare meals without actually calculating each gram of carbohydrate. But for the first few months you need to pay particular attention to stay within your carbohydrate limit.

Most meats, fish, fowl, and all fats are free foods; meaning there is no limit on the amount you are allowed to eat. Eggs, cheese, and lettuce contain very small amounts of carbohydrate. Use the Net Carbohydrate Counter in Appendix D to calculate the amount of net carbohydrate in foods eaten. The term "net carbohydrate" refers to carbohydrate that is digestible, provides calories, and raises blood sugar. Dietary fiber is also a carbohydrate, but it does not raise blood sugar or supply calories, so it is not included. Most plant foods will contain both digestible carbohydrate and fiber. To calculate the net carbohydrate content, you subtract the fiber from the total. The Carbohydrate Counter in Appendix D lists net carbohydrate on various whole foods. You can figure out the net carbohydrate content of packaged foods yourself. The Nutrition Facts label on packages show the amount of calories, fat, carbohydrate, protein, and other nutrients per serving. Under the "Total Carbohydrate" heading you will see "Dietary Fiber." To calculate the net carbohydrate content, subtract the grams of fiber listed, from the grams of total carbohydrate.

The Carbohydrate Counter lists the most common vegetables, fruits, dairy, grains, nuts, and seeds. To find foods not on the list, including many popular packaged and restaurant foods, go online to www.calorieking.com. On this website, type in the food you are looking for and you will get a listing of everything included on a Nutrition Facts label. To find the net carbohydrate content you must go through the same steps you do with any Nutrition Facts label and subtract the

Nutrition Facts
Serving Size 1 box (28g)

Amount Per Serving	
Calories	110
Calories from Fat	10
	% Daily Value*
Total Fat 1g	**2%**
Saturated Fat 0g	**0%**
Trans Fat 0g	
Polyunsaturated Fat 0g	
Monounsaturated Fat 0.5g	
Cholesterol 0mg	**0%**
Sodium 170mg	**7%**
Potassium 4mg	**1%**
Total Carbohydrate 24g	**8%**
Dietary Fiber 1g	**4%**
Sugars 10g	
Protein 1g	

Vitamin A 8%	Vitamin C 8%
Calcium 8%	Iron 20%
Vitamin D 8%	Thiamin 20%
Riboflavin 20%	Niacin 20%
Vitamin B_6 20%	Folic Acid 20%
Vitamin B_{12} 20%	Zinc 20%

*Percent Daily Values are based on a 2,000 calorie diet.

This product contains 24 grams of total carbohydrate and 1 gram of fiber. Total net carbs is 23 grams.

fiber from total carbohydrate listed. There are several websites that provide the carbohydrate count on various foods. Another good one is www.carb-counter.org.

In order to stay under your carbohydrate limit for the day, you will want to eliminate or dramatically reduce all high-carb foods in the diet. For instance, a slice of white bread contains 12 grams of carbohydrate. If you are on the Low-Carb 25 Gram Diet, just two slices will bring you to your day's limit. Since all vegetables and fruits contain carbohydrate, you would be restricted to eating only meat and fat for the rest of the day in order to stay under your 25 gram limit—which is not a good idea. A single medium-size baked potato contains 33 grams of carbohydrate—more than a day's allotment. An apple has 18 grams, an orange 12 grams, and a medium-size banana 24 grams. Breads and grains contain the highest amount of carbohydrate. A single 4-inch pancake without any syrup or sweeteners has 13 grams, a 10-inch tortilla has 34 grams, and a plain 4½-inch bagel has 57 grams. Candy and desserts are even higher in carbohydrate and provide almost no nutritional value, so they should be completely eliminated from the diet. All breads and most fruits are very limited if not totally eliminated, especially on the 25 and 50 gram diets.

Vegetables, however, have much lower carbohydrate content. One cup of asparagus has 2 grams, a cup of raw cabbage 2 grams, and a cup of cauliflower 3 grams. All lettuce is very low in carbohydrate: a cup of shredded lettuce has only about 0.6 gram. You can easily fill up on green salad and other low-carb vegetables without worrying too much about going over your carbohydrate limit.

Even on the Low-Carb 25 Gram Diet a limited amount of fruit can be consumed. Fruits with the lowest carbohydrate content are berries such as blackberries (½ cup 3.5 grams), boysenberries (½ cup 4.5 grams), raspberries (½ cup 3 grams), and strawberries (½ cup, sliced 4.8 grams). Any fruit, vegetable, or even grain product can be eaten, as long as the portion size is not so big that it puts you over your carbohydrate limit. Since most fruits, starchy vegetables, and breads are high in carbohydrate, it is best to simply avoid them altogether.

Let's look at a typical daily meal plan for the Low-Carb 25 Gram Diet. Net carbs for each item are listed in parentheses.

Breakfast

Omelet with 2 eggs (1.2 g), 1 ounce of cheddar cheese (0.4 g), ½ cup sliced mushrooms (1.2 g), 2 ounces of diced sugar-free ham (0 g), and one teaspoon of chopped chives (<0.1 g), cooked in 1 tablespoon of coconut oil (0 g). Net carbohydrate count 2.8 grams.

Lunch

Tossed green salad with 2 cups shredded lettuce (1.2 g), ½ cup shredded carrot (4 g), ¼ cup diced sweet bell pepper (1.1 g), ½ medium tomato (1.7 g), ¼ avocado (0.9 g), ½ cup shredded cabbage (1.6 g), 3 ounces chopped roasted chicken (0 g), 1 tablespoon roasted sunflower seeds (1 g), topped with 2 tablespoons of olive oil-based Italian dressing, without sugar (1 g). Net carbohydrate count 12.5 grams.

Dinner

One or more pork chops (0 g), 1 cup cooked asparagus (2.4 g) with 1 teaspoon of butter (0 g), 2 cups cooked cauliflower (3.2 g) topped with 1 ounce of Colby cheese (0.7 g) with various herbs and spices (<0.1 g) to enhance flavor. Net carbohydrate count 6.3 grams.

Total net carbohydrate consumed in the above three meals is 21.6 grams, which is 3.4 grams under the 25 gram daily limit. As you see from this example, the diet provides a variety of nutritious foods. In a Low-Carb 50 Gram Diet, 28.1 grams of net carbs could be added to the above. This could be in the form of higher-carb vegetables, fruits, or even a small amount of whole grains.

A Low-Carb 100 Gram Diet is very lenient in comparison to the other two diets. It includes essentially all types of foods. Simply reducing portion sizes or frequency of eating starchy vegetables, fruits, grain products, and even occasional treats can easily keep total carbohydrate consumption within bounds.

In comparison, let's look at the carbohydrate content of some typical unrestricted meals. A typical breakfast might include a 1 cup serving of Frosted Flakes cereal (35 g) with ½ cup serving of 2% milk (12.5 g). Total carbohydrate count comes to 47 grams. A single serving of this cold cereal, which is very typical in carb content, exceeds the 25 gram limit and eats up almost the entire carbohydrate allotment of the 50 gram limit. Obviously, cold cereals are not a good option for those following a low-carb eating plan.

Most people realize that cold breakfast cereals are not the healthiest of foods. People eat them because they are convenient, quick, and generally tasty. People certainly shouldn't eat them for their nutritional content. Hot whole grain cereal is considered a better choice. While a bowl of hot oatmeal is more nutritious than an equal portion of cold cereal, the carbohydrate content is about the same. A one cup serving of cooked oatmeal (21.3 g), with 1 tablespoon of sugar (12 g) and ½ cup of 2% milk (12.5 g) provides a total carbohydrate count of 45.8 grams.

A typical lunch might include a MacDonald's Big Mac hamburger (42 g), one medium fries (43.3 g), and a 12-ounce soda (39.9 g) providing a whopping 125.2 grams of carbohydrate, more than the daily limit of any of the three diet programs.

A typical dinner might include three medium-size slices of pepperoni pizza (97.2 g) and a 12-ounce soda (39.9 g), providing 137.1 grams of carbohydrate.

Most typical meals are carbohydrate-rich. Consequently, the average American (or European or Australian) consumes in excess of 300 grams of carbohydrate a day. The best way to avoid excess carbohydrate is to make your meals at home using fresh, low-carb ingredients.

Does this mean you can't have pizza anymore? You will have to make some difficult decisions. Do you want pizza or do you want dementia? It's your choice. You must decide if eating a pizza is more important to you than your ability to think clearly and remember who your family and friends are and to not be totally dependent on someone else for all your needs. If you are thinking that eating pizza, or ice cream, or soda, or whatever is not going to hurt, then you are addicted to those foods. You are in denial. The sure sign of addiction is to ignore sound reason in favor of satisfying cravings. You need this diet to break those addictions.

This low-carb eating plan really doesn't forbid any type of food; it only sets limits on how much you eat. So, you can eat pizza occasionally, but restrict the portion size and make adjustments in the other foods you eat so that your daily carbohydrate consumption remains within the limits established by your diet program.

It is not a good idea to be too indulgent by eating one high-carb meal in anticipation of eliminating all carbs from the other two meals to make up for it. Let's assume you are on the Low-Carb 50 Gram Diet and you splurge by eating a piece of pie with 46 grams of carbohydrate. That leaves you with just 4 grams of carbs for the rest of the day. You would have to eat almost nothing but meat for two meals to make up for it. Even if you managed to do this, it is not a good idea. The 46 grams of carbohydrate consumed all at once is going to unleash a metabolic tidal wave in your body. The reason for limiting carbohydrate consumption in the first place is to avoid large influxes of sugar into your bloodstream, as this is what throws the body out of whack. It is best to divide your carbohydrate consumption over all three meals so that no single meal contains more than half of a day's total allotment.

Obviously you cannot gorge yourself on pizza or ice cream as you may have as a teenager. The body is very sensitive to carbohydrates. A single candy bar can be very destructive. The sugar it contains is enough to block the formation of ketone bodies and significantly lower ketone levels, not to mention what it does to blood sugar levels.

Often a caretaker who is responsible for someone with advanced neurodegenerative disease will say, "Oh, but he likes ice cream so much, I can't deny him." Well of course he likes ice cream, everybody likes ice cream. By feeding high-carb foods to someone who is suffering from neurodegeneration, you are contributing to their illness and continual mental decline. You are not doing him any favors. Replace the ice cream with a low-carb alternative, such as a bowl of sliced strawberries and cream. There are also many low-carb versions of favorite foods available at the grocery store.

Food preferences can and do change. As you begin to eat more vegetables, especially when combined with butter, cheese, and rich sauces, they will become more satisfying than the junk foods you used to eat.

You are encouraged to eat at least one fresh, raw salad every day. A variety of tossed green salads can be made by simply changing the type of vegetables, toppings, and dressings you use.

Homemade salad dressings are generally the best. If you use a store bought dressing, avoid those with added sugar. Check the Nutrition Facts label for carbohydrate content. See Chapter 20 for dressing recipes.

Very simple dinners may consist of a main course of your favorite meat—roast beef, roasted chicken, lamb chop, baked salmon, lobster, etc.—served along with a side dish or two of raw or cooked vegetables, such as steamed broccoli topped with butter and melted cheddar cheese.

You will find a few low-carb recipes in Chapter 20 to get you started. With the popularization of low-carb dieting, there has been an explosion of low-carb recipes. There are many dozens of low-carb cookbooks available at the bookstore or library and many hundreds of low-carb recipes on the Internet. Just do a search for "low-carb recipes" and you will find a number of websites with free recipes. You must check the total carbohydrate content of each recipe. Not all recipes that claim to be "low-carb" are really that low. Many are reduced carb versions of standard favorites, but still deliver a substantial amount of carbohydrate.

You are encouraged to eat full-fat foods, butter, cream, coconut oil, the fat on meat, and chicken skin. Fat is good for you. Fat satisfies hunger and prevents food cravings. Desires for sweets will greatly diminish. Because fat is filling, hunger can be satisfied with less food, so total calorie consumption may decline somewhat. Those who are overweight may even see a reduction in weight. Underweight and undernourished people usually don't have a problem with losing weight, but the added fat in their diet helps them to regain weight to a more healthy level.

Eating out can be a little challenging but has gotten much easier over the years. Because of the popularity of low-carbing, many restaurants now offer low-carb options. Most every restaurant that sells hamburgers, including all the popular fast food restaurants, offer bunless hamburgers. These hamburgers include everything you would expect in a regular hamburger but are wrapped in a blanket of lettuce without the bun. Even if this item isn't listed on the menu, most restaurants will be happy to make it for you on request.

KETOSIS TEST STRIPS

Once a ketogenic diet is started, it takes a few days for blood levels of ketones to build up. While we always have some ketones in our blood, the levels are usually too low to be of any therapeutic value. During starvation, fasting, or carbohydrate restriction, ketone production increases. Once the liver's stores of glucose are depleted, ketone production shifts into high gear. After two or three days you will be able to measure the relative amount of ketones in the blood using a urine ketosis test strip, also known as a lipolysis test strip.

One end of the test strip is dipped into a fresh specimen of urine. The strip changes color depending on the ketone concentration in the urine. With the test strip a person can tell if their blood ketone level is "none," "trace," "small," "moderate," or "large." The test is helpful in that it indicates that the dietary changes are producing ketones, and to what degree. As you add more carbohydrate into the diet, ketone levels drop. To increase ketosis you can reduce carbohydrate consumption.

Generally, the Low-Carb 25 Gram Diet will produce a measurable reading on the test strips. The Low-Carb 50 Gram Diet may or may not produce a reading depending on how carb sensitive a person is. The Low-Carb 100 Gram Diet will generally not register on the test strips. The fact that the test strips may indicate none does not mean the blood is devoid of all ketones. It means that the ketone level is too low to be detected using the strips. Ketones will, however, be in the blood at a slightly higher level than normal.

Adding coconut oil to these diets will enhance ketone levels. Coconut oil on its own, regardless of the diet, will produce some level of ketosis, depending on the amount consumed. Coconut oil will elevate each of the Low-Carb Diets to a higher level of ketosis. Even the Low-Carb 100 Gram Diet, with coconut oil added, can produce a measurable reading.

Heavy water consumption may affect the readings. Although blood ketosis levels may be elevated, drinking a lot of water will dilute the urine, which will in turn, dilute the reading. So you can be in moderate or high ketosis even though the test strips may indicate only trace or none.

Although not required, the test strips can be helpful in encouraging compliance to the program and maintaining carbohydrate restriction. Ketosis test strips are sold in pharmacies. A popular brand is Ketostix.

BASIC FOOD CHOICES

Meats

You can eat all fresh meats—beef, pork, lamb, buffalo, venison, and game meats. All cuts of meat such as steaks, ribs, roasts, chops, and ground beef, pork, and lamb can be consumed. Red meat from organically raised, grass-fed animals without hormones and antibiotics is preferred. Leave the fat on the meat and eat it. Fat is necessary for proper protein metabolism and enhances the flavor of the meat.

Processed meats that contain nitrates, nitrites, MSG, or sugar should be avoided. This includes most lunch and processed meats like hot dogs, bratwurst, sausage, bacon, and ham. However, processed meats with only herbs and spices added are allowed. Read the ingredient labels. If they don't contain chemical additives or sugar they are likely okay to use. If they contain only a small amount of sugar and no other chemicals, you may still use them if you take in account the sugar and add it to your total carbohydrate allotment for the day. If you eat breaded meats or meatloaf you must account for the carbohydrate content.

All forms of fowl are allowed—chicken, turkey, duck, goose, Cornish hen, quail, pheasant, emu, ostrich, and all others. Do not remove the skin; eat it along with the meat. It is often the tastiest part. All eggs are allowed.

All forms of fish and shellfish are allowed—salmon, tuna, sole, trout, catfish, flounder, sardines, herring, crab, lobster, oysters, mussels, clams, and all others. Wild-caught fish is recommended over farm raised. Fish roe or caviar is also allowed.

Most *fresh* meats do not have carbohydrate. They are free foods, so you can eat them without doing any calculations on carbohydrate content. The only exceptions are some shell fish and eggs, which do contain a small amount of carbohydrate. A large chicken egg, for instance, contains about 0.6 grams of carbohydrate.

Processed meats are not free foods. They often have added carbohydrate, so you will need to calculate the carb content using the Nutrition Facts label on the package.

One of the things many people miss when they go on a low-carb diet is the crispy snacks they used to eat—the pretzels, chips, crackers. These, of course, are too high in carbohydrate and often contain unwanted additives such as iron and high fructose corn syrup. A zero-carb alternative is fried pork rinds, sometimes also called pork skins. Pork rinds are made from the layer of fat under the animal's skin. As the fat is rendered off, only the protein matrix is left. These crispy treats can be eaten as snacks, used in place of croutons in salads, crushed and used as breading in frying fish or chicken, or as a topping on casseroles or other dishes.

Dairy

Some dairy products are relatively high in carbohydrate while others are low. A cup of whole milk contains 11 grams of carbohydrate; 2% has 11.4 grams and 1% has 12.2 grams. As you can see, as the fat content decreases, carbohydrate content increases.

A cup of full-fat plain yogurt contains 12 grams of carbohydrate and a cup of fat-free yogurt 19 grams. Sweetened vanilla low-fat yogurt has 31 grams and fruited low-fat yogurt 43 grams.

Most hard cheeses are very low in carbohydrate. Soft cheeses have a little higher carb count but are still not bad. Good cheese choices include cheddar, Colby, Monterey, mozzarella, gruyere, Edam, Swiss, feta, cream cheese (plain), cottage cheese, and goat cheese. An ounce of cheddar cheese has only 0.4 grams. A full cup of cheddar cheese contains a mere 1.5 grams. A cup of cottage cheese has 8 grams; a tablespoon of plain cream cheese contains 0.4 grams. Whey cheese and imitation cheese products have a much higher carb content and should be avoided.

Heavy cream has a little over 6 grams per cup. Half and half contains 10 grams per cup, so you would want to stick with full-fat cream. A tablespoon of sour cream has 0.5 grams.

You can eat most cheeses and creams without overloading on carbs, but be careful with milk and yogurt. Sweetened dairy products like eggnog, ice cream, and chocolate milk should be avoided.

Fats and Oils

Fats and oils contain no carbohydrate, so they are free foods and you can eat as much as you like. Some fats are healthier than others. Choose fats from the "Preferred Fats" category below. All of these oils are safe for food preparation. Steer away from the "Non-Preferred Fats" and never use them in cooking. Completely avoid the "Bad Fats," all foods that contain them, and foods cooked in them such as fries and battered fish.

Preferred Fats

Coconut Oil
Palm Oil/Palm Fruit Oil
Palm Shortening
Red Palm Oil
Palm Kernel Oil
Extra Light Olive Oil
Extra Virgin Olive Oil
Macadamia Nut Oil
Avocado Oil
Animal Fat (lard, tallow, meat drippings)
Butter
Ghee
MCT Oil

Non-Preferred Fats

Corn Oil
Safflower Oil
Sunflower Oil
Soybean Oil
Cottonseed Oil
Canola Oil
Peanut Oil
Walnut Oil
Pumpkin Seed Oil

Bad Fats

Margarine
Shortening
Hydrogenated Vegetable Oils

Vegetables

You are encouraged to eat plenty of vegetables. Most vegetables are relatively low in carbohydrate. You can easily get the government's recommended five servings without going over 25 grams of carbohydrate. Serving sizes are generally about ½ cup. A half cup each of cooked cabbage, asparagus, broccoli, mushrooms, and green beans provides a total of less than 9 grams of carbs. You should eat at least twice this amount every day along with other appropriate low-carb foods.

Salad greens provide the greatest bulk with the least amount of carbs. Lettuce has less than 1 gram of carbohydrate per cup. A tossed salad consisting of two cups of lettuce, 1 cup of mixed low-carb vegetables, and ½ cup of medium-carb vegetables plus a tablespoon or two of Italian dressing could easily come to under 9 grams of carbs. You can add on cheese and meat without seriously affecting the total carb count. At least one raw salad daily is highly recommended.

Although you are encouraged to eat both raw and cooked vegetables, raw vegetables are preferred. When vegetables are cooked, starches and cellulose (fiber) are broken down somewhat and are more easily converted into sugar. For this reason, cooked vegetables tend to raise blood sugar levels more than raw vegetables.

Vegetables are listed below according to their relative carbohydrate content. Vegetables with 6 grams of carbohydrate or less per cup are listed in the low-carb group. Some of these vegetables, particularly the leafy greens, have much less than 6 grams. The average carbohydrate content for the vegetables in the low-carb list is about 3 grams per cup. Most of the vegetables you eat should come from this group.

The medium-carb vegetable group has between 7 and 14 grams of carbohydrate per cup. These vegetables should be eaten in moderation. Eating too many can easily go over the 25 gram diet limit and possibly even the 50 gram diet limit. A cup of chopped onions contains 14 grams of carbohydrate. However, it isn't often you would want to eat this much onion. A couple of tablespoons or less is more likely. A tablespoon of chopped onion has less than 1 gram of carbs.

High-carb starchy vegetables are packed with carbohydrate. One medium-sized baked potato delivers a whopping 33 grams of carbohydrate. While no vegetable is strictly off-limits, it makes sense that you would want to avoid eating these types of vegetables as a general rule, especially if you are on the 25 gram diet. One serving can eat up an entire day's worth of your carbohydrate allowance. Even in the 50 gram diet, eating a single serving would severely limit your food choices for the rest of the day. The 100 gram diet may include some starchy vegetables, but again, they should be limited to just one meal at most, and even then to one serving.

Most types of winter squash are high in carbohydrate. Two exceptions are pumpkin and spaghetti squash, which have about half the amount of carbohydrate as other squashes. Spaghetti squash gets its name from the fact that after it is cooked, it separates into strings resembling spaghetti noodles. These "noodles" can be used as a replacement for noodles in some pasta dishes. For example, a low-carb spaghetti dish can be made by topping the spaghetti squash noodles with meat and sauce.

Fresh corn is listed in the high-carb category. Technically, corn is not a vegetable, it is a grain, but it is typically eaten like a vegetable. Corn contains over 25 grams of carbohydrate per cup.

Low-Carb Vegetables (less than 6 g/cup)

Artichoke
Avocado
Asparagus
Bamboo Shoots
Bean Sprouts (mung bean)
Beet Greens
Bok Choy
Broccoli
Brussels Sprouts
Cabbage
Cauliflower
Celery
Celery Root/Celeriac
Chard
Chives
Collard Greens
Cucumber
Daikon Radish
Eggplant
Endive
Fennel
Green Beans
Herbs and Spices
Jicama

Kale
Lettuce (all types)
Mushrooms
Napa Cabbage
Okra
Kohlrabi
Peppers (hot and sweet)
Radish
Rhubarb
Sauerkraut
Scallions
Seaweed (nori, kombu, and wakame)
Sprouts (alfalfa, clover, broccoli, radish)
Sorrel
Spinach
Snow Peas
Summer Squash
Taro leaves
Tomatillos
Tomato
Turnips
Water Chestnuts
Watercress
Wax Beans
Zucchini

Medium-Carb Vegetables (between 7-14 g/cup)
Beets
Carrot
Leeks
Onion
Parsnip
Pumpkin
Rutabaga
Soybean (edamame)
Spaghetti Squash

High-Carb Starchy Vegetables (over 15 g/cup)
Chickpeas (garbanzo)
Corn (fresh)
Dry Beans (pinto, black, kidney, etc.)
Jerusalem Artichoke
Lima beans
Lentils
Peas
Potato
Sweet Potato
Taro root
Winter Squash (acorn, butternut, etc.)
Yams

Fruits

A few fruits can be incorporated into the diet if eaten sparingly. Berries have the lowest carbohydrate content of all the fruits. Blackberries and raspberries contain about 7 grams per cup. Strawberries, boysenberries, and gooseberries have a little more, about 9 grams per cup. Blueberries, however, have a much higher carb content, nearly 18 grams per cup. Lemons and limes are also low in carbs, containing less than 4 grams per fruit. Most other fruits typically deliver about 15 to 30 grams of carbohydrate per cup.

With careful planning you can incorporate some low-carb fruits into even the 25 gram diet. More fruit can be added to the 50 and 100 gram diets. Because of their high sugar content, fruits should always be eaten in moderation. Choose fresh fruits over canned or frozen. With fresh fruit you know exactly what you are getting. Canned and frozen fruits often have added sugar or syrup.

Dried fruit is extraordinarily sweet because the sugar is concentrated. For example, a cup of fresh grapes contains about 26 grams of carbohydrate while a cup of dried grapes (raisins) contains 109 grams. Dates, figs, currants, raisins, and fruit leathers are so sweet that they are little more than candy.

Low-Carb Fruits

Boysenberries	Lemon	Raspberries
Blackberries	Lime	Strawberries
Gooseberries	Cranberries (unsweetened)	

High-Carb Fruits

Apple	Grapes	Passion fruit
Apricot	Guava	Peach
Banana	Kiwi	Pear
Blueberries	Kumquat	Persimmon
Cherries	Mango	Pineapple
Currants	Melons	Plum
Dates	Mulberries	Prunes
Elderberries	Nectarine	Raisins
Figs	Orange	Tangerine
Grapefruit	Papaya	

Nuts and Seeds

At first, you might think of nuts and seeds as being high in carbohydrate, but surprisingly they are only a modest source. For example, one cup of sliced almonds contains only a little more than 7 grams of carbohydrate. A single whole almond supplies about 0.10 gram of carbohydrate.

Most tree nuts deliver about 6-10 grams of carbs per cup. Cashews and pistachios pack a higher carbohydrate punch of 40 and 21 grams per cup respectively.

Seeds are generally more carbohydrate rich than nuts. Both sesame seeds and sunflower seeds contain about 16 grams per cup.

Black walnut, pecan, and coconut contain the lowest carbohydrate content of all the common nuts and seeds. One cup of shredded raw coconut has less than 5 grams of carbohydrate. One cup of dried, desiccated, unsweetened coconut has 7 grams. Canned coconut milk has about 6 grams per cup. In comparison, whole dairy milk with 11 grams per cup. Coconut milk can make a suitable lower carb substitute for dairy milk in most recipes.

All nuts and seeds can be used as toppings on vegetables and salads if the serving size is limited to a tablespoon or two. When eaten as a snack it is best to stick with the low-carb nuts. The nuts in the low-carb category below contain less than 10 grams of carbohydrate per cup. Those in the high-carb list have 11 grams or more per cup.

Low-Carb Nuts and Seeds

Almond	Coconut	Macadamia
Black walnut	English Walnuts	Pecan
Brazil nuts	Hazelnut (Filberts)	

High-Carb Nuts and Seeds

Cashew	Pistachio	Soy Nuts
Peanut	Pumpkin Seed	Sunflower Seed
Pine nuts	Sesame Seed	

Breads and Grains

Breads and grains are among the highest sources of carbohydrate. On the 25 and 50 gram diets you will generally need to eliminate all breads, grains, and cereals. This includes wheat, barley, cornmeal, oats, rice, amaranth, arrowroot, millet, quinoa, pasta, couscous, cornstarch, and bran. A single serving can eat up all or most of the day's carbohydrate allotment. A large soft pretzel contains 97 grams of carbohydrate; a cup of Froot Loops breakfast cereal supplies 25 grams, and a cup of Raisin Bran cereal contains 39 grams. A cup of Cream of Wheat with a half cup of milk and a spoonful of honey comes to 48 grams of carbohydrate.

Whole grain breads and cereals are more nutritious and have a much higher fiber content than refined breads; however, the carbohydrate content is almost the same. A slice of whole wheat bread delivers about 11 grams of carbohydrate, while a slice of white bread has 12 grams. Not a big difference.

A small amount of flour or cornstarch can be used to thicken gravies and sauces. One tablespoon of whole wheat flour contains 4.5 grams of carbohydrate. A tablespoon of cornstarch contains 7 grams. This must be calculated into your daily total carbohydrate allotment, so you don't want to use too much. Cornstarch has greater thickening power than wheat or other flours so a smaller amount can be used to accomplish the same effect.

A non-carb thickening option is to use cream cheese, which will impart a cheesy flavor to the gravy or sauce. Another non-carb and tasteless thickener is xanthan gum, a soluble vegetable fiber commonly used as a thickening agent in processed foods. A similar product is ThickenThin not/Starch thickener. This product can be used to thicken sauces the way cornstarch or flour do, and since it is made from fiber it has no net carbs. Both ThickenThin not/Starch and xanthan gum powder are available at health food stores and online.

Beverages

Beverages are among the biggest contributors to diabetes and obesity. Most beverages are loaded with sugar and provide little or no nutrition. Sodas and powdered drinks are no more than liquid candy. Even fruit juices and sports drinks are primarily sugar water. One cup of orange juice contains 25 grams of carbs. Vegetable juices are not much better. Many beverages contain caffeine, which is addicting and encourages the overconsumption of sugary beverages. Many people habitually down five, six, or 10 cups of coffee or cans of cola a day. Some people don't even drink water, relying solely on beverages of one type or another for their daily fluid needs. You should avoid all caffeinated beverages. Caffeine mimics the effect of sugar on blood glucose levels by stimulating insulin release. It also blocks transport of glucose across the blood-brain barrier.[4]

The absolute best beverage for the body is water. When the body is dehydrated and needs fluids, it requires water, not a Coke or a cappuccino. Water satisfies thirst better than any beverage without the added baggage of sugar, caffeine, or chemicals.

Water is by far the best option and I encourage you to make it your first choice. You can spike the water—or club soda, which is basically carbonated water without sweetening or flavoring—with a little fresh lemon or lime juice to give it flavor. Another option is unsweetened essence-flavored seltzer water. Unsweetened herbal teas and decaffeinated coffee are essentially carb-free. Stay away from all artificially sweetened low-calorie soft drinks. Artificial sweeteners carry health risks and keep sugar cravings alive and active.

Dehydration increases blood sugar concentration and exacerbates insulin resistance. Most people are slightly dehydrated most of the time. People often ignore their body's internal signals of thirst until dehydration is well under way. This situation is compounded in the elderly because the sense of thirst declines with age. Most people, especially the elderly, would benefit by taking greater effort to drink approved beverages more often. As a rule of thumb, you should drink at least eight 8-ounce (240 ml) servings of water daily. In the summer or when temperatures are hot you may need to increase this to 10-12 servings a day or more.

Condiments

Condiments include herbs, spices, garlic, salt, seasonings, salt substitutes, vinegar, mustard, horseradish, relish, hot sauce, fish sauce, and the like. Most condiments are allowed because they are used in such small quantities that the amount of carbohydrate consumed is insignificant. There are a couple of exceptions however. Ketchup, sweet pickle relish, barbeque sauce, and some salad dressings are loaded with sugar. In many cases you can find low-carb versions. You need to read the ingredient and Nutrition Facts labels on all prepared foods.

Most salad dressings are made with polyunsaturated vegetable oil. A better choice is an olive oil-based dressing or a homemade dressing. See Chapter 20 for dressing recipes and ideas. Vinegar and olive oil or vinegar and water make excellent dressings. Vinegar is especially good because it has shown to improve insulin sensitivity and to lower blood sugar levels by as much as 30 percent after a high-carb meal.[5] The effects of vinegar have been compared favorably to metformin, a popular medication used for blood sugar control.[6] Incorporating a little vinegar into your diet would be beneficial.

Sugar and Sweets

It is best to avoid *all* sweeteners and foods that contain them, especially on the 25 and 50 gram diets. One of the signs of carbohydrate addiction, and a potential or existing blood sugar problem, is a craving for sweets. The so-called "natural" sweeteners such as honey, molasses, sucanat (dehydrated sugarcane juice), fructose, agave syrup, and such are no better than white sugar. All foods containing artificial sweeteners and sugar substitutes such as aspartame, Splenda, xyitol, sorbitol, and stevia should also be avoided. Stevia is an herbal extract that is used as a no-calorie sweetener. Although it is considered to be a healthier alternative to most other sweeteners, it keeps sugar cravings alive and interferes with ketone production.

Lisa had been on the Low-Carb 25 Gram diet for several weeks but her ketone levels, as measured by ketosis test strips, were only at the "trace" to "small" level. Her husband, who was eating the exact same foods, had a ketone reading at the "high" level. The only difference in their food consumption was that Lisa routinely drank water sweetened with stevia. Before starting the new diet she was addicted to sugar and was controlling the addiction, or so she thought, by drinking stevia-sweetened water. Suspecting stevia to be the problem, she discontinued using it and her ketone levels rose abruptly.

All sweeteners, even the natural ones, feed sugar addiction. When the tongue senses sweetness, it doesn't make a difference if it is from granulated sugar, Splenda, or stevia; cravings for sweets are maintained. When you are tempted, your willpower will be tested. Once you break down and eat a forbidden sweet, it will be easier to repeat the action the next time temptation arises and, before you know it, you are hopelessly trapped in the clutches of carbohydrate addiction.

Once you break your addiction to sugar, sweets lose their control over you. They become less appealing. You can take them or leave them. They no longer control you; you control them. If you do indulge, you decide when and where. You are in charge.

In packaged foods, sugar can appear under a variety of names. Listed below are some of the different names for various types of sugar.

Agave
Barley malt
Brown rice syrup
Corn syrup
Date sugar
Dextrin
Dextrose
Dulcitol
Fructose
Fruit juice
Glucose
High fructose corn syrup
Honey
Lactose
Levulose
Maltodextrin
Maltose
Mannitol
Maple sugar
Maple syrup
Molasses
Saccharose
Sorbitol
Sorghum
Sucanat
Sucrose
Treacle
Turbinado
Xylitol
Xylose

Snacks

Occasionally you may want a snack between meals. Often when a person starts to feel hungry in the middle of the day, the reason isn't because of hunger but thirst. Simply drinking a glass of water is enough to satisfy these feelings.

If water isn't satisfying enough, there are some low-carb options. Vegetables such as cucumber, daikon radish, and celery make good snacks. Celery sticks can be filled with peanut butter or cream cheese. One tablespoon of peanut butter has 2 grams of carbs and a tablespoon of plain cream cheese 0.4 grams.

If you crave a crispy snack, pork rinds with zero carbs can fit the bill. Another crispy snack is nori—a seaweed. Nori is popular in Japanese cooking and is used as the wrapper for sushi. It is commonly sold dried and roasted in paper thin 8 x 8-inch (20 x 20-cm) sheets. Nori has a mild salty seafood flavor. It can be cut into bite-size squares and eaten like chips. It is usually purchased in a package containing 10 sheets. One sheet has essentially zero carbs.

Low-carb nuts such as almonds, pecans, and coconut make good snacks. A quarter of a cup of these nuts supplies about 2.5 grams of carbohydrate.

Meat, cheese, and eggs are other good snack foods. A 1-ounce slice of cheese has about 0.5 grams of carbs. Eggs have about the same. Meat has none, unless it is processed. Some simple snacks are deviled eggs, or string cheese, and cucumber "boats" filled with tuna salad, and sliced cheese and ham rolled together with a little mustard or sour cream or rolled around some fresh sprouts.

Store-bought protein bars are popular with low-carbers. I don't recommend them. They are nothing more than glorified candy bars and sweetened with artificial sweeteners or sugar substitutes. They are just a form of processed junk food.

DIETARY SUPPLEMENTS

At first glance, because many foods are restricted, including some healthy foods, it may seem that the diet could be lacking in nutrients. That is not the case. This diet supplies all the nutrition a person needs to be healthy.

For some reason, people tend to assume that meat and fat are nutritionally poor foods. That is far from the truth. Meat provides plenty of nutrition. In fact, it is an excellent source of many vitamins and minerals, supplying some essential nutrients not easily obtainable from plant sources, such as vitamins A, B_6, and B_{12} as well as CoQ10, zinc, and other nutrients. Fat, as discussed earlier, enhances the absorption of vitamins and minerals. In fact, this diet will supply you with far more nutrients than you had when the bulk of your diet consisted of low-fat, empty calorie foods.

This is not a meat diet. Make note of that. It includes plenty of natural, whole plant foods, both raw and cooked. The amount of meat you eat on this diet may increase slightly (perhaps 5 percent of total calories) to replace some of the carbohydrate you remove, but most of the added nutrition will come from a better quality, nutritionally dense source of carbohydrate—fresh vegetables. You will be eating more vegetables than you probably have in your entire life. You could call this a vegetable-based diet supplemented with ample fat and adequate protein.

You do not need to take dietary supplements to make up for any missing nutrients because there aren't any that are missing. If you are already taking supplements and would like to continue them, you can.

Despite everything that has just been said, I do recommend certain supplements *at the start of the diet.* This isn't a requirement, but it is strongly suggested. The reason for this is that most people are deficient in many essential and supportive nutrients, especially older people. Adding certain vitamins and minerals will help to make up for nutritional deficiencies and speed your progress. The supplements should be taken for the first two to three months of the program. By then, nutrient reserves should be restored and the foods in the diet should provide adequate nutrition so that supplementation is no longer necessary.

The nutritional supplements I recommend will support fat metabolism, enhance insulin sensitivity, calm inflammation, and encourage neuron repair. The first recommendation is an iron-free all-purpose multiple vitamin and mineral supplement containing vitamins A, B_1 (thiamin), B_2 (Riboflavin) B_6, and B_{12}, folic acid (folate), niacin, manganese, zinc, and other basic nutrients. It should supply the RDA of each nutrient. Make sure it contains no iron. If you cannot find an iron-free multiple vitamin and mineral supplement at your local store, you can get it over the Internet. In addition to the nutrients in the multiple vitamin and mineral supplement, add the following even if they are already included in the supplement:

Alpha-lipoic acid 400 mg
CoQ10 100 mg
Magnesium 300 mg
Vitamin C 500 mg
L-Carnitine 2,000 mg
Curcumin 450 mg

In addition to the above supplements it is recommended that you also take 1 tablespoon of red palm oil or 250 mg of palm tocotrienols. Take the dietary supplements once a day at mealtime. After two to three months you may discontinue taking these supplements if you so desire, but it is recommended that you continue taking the red palm oil indefinitely. Red palm oil is a food that is rich in a wide variety of vitamins and phytonutrients that support good health.

The best way to take the red palm oil is to simply use it as a cooking oil and prepare your meals with it. Taken alone by the spoonful it has a strong flavor that most people find difficult to tolerate, but when used to cook eggs, meat, or vegetables, it enhances the flavor of the foods and is very pleasant. It can also be added to soups, stews, gravies, and sauces.

An alternative to the liquid red palm oil is to take it in gel capsule form, sold as Palmvitee. Take 250 mg of this red palm oil supplement daily.

Stop Alzheimer's Now At A Glance

Below is an overview of the most important topics concerning the treatment of neurodegenerative diseases with ketone/low-carb therapy. The numbers within the parentheses indicate the pages in this book where each topic is discussed in detail.

Like the rest of the body, the brain has the ability to heal itself from injury and disease (pp. 21-24). New brain cells replace old or injured cells throughout a person's life. In this way the brain can overcome periodic stress and injury and remain healthy and alert for a lifetime.

Although genetics may play a role in some cases, the primary factors that influence brain health are diet (pp. 49-52, 61-65, 208-217, 218-232), brain trauma (pp. 69-73), drugs (pp. 74-87), chronic stress (pp. 85-86), environmental toxins (pp. 88-99), toxic metals (pp. 100-114), and infections (pp. 115-128), particularly dental infections (pp. 129-138). Any one of these factors can prematurely age the brain, but generally a combination of them over an extended period of time is needed to degrade the brain to the point that neurodegenerative disease develops.

While each of these factors can promote excessive oxidation, runaway inflammation, and the deposition of abnormal proteins, the most devastating consequence is the disruption in energy or glucose metabolism. Energy is vital to properly maintain brain function, cope with stress, repair damaged tissues, and stimulate new cell growth. Without adequate energy, brain cells starve, degenerate, and die.

The primary way energy production is hampered is by insulin resistance (pp. 61-65). Insulin resistance throughout the body produces type 2 diabetes. Insulin resistance in the brain produces what is called type 3 diabetes. Type 2 diabetes promotes brain insulin resistance and is a high risk factor for many neurodegenerative diseases. Alzheimer's is referred to as type 3 diabetes (pp. 58-60, 66-68).

Ketones are produced from fat and provide the brain with an alternative source of fuel that bypasses the defect in glucose metabolism. Insulin resistance does not affect ketone energy metabolism. Ketones are a more concentrated and efficient source of energy (pp. 158-170). They are described as the body's superfuel. Ketone bodies also provide the lipid building blocks for the synthesis of new brain cells (pp. 167-168). Ketones allow the brain to maintain normal function and stimulate maintenance and repair. Ketone production is amplified by a high-fat, very low-carbohydrate diet.

Dietary fat (pp. 177-191) and cholesterol (pp. 139-157) are essential for healthy brain function. The high fat ketogenic diet has proven successful in the treatment of epilepsy for over 90 years. Severe cases of epilepsy which have

Continued on next page.

resisted all forms of drug treatment have responded well to ketone therapy and in many cases resulted in complete cures.

Likewise, the ketogenic diet has proven to be useful in treating other neurological disorders such as Alzheimer's, Parkinson's, ALS, Huntington's, traumatic brain injury, stroke, narcolepsy, and migraines as well as cancer and type 1 and type 2 diabetes (pp. 166-170). This provides a very effective therapeutic tool that can successfully prevent and treat neurodegenerative disease. The primary drawback to the ketogenic diet is the difficulty of preparing palatable meals consisting primarily of fat.

A special group of fats known as medium chain triglycerides (MCTs) stimulate the body's production of ketones (pp. 164-165), producing the therapeutic effects of the ketogenic diet with less dietary constraints. MCTs without any dietary restrictions have shown to significantly improve the memory of Alzheimer's patients (p. 172). These studies have led the FDA to approve a "drug" (available by prescription) containing nothing more than MCTs for the specific purpose of treating Alzheimer's disease (p. 176).

The primary drawback with this MCT "drug" is that it raises ketone levels in the body for only about 3 hours per dose and only one dose is taken each day. Much more than that causes nausea and diarrhea.

MCTs are derived from coconut oil, which contains the richest natural source of these special fats (pp. 172-176). Unlike the MCT drug, which consists of only one type of MCT, coconut oil contains a full spectrum of MCTs that work synergistically together. One dose of coconut oil can raise blood ketone levels for 8 hours. Doses can be repeated during the day without experiencing the discomforting side effects associated with the drug. Coconut oil is more effective than the drug because it can keep ketone levels elevated throughout the day. When combined with a low-carbohydrate diet, ketone levels are enhanced and can be maintained both day and night, allowing them to energize the brain and stimulate continuous healing (pp. 206-207).

Coconut oil not only raises blood ketone levels but it also helps fight infections (pp. 193-195), improves oral health (pp. 198-201), protects against environmental toxins (pp. 201-203), and mitigates symptoms of insulin resistance and diabetes (pp. 203-205), thus counteracting many of the factors that contribute to neurodegeneration. Coconut oil based ketone therapy has proven successful in reversing symptoms associated with Alzheimer's disease (pp. 11-15, 170-176).

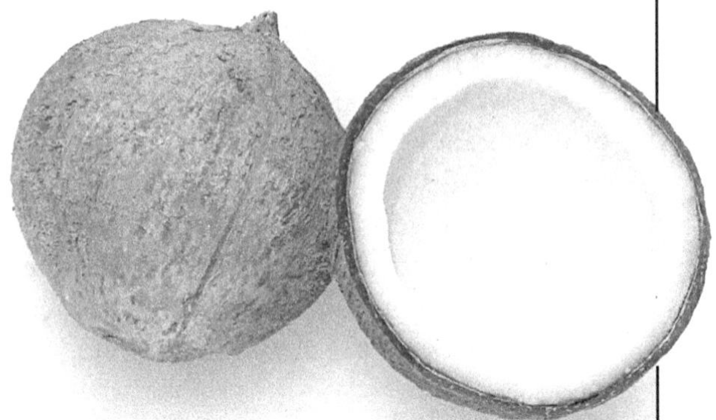

19 The Alzheimer's Battle Plan

THE BASIC STEPS

This chapter brings together the information discussed in previous chapters and condenses it into a concise program, which I refer to as The Alzheimer's Battle Plan. Although the name "Alzheimer's" is used, the program works for Parkinson's, ALS, MS, Huntington's, and many other neurodegenerative disorders.

If you skipped to this chapter without reading any of the previous chapters, you may not understand the reasons for each step. That is okay, so long as the steps are followed as directed, but you are encouraged to read the entire book to gain the reasoning and motivation for following the program as outlined. The hows and whys of each step listed below are not given in full detail here; for that you will need to read the previous chapters.

The most important steps in this program are Steps 1 and 2. Step 1: Ketone Therapy is crucial for the success of the program. It provides the foundation upon which the program is based. Step 2: Low-Carb Diet is also essential because it addresses an underlying flaw in brain metabolism. It will enhance ketone production and is necessary for balancing blood sugars and putting a stop to the destructive processes that are destroying the brain.

The remaining steps are not as essential but they will *greatly* enhance the effectiveness of the first two steps and speed the healing process. So they are highly recommended.

Step 1: Ketone Therapy

The first step in the Alzheimer's Battle Plan is to raise ketone levels. You do this by consuming at least 5 tablespoons (74 ml) of coconut oil every day. Please note that a tablespoon is a unit of measurement and equals 14.8 ml of liquid. The tablespoon referred to here is not the same as the tablespoon commonly used for eating. The oil should be taken with food. It can be used in food preparation or taken separately by the spoonful like a dietary supplement. Two tablespoons of coconut oil should always be consumed at breakfast. In the morning, ketone levels will be at their lowest, so this step is very important. The remaining 3 tablespoons can be divided up between lunch and dinner in any manner you desire. You could take 1 tablespoon for lunch and 2 for dinner or 2 for lunch and 1 for dinner or 1½ for both lunch and dinner. Just make sure you get at least 5 tablespoons spaced throughout the day. If a meal is skipped, it is a good idea to take a tablespoon of oil anyway to maintain ketone levels.

You can take more than 5 tablespoons of coconut oil a day. There is no harm in it, but you will also be consuming other fats and oils in your diet as well. Be aware that consuming too much oil of any type can loosen the bowels, requiring multiple trips to the restroom.

Five tablespoons of coconut oil is recommended for treating those who have clear symptoms of neurodegeneration. For prevention, 2-3 tablespoons daily is adequate.

Taking 2 tablespoons of oil at one sitting can be difficult if it is not incorporated into a meal. Chapter 20 provides recipe ideas that make taking the oil relatively easy. See the Daily Dose of Coconut Oil section for ideas.

Step 2: Low-Carb Diet

The next step is to adopt a low-carb eating plan. Choose the plan that matches your fasting blood glucose level.

Low-Carb 25 Gram Diet. If fasting blood glucose is 126 mg/dl (7 mmol/l) or greater, carbohydrate consumption is limited to a maximum of 25 grams per day. No single meal should exceed half of the day's total carbohydrate allowance (12.5 grams).

Low-Carb 50 Gram Diet. If fasting blood glucose is 101-125 mg/dl (5.6-6.9 mmol/l), carbohydrate consumption is limited to a maximum of 50 grams per day. No single meal should exceed half of the day's total carbohydrate allowance (25 grams).

Low-Carb 100 Gram Diet. If fasting blood glucose is 91-100 mg/dl (5.0-5.5 mmol/l), carbohydrate consumption is limited to a maximum of 100 grams per day. No single meal should exceed half of the day's total carbohydrate allowance (50 grams).

If you don't know your fasting blood glucose, go to your doctor and get it checked, otherwise follow the Low-Carb 25 Gram Diet. Almost everyone who has a diagnosed neurodegenerative disease will follow either the 25 or 50 gram diet plan in the beginning. As health and blood sugar readings improve, a higher carb diet may be adopted, the maximum being 100 grams per day.

Step 3: Oral Health

Have a dental examination and correct any existing infections. Oil pull for 15-20 minutes at least once a day, preferably before meals. This should become a daily habit just like brushing your teeth.

Step 4: Dietary Supplements

Most people do not get the recommended amount of vitamins and minerals they need for optimal health. This is especially true for those suffering from neurodegenerative disease. Although the diet provides adequate nutrition, dietary supplements are recommended for the first two to three months to bring nutrient reserves up to normal. Take the following daily:

- Iron-free multiple vitamin and mineral supplement that supplies the RDA of all the major nutrients except iron.
- Alpha-lipoic acid 400 mg
- CoQ10 100 mg
- Magnesium 300 mg
- Vitamin C 500 mg
- L-Carnitine 2,000 mg
- Curcumin 450 mg

Step 5: Red Palm Oil

Red palm oil provides a rich source of natural protective antioxidants that are helpful in fighting oxidative stress and calming inflammation. Take 1 tablespoon of red palm oil daily. It can be taken any time of the day. It is best consumed with foods and makes a good cooking oil. An option to eating the liquid oil is to take it in capsule form. If you do this, you need to take at least 250 mg per day. One popular brand is called Palmvitee and is marketed as a tocotrienol or vitamin E and antioxidant supplement. The supplement should be taken with foods.

Step 6: Fish

Eat one or two 4-ounce servings of fish per week or take 1 gram of krill oil. Fish is beneficial because it provides DHA, an important fatty acid necessary for healthy brain function, and supplies precursors for the production of prostaglandins that help reduce inflammation.

Step 7: Vitamin D

Get daily sun exposure to maintain proper vitamin D levels. During the winter when sun exposure is reduced, you can get your vitamin D requirements by consuming 1 tablespoon a day of cod liver oil or a vitamin D_3 supplemnet (2,000-5,000 IU/day). Taking the cod liver oil can satisfy both the fish oil and vitamin D requirement. However, it is still recommend that you get as much sun exposure as possible without overdoing it.

Step 8: Exercise

Exercise regularly three to seven days a week, 30-60 minutes at each session. Any type of exercise is beneficial—walking, jogging, swimming, aerobics, resistance training, hiking, etc. as long as it is vigorous enough to increase heart rate and respiration over the course of the session. Start off slowly for the first few weeks and gradually increase frequency, speed, and time as endurance builds. A good starting point is to walk for 30 minutes three times a week. Outdoor activities are an excellent way to get your daily sun exposure at the same time.

Basic Dietary Guidelines

Focus on eating fresh, whole foods, preferably organically produced. Eat plenty of low-starch vegetables with adequate meats, fish, poultry, and eggs supplemented with full-fat dairy, nuts, fruits, and, as allowed, a limited amount of whole grains and higher starch vegetables.

Avoid as much as possible prepackaged, processed foods. Most packaged foods contain ingredients that are unhealthful and may contribute to neurodegeneration. Reading ingredient labels should become second nature to you. Ingredients that you should take special care to avoid are hydrogenated or partially hydrogenated vegetable oil, shortening, margarine, nitrites, nitrates, monosodium glutamate (MSG), aspartame, ferrous sulfate (iron), sodium aluminum phosphate, aluminum ammonium sulfate, calcium aluminum silicate, sodium aluminosilicate, and powdered or dehydrated milk, butter, cheese, and eggs. Additives that often contain MSG include hydrolyzed vegetable protein, sodium caseinate, calcium caseinate, yeast extract, autolyzed yeast, soy protein isolate, textured protein, and natural flavor.

All products made with refined or white wheat flour contain ferrous sulfate (iron). This includes pizza, donuts, crackers, chips, cookies, pie crust, cake, pancake and muffin mixes, bread, rolls, egg rolls, hot and cold breakfast cereals, toaster pastries, pasta, pretzels, tortillas, canned soup, breaded fish, and macaroni and cheese, to mention just a few. Whole wheat products do not contain added iron. While grains are generally restricted in this program, if you do eat them it is best to eat whole grains without added iron.

Sugar and artificial sweeteners of all types and especially aspartame, fructose, high fructose corn syrup, and agave syrup should be avoided. It would also be a good idea to avoid any product that contains refined vegetable oils, which would include corn, soybean, safflower, cottonseed, canola, sunflower, and peanut oils. If these oils are used in processed foods, they are probably rancid. They should never be used as cooking oils. Better choices for food preparation are olive, coconut, palm, and macadamia nut oils.

Avoid caffeinated beverages, sodas, powdered drink mixes, fruit and vegetable juices, and even zero calorie drinks sweetened with aspartame or other artificial sweeteners. Water is the healthiest beverage. You should drink at least 2-3 quarts of water daily and increase this to 3-4 quarts a day during the summer when the body's water loss is higher. If you sweat a lot during exercise you may need even more.

BEFORE STARTING THE PROGRAM

Get A Medical Checkup

Regardless of your age or level of health, I recommend that you get a medical checkup before starting the program. The reason for this is partly to make sure you are physically capable of making a dramatic change to your diet but more importantly to get a record of your current level of health.

Record your blood pressure. Get your blood chemistries done so that you have a record of your fasting blood glucose level, high sensitivity C-reactive protein (hs-CRP), triglycerides, HDL, Total Cholesterol/HDL ratio, and Triglyceride/HDL ratio. Your fasting blood glucose is important because it determines which of the three Low-Carb Diets you will start on.

All of these measurements are needed in order to establish a baseline for comparison. After several weeks on the program you will have your blood work done again so you can compare your results and evaluate your progress. This step is very important! It will provide you with the proof that the program is improving your overall health and that the increased fat you will be consuming is not causing you any harm, but is promoting better health. It also provides documented proof you can show to your doctor or to anyone who is skeptical about this program. These records will also help to encourage you to keep with the program and continue progressing and improving.

A common concern about replacing carbohydrates with fat and protein is how it is going to affect cholesterol levels. If you have read Chapters 12, 13, and 14, then you know this is not a problem. Cholesterol numbers will improve. All blood markers will improve. Memory will improve.

Don't worry about *total* cholesterol or even the so-called "bad" LDL cholesterol. Recent research now shows that there are two types of LDL cholesterol: a "good" LDL and a "bad" LDL. Most tests don't differentiate between the two and lump them together under LDL, so this reading is useless.

Be aware that total cholesterol may rise a bit or fall—it doesn't matter either way. Total cholesterol is not a good predictor of heart disease or ill health.

Do not wait until a week or two after you start the program to have your blood work done. ***It must be done before you start.*** If you wait until after you start the program, you may see some values that are not to your liking and complain that the program is not working. For example, your HDL may be low, around 35 mg/dl, and you may blame the new diet for the low reading. Yet when you started the program your HDL may have been only 25 mg/dl. So although it is low, it has improved. But you would never know this unless you have a record of this marker before going on the program.

Stay on the program for at least six to eight weeks and then go back and get your blood work done again. The longer you are on the program the better will be your results. It is important that you get your blood work done by the same doctor and that he or she use the same laboratory, as results may vary somewhat from lab to lab.

Use the chart on the following page to see where you stand and evaluate your progress. Here is what you can expect to happen. Your blood pressure, if too high at the start of the program, will be lower. Triglycerides will be lower, HDL cholesterol will be higher, both your total cholesterol/HDL and triglyceride/HDL ratios will be lower, your level of inflammation (C-reactive protein) will be lower. All of these changes are positive and indicate better blood sugar control, improved

Blood Test Reference Values

Blood Pressure (mm Hg)

Systolic (top number)	Diastolic (bottom number)	Category
<90	<60	Low
90-99	60-65	Low Normal
100-130	66-85	Normal
131-140	86-90	High Normal
141-159	91-99	High
>159	>99	Very High

Fasting Glucose

mg/dl	mmol/l	Category
75-90	4.2-5.0	Normal
91-100	5.0-5.5	Borderline High
101-125	5.6-6.9	High (early diabetes)
>125	>6.9	Very High (established diabetes)

High Sensitivity C-Reactive Protein (hs-CRP)

mg/l	Category
< 1.0	Optimal
1.0 to 3.0	Average
3.1-10	High
>10	Very High

Blood Lipids

HDL Men

mg/dl	mmol/l	Category
<40	<1.0	Low
40-60	1.0-1.6	Average
>60	>1.6	Optimal

HDL Women

mg/dl	mmol/l	Category
<50	<1.3	Low
50-60	1.3-1.6	Average
>60	>1.6	Optimal

Total Chol/HDL Ratio

Ratio	Category
<3.3	Optimal
3.3-5.0	Normal
>5.0	High

Trig/HDL Ratio

Ratio	Category
<2	Optimal
2-4	Normal
>4	High

Triglycerides

mg/dl	mmol/l	Category
<150	<1.7	Normal
150-199	1.7-2.2	Borderline High
200-499	2.3-5.6	High
>499	>5.6	Very High

In the United States, blood sugar and cholesterol readings are usually given in milligrams per deciliter (mg/dl). In Europe they are commonly given as millimoles per liter (mmol/l).

insulin sensitivity, reduced risk of heart disease, better circulation, less oxidative stress, reduced inflammation, and better overall health. All these changes show that the program is working! Keep going. The numbers will continue to improve.

Get your blood work done as soon as possible, even before you finish reading this book. You want to have this data available so that you can begin the program as soon as possible. But do not start until the blood work is completed.

C-reactive protein (CRP) is a protein found in the blood that indicates the presence of inflammation. Normally there is no CRP in blood. A measure of 1.0 mg/l or less is desirable. When CRP is above 10 mg/l, it suggests an active infection or chronic inflammation.

There are two types of blood tests for CRP. Both tests measure the same molecule, but one test is more sensitive than the other. The *high sensitivity CRP* or hs-CRP is the test you want. It measures very small amounts of C-reactive protein in the blood and is used most frequently as a means to assess potential risks for heart problems, which are commonly associated with low-grade chronic inflammation. High sensitivity CRP is generally measured in the range of 0.5 to 10 mg/l. The regular CRP test is ordered for patients at risk for acute infections or chronic inflammatory diseases and measures a range from 10 to 1000 mg/l. The scale on the previous page is based on recommendations by the American Heart Association to assess risks for heart disease.

Take the Cognitive and/or Parkinson's Tests

Often, small improvements in mental or motor skills function can go unnoticed. Like with the blood tests, you wouldn't know how well the program is working unless you had a means by which to evaluate these often small changes. Before starting the program it is advisable to complete the Mental Status Test and/or the Parkinson's Disease Rating Scale found in Appendices A and B respectively.

Those who have a confirmed diagnosis or suspect they are developing dementia or Alzheimer's disease should take the Mental Status Test. It may also be of value to take the clock test as well. In this test the subject draws a clock face from memory. This test is highly recommended because it gives a graphic demonstration of cognitive ability and later of improvement.

Those who are affected with Parkinson's-like symptoms should be evaluated using the Parkinson's Disease Rating Scale. If cognitive problems also appear to be present, the Mental Status Test should be taken as well.

Anytime after the first six to eight weeks of the program, the tests can be repeated. Compare the before and after results. There should be a measureable difference. Generally, the greatest improvement will be seen in those people who started with the lowest test scores. Test scores that were normal or close to normal to begin with may not show much improvement because of the greater difficulty in detecting very minor fluctuations in brain function.

The results of these tests should be encouraging and demonstrate the effectiveness of the program. Neurodegeneration is a progressive process. Those affected don't normally improve on their own but continue to gradually decline over time. Even just stopping or slowing the progression of the disease is a positive sign.

Discontinue Medications

Before jumping into the program, discontinue all non-essential medications. This includes cholesterol-lowering drugs. The diet balances blood sugar and insulin; so, once you begin the program diabetic medications and insulin become unnecessary. As you start the diet, if you have high blood pressure, it will come down naturally. If you continue taking blood pressure medications while you are on the program, your blood pressure may dip too low. This is not a good thing. For a detailed list of drugs you should not be using, see Appendix C.

If there are some drugs that you feel you must have and are hesitant about stopping, you may gradually wean yourself off them. Have your doctor monitor your progress and adjust the dosages as needed.

Herbs and dietary supplements may be continued if you so desire, but in most cases they are not necessary.

Prepare Your Pantry

One of the downfalls with sticking to the dietary guidelines in this program is succumbing to temptation from easily accessible restricted foods. Just knowing a favorite treat is sitting and waiting to be eaten can be too overpowering to resist. Removing the temptation is the simplest and best solution.

If possible, all foods that are not allowed on the diet should be removed from the house or at least from easy access. Give all the high-carb foods to friends or neighbors or just throw them away. If there are other people living in the house who have no dietary restraints, it will make the diet a bit harder. Perhaps restricted foods can be put in a place where no one except the one who eats them can get them.

Next, you need to stock your refrigerator and cupboards with the types of foods that are allowed on the diet. Have them available at all times so that there is less of a temptation to resort to seeking restricted foods. Purchase plenty of coconut oil. Have all your dietary supplements and ketosis test strips on hand.

Before starting the program, review acceptable foods and develop several meal plans. Calculate the carb content for each meal and arrange them to fit within the day's total carb allotment. Get into the habit of planning meals and snacks before going to the grocery store so you have everything on hand. If you shop for groceries once a week, it is a good idea to plan each meal for the week before shopping. Otherwise you may find yourself grabbing the first thing you find in the refrigerator or pantry, which may boost your carbs over the daily limit.

The Induction Diet

The purpose of the Induction Diet is to prepare you both physically and mentally for the full Alzheimer's Battle Plan program. Because the dietary changes you are about to make may be significant, jumping straight into the program can be difficult. The Induction Diet allows you time to ease into the program, become accustomed to eating more fat, and learn how to prepare and enjoy eating the low-carb way.

After visiting your doctor and getting your blood work done, you should start immediately adding coconut oil into your diet. You are encouraged to do this one to three weeks before officially beginning the Alzheimer's Battle Plan program.

Go to your local health food store or online and purchase a jar of coconut oil. It doesn't matter what brand or type of coconut oil you use. Most of the brands will be labeled as "Virgin," "Extra Virgin," or "Expeller Pressed." Any of them will do. Start using the oil in your everyday cooking now. In recipes that call for butter, margarine, vegetable oil, or shortening, use coconut oil instead. Try to consume at least 1 tablespoon of coconut oil every day with your foods.

The reason for this recommendation is that many people have cut back on fat consumption due to the hysteria in our society against eating fat. Because people have reduced their fat intake, their digestive systems are not accustomed to the amount of fat that is required in the Alzheimer's Battle Plan. Adding fat into the diet may cause some people to experience nausea or runny stools. To avoid this, it is advised that you start now to prepare your digestive system for the increased fat by adding 1 tablespoon of coconut oil in your daily diet. When fat consumption increases, your body naturally steps up production of fat-digesting enzymes. As your body adjusts to the added fat, you can increase your fat consumption without experiencing any side effects.

If 1 tablespoon of coconut oil causes nausea or diarrhea (which is rare), cut back to ½ tablespoon daily. If you can handle 1 tablespoon of coconut oil without problems, after a few days increase your daily dosage to 2 tablespoons. If 2 tablespoons are too much for your digestive tract at this time, go back to 1 tablespoon for another week or so and then try again. Gradually work toward consuming 3 tablespoons of coconut oil daily. Most people are able to add 2 tablespoons of coconut oil immediately into their diet without experiencing any problems whatsoever. However, everyone is different; some will experience a little diarrhea with 1 tablespoon while others can take 5 or 6 tablespoons right from the start without problem. Everyone can build up their tolerance for oil by gradually working it into their diet. You should start doing this now. Getting the body accustomed to processing a higher intake of fat is the primary purpose for the Induction Diet.

As you are adjusting to the increased fat intake from the coconut oil, experiment with preparing low-carb meals. This is a good time to practice cooking and eating the low-carb way. It will help you to build up a file of tested low-carb recipes and meal plans that you enjoy as well as give you experience in preparing meals this way. Start by preparing at least one or two low-carb meals a day.

After one to three weeks of using coconut oil and testing meal plans, jump into the Alzheimer's Battle Plan program full speed. Even if 5 tablespoons of coconut oil give you diarrhea (four or more bowel movements per day), start the program. Cut back on the coconut oil to the point where diarrhea is not a problem and over time gradually work up to 5 tablespoons. This may take several additional weeks depending on how sensitive you are to fats. Keep in mind that emptying the bowels once or twice a day does not indicate diarrhea; this is how a healthy colon should work. Your bowels will be working better and possibly more often on this diet.

The body is better able to digest fat if it is eaten along with other foods. When you start the diet, consume the coconut oil as part of your meals. Over time as your body adapts to the increased fat intake, you can, if you desire, take the oil by the spoonful like a dietary supplement.

WHAT TO EXPECT

This program will improve not only brain health but overall health as well. Poor quality empty calorie foods are replaced with higher quality, nutrient dense foods. This may have a dramatic affect on the body. Many people notice a marked increase in energy and vitality as they adopt the new eating regimen. Others may temporarily experience some discomforting symptoms initially before they start to feel better. Knowing what to expect will help prepare you for the transformation that will occur.

As you change your eating habits and the types of foods you eat, you will be increasing the amount of fiber consumed and reducing easily digestible starch and sugar. Fat consumption will likely be higher than it was previously. All this can have a marked impact on digestive function. The frequency and consistency of bowel movements will change. Generally, you can expect stools to be softer and more frequent. A healthy digestive tract should evacuate between one to three times daily. Any less than that indicates constipation. Doctors may say that one bowel movement every one to three days is average or normal, but *normal* does not mean *healthy*. As you eat healthier foods, expect to become more regular.

Eliminating starchy foods, sugar, caffeine, alcohol, and unnecessary medications can cause withdrawal symptoms. These substances can be just as addictive as hard drugs. While physical symptoms may not be as dramatic, psychological symptoms and cravings can be trying. Fortunately, the fats, meats, and rich sauces that are allowed on the diet can help curb cravings and temper feelings of deprivation and dependence. Before long, the power these substances once held over you will fade away.

Coconut oil's antimicrobial effects, along with improved immune efficiency due to the diet, may cause what is called a "die-off reaction," also known as a Herxheimer reaction. This occurs when large numbers of bacteria or other microorganisms are killed and their toxins are dumped into the bloodstream. The death of the bacteria and associated toxins occurs faster than the body can remove them. In response, the body shifts into a heightened state of detoxification and elimination. As a consequence, symptoms resembling illness may become manifest. Symptoms may include one or more of the following: fever, chills, headache, muscle or joint pain, nausea, diarrhea, vomiting, skin outbreaks, itchiness, anxiety, irritability, insomnia, fatigue, and nasal congestion. In fact, any symptom or combination of symptoms can arise.

This cleansing reaction is often misdiagnosed as an illness or an allergic reaction. While the symptoms may be discomforting, they are not indications of an illness and do not need any special treatment or medications. The body is simply doing what it needs to do to cleanse itself. For example, if the sinuses are eliminating a great deal of mucus, they are doing so in order to rid the body of toxins. Taking a decongestant stops the removal of these toxins, preventing them from exiting the body. Likewise, anti-diarrhea medications prevent the elimination of toxins from the bowel. Antibiotics won't do any good because the bacteria are already dead; these drugs may actually depress the immune system and slow down the cleansing process. These symptoms are temporary. Let the process run its course. Cleansing reactions can last anywhere from one day to two weeks, and sometimes even longer. Three to four days is typical.

Since this new eating plan is probably far healthier than anything you have ever experienced in your life, you will begin to notice many positive changes in your health. Blood chemistries will improve, and blood sugar will come under control. Better memory, clearer thinking, happier, positive outlook on life, increased energy, improved digestion, better eyesight, fewer and less severe infections, deeper and more restful night's sleep, and a general overall feeling of better health will follow.

EVALUATE PROGRESS

After following the program for six to eight weeks, go back to your doctor and have your blood chemistries retested. You should see dramatic improvement in all measurements.

If you don't see the improvements you were expecting, reevaluate your eating patterns and make sure you are following the diet correctly. Are you actually calculating the exact amount of carbohydrate you eat at every meal? If you are only guessing, that may be your problem. We generally tend to underestimate carbohydrate content of foods eaten. That is why it is so important during the first few months of the program that you calculate carbohydrate content precisely for each meal. If you are calculating correctly, then you may need to restrict your carbohydrate intake more. If you were doing the Low-Carb 50 Gram diet, then go to the Low-Carb 25 Gram program.

You can adjust the diet over time. For example, if you are successfully following the Low-Carb 25 Gram Diet (fasting blood glucose 126 mg/dl or 7 mmol/l and greater) and your fasting blood glucose reading has dropped below 126 mg/dl (7 mmol/l), then you can move to the Low-Carb 50 Gram Diet. Likewise, if you were following the Low-Carb 50 Gram diet (fasting blood glucose between 101 and 125 mg/dl or 5.6 and 6.9 mmol/l) and your fasting blood glucose reading has dropped below 101 mg/dl (5.6 mmol/l), then you can move to the Low-Carb 100 Gram Diet.

Also, retake the tests for cognitive and Parkinson's evaluation, as well as the clock test if it was taken earlier. Compare results with initial tests. Improvement should be evident.

After being on the program for at least six months, have your blood chemistries tested a third time and compare results. Blood tests can be retaken every 6 to 12 months to monitor progress.

Retake the written tests. Compare with the earlier results. Continued improvement should be evident if the program has been followed as outlined.

Each person will progress at their own rate. Here is an example of someone who successfully followed the program. It will give you an idea of what to expect. Charles Brewer, age 69, was troubled by lapses of memory which he described as periodic episodes of "brain fog." When asked simple questions, such as his address or phone number, his mind would often go blank. Yet hours later he could remember these details without difficulty. He started the program with a fasting blood sugar level of 162 mg/dl (9.0 mmol/l), indicating a diagnosis of diabetes and putting him in the Low-Carb 25 Gram Diet phase. His blood chemistries indicated he was at high risk for heart attack and stroke. He kept his total carb intake down to 25 grams or less for three months. In that time, all of his numbers improved, many of them moving into the "optimal" range. His blood sugar is coming under control, risk of heart disease has declined dramatically, and his episodes of brain fog are now a thing of the past. Brewer's numbers are shown below.

Before	Category	After	Category
Fasting Blood Glucose 162 mg/dl (9.0 mmol/l)	very high	106 mg/dl (5.9 mmol/l)	high but declining
C-Reactive Protein 4.8 mg/dl	high	0.5 mg/dl	optimal
HDL Cholesterol 45 mg/dl (1.2 mmol/l)	average	91 mg (2.4 mmol/l)	optimal
Total Chol/HDL Chol 6.0	high	3.0	optimal
Triglyceride 204 mg/dl (2.3 mmol/l)	high	66 mg/dl (0.7 mmol/l)	normal
Trig/HDL Ratio 4.5	high	0.73	optimal
Blood Pressure 150/95	high	130/80	normal

CONTINUED SUPPORT

The Internet has many websites offering low-carb advice, encouragement, and recipes that can be of tremendous benefit. Perhaps the best resource is the Atkins website, www.atkins.com, which has numerous recipes, a chat group, a carb counter database so you can look up the net carbs for a variety of foods, the latest research on low-carb eating, and blogs for support, encouragement, and sharing success stories, as well as other aids. The recipes are numerous and creative and all include the net carb content.

If you would like to learn more about the health benefits of coconut and palm products my website, www.coconutresearchcenter.org, offers a variety of interesting articles, research findings, nutritional facts, news, and success stories from people who are overcoming debilitating health problems.

20 Recipes

At first, learning how to cook the low-carb way may seem like a daunting task. However, it isn't as hard as it may appear. While some low-carb recipes are complicated and time-consuming, much of the cooking is as simple as frying a lamb chop and steaming some zucchini. What could be easier than that?

If you are new to low-carb cooking, I strongly urge you to read this entire chapter. Whether you use any of the recipes or not, this chapter will show you how to make low-carb cooking simple and easy. It will also show you how to incorporate coconut oil into your everyday life. The recipes provided here are just a few examples of low-carb cooking. For more ideas, check out the books and recipes available at your library, book store, and the Internet.

One of the biggest challenges to the program outlined in this book is consuming five tablespoons of coconut oil daily. The first part of this chapter provides numerous methods of consuming coconut oil in a palatable way. Recipes later on explain how to add the oil during meal preparation.

DAILY DOSE OF COCONUT OIL

The program in this book recommends consuming at least 5 tablespoons (74 ml) of coconut oil daily, taken in divided doses during breakfast, lunch, and dinner. This would mean that each meal would contain between 1 and 2 tablespoons (15-30 ml) of coconut oil.

This is a lot of oil to consume during the day and often takes a little creative planning to accomplish in a palatable manner. The best way to take the oil is to use it in food preparation. Cook your foods in the oil or use it as a salad dressing or as a topping on vegetables. Below you will find a number of ideas you can use to get your daily dose.

By the Spoonful

The simplest way to take the oil is by the spoonful, like a dietary supplement. Many people do this. However, others have a harder time because they find putting pure oil into their mouths difficult. They are not accustomed to the taste and texture. It does take some getting used to and over time most people can do it this way without problem. A good quality "virgin" coconut oil has a mild coconut flavor that tastes good enough to eat off the spoon. All brands are different however. Some brands have a much stronger flavor (sometimes tainted with smoke during processing), which can be overpowering. Choose the brand of coconut oil you use carefully. Try several brands and select the one that tastes best to you. If you don't like the taste of virgin coconut oil, you can use the tasteless "expeller pressed" coconut oil.

If consuming coconut oil by the spoonful is difficult for you, one way to make it easier is to enhance the flavor using food extracts and flavorings. A little cinnamon oil mixed with the coconut oil gives it a remarkably pleasant taste that most people find very enjoyable. It's almost like candy. Here are some recipes.

- 1 tablespoon coconut oil mixed with 1-2 drops of cinnamon oil
- 1 tablespoon coconut oil mixed with 1-2 drops peppermint oil
- 1 tablespoon coconut oil mixed with 3-6 drops coconut flavoring

This last one may sound redundant, but the coconut flavoring gives the oil a richer, dessert-like coconut flavor. Experiment with other food flavorings available in the herb and spice section of the grocery store. You want to use only those products produced as flavorings for baking and food preparation, you don't want to use anything with added sugar. Oil-based extracts work better than alcohol-based flavorings. If you use an alcohol-based extract, combine the extract with the coconut oil in a small stovetop safe pan and heat for a minute or two to drive off the alcohol.

Mini Soups

Another way to incorporate 1-2 tablespoons of coconut oil into your diet in a relatively easy manner is to make Mini Soups. I call them Mini Soups because only a small amount is consumed at any one time. This is basically a flavorful soup combined with coconut oil. The taste, texture, and smell of the soup makes the oil easy to consume. Each serving amounts to only ¼ cup (60 ml) so it doesn't take the place of or interfere with meals. It is eaten before meals, much like an appetizer. The sole purpose of the Mini Soup is not to serve as a meal but to provide a tasty medium in which to consume the coconut oil. Red palm oil may be consumed this way too, if desired.

Multiple servings of the soup are made in advance and refrigerated or frozen. To each serving is added 1-2 tablespoons of coconut oil. Over the course of several days the soup is gradually consumed. The soup is not eaten at every meal, but only when meals do not provide enough coconut oil to meet the daily minimum. The soups will keep in the refrigerator for several days and for several months when frozen.

Recipes for several soups are given below. Please note, coconut oil is not used in these recipes. *You add the oil to each serving just before consuming it.* This way you can add 1, 1½, 2 tablespoons or whatever amount of coconut oil you need for that particular meal. One serving is ¼ cup of soup, *plus* the added coconut oil. The number of net carbs is given in each recipe. You need to account for these carbs in your daily total.

Beef Soup

¼ pound (120 g) ground beef
½ cup (50 g) chopped vegetables*
1¼ cups (300 ml) water
¼ teaspoon onion powder
¼ teaspoon paprika
¼ teaspoon marjoram
Salt and pepper to taste

Put ground beef, vegetables and water in a quart saucepan. Bring to a boil, reduce heat and simmer for about 15 minutes. While cooking, break ground beef into small pieces. Add onion powder, paprika, and marjoram, cook for 1 minute and remove from heat. Add salt and pepper to taste. Let cool and store in an airtight container in the refrigerator. Makes six ¼ cup servings.

*Use two or more of the following vegetables: onion, carrot, mushroom, celery, green beans, bell peppers, okra, and asparagus.

Net carbs: 0.5 grams per ¼ cup serving.

Beef Salsa Soup

¼ pound (120 g) ground beef
½ cup (50 g) chopped vegetables*
1¼ (300 ml) cups water
2 tablespoons (30 ml) salsa
Salt and pepper to taste

Put ground beef, vegetables, water, and salsa in a quart saucepan. Bring to a boil, reduce heat and simmer for about 15 minutes. While cooking, break ground beef into small pieces. Remove from heat and add salt and pepper to taste. Let cool and store in an airtight container in the refrigerator. Makes seven ¼ cup servings.

*Use two or more of the following vegetables: onion, carrot, mushroom, celery, green beans, bell peppers, okra, and asparagus.

Net carbs: 0.6 gram per ¼ cup serving.

Pork Soup

¼ pound (120 g) ground or chopped pork
½ cup (50 g) chopped vegetables*
1¼ (300 ml) cups water
¼ teaspoon onion powder
¼ teaspoon thyme
Salt and pepper to taste

Put ground pork, vegetables, and water in a quart saucepan. Bring to a boil, reduce heat and simmer for about 15 minutes. Add onion powder and thyme, cook for 1 minute and remove from heat. Add salt and pepper to taste. Let cool and store in an airtight container in the refrigerator. Makes six ¼ cup servings.

*Use two or more of the following vegetables: onion, carrot, mushroom, celery, green beans, bell peppers, okra, and asparagus.

Net carbs: 0.5 grams per ¼ cup serving.

Chicken Soup

1 cup (120 g) chicken, chopped
½ cup (50 g) chopped vegetables*
1¼ (300 ml) cups water
⅛ teaspoon celery seed
¼ teaspoon ground sage
Salt and pepper to taste

Put chicken, vegetables, and water in a quart saucepan. Bring to a boil, reduce heat and simmer for about 15 minutes. Add celery seed and sage, cook for 1 minute and remove from heat. Add salt and pepper to taste. Let cool and store in an airtight container in the refrigerator. Makes six ¼ cup servings.

*Use two or more of the following vegetables: onion, carrot, mushroom, celery, green beans, bell peppers, okra, and asparagus.

Net carbs: 0.5 grams per ¼ cup serving.

Clam Chowder

1 can (10 oz/300 ml) minced clams, with juice*
¼ cup (25 g) onion, chopped
⅛ teaspoon celery seed
⅛ teaspoon black pepper
1 cup (240 ml) heavy cream
2 teaspoons (10 ml) fish sauce

Drain juice from clams into saucepan and put the clams aside. Add onion, celery seed, and pepper to the juice in the saucepan and bring it to a boil, reduce heat and simmer for about 10 minutes or until onions are tender. Add cream, fish sauce, and clams. Cook for 2 minutes. Let cool and store in an airtight container in the refrigerator. Makes about 10 servings.

*Oysters may be substituted for the claims if desired.

Net carbs: 1 gram per ¼ cup serving.

Fish Chowder

¼ cup (25 g) onion, chopped
⅛ teaspoon celery seed
⅛ teaspoon black pepper

¼ pound (120 g) chopped fish*
1 cup (240 ml) heavy cream
2 teaspoons (10 ml) fish sauce

In a saucepan bring water to a boil. Add onion, celery seed, and pepper, reduce heat, and simmer for 8-10 minutes or until onions are tender. Add fish and cream and simmer for an additional 5 minutes. Let cool and store in an airtight container in the refrigerator.

*Use any type of low-mercury fish such as sole, catfish, salmon, trout, flounder, haddock, mackerel, perch, or tilapia. You can also use shellfish such as scallop, or crab.

Net carbs: 1 gram per ¼ cup serving.

Creamy Chicken Soup

1 cup (120 g) chicken, chopped
½ cup (50 g) chopped vegetables*
¾ cup (180 ml) chicken broth or water
½ cup (120 ml) heavy cream
⅛ teaspoon onion powder
⅛ teaspoon celery seed
¼ teaspoon thyme
⅛ teaspoon salt
⅛ teaspoon black pepper

Put chicken, vegetables, and water in a saucepan. Bring to a boil, reduce heat and simmer for about 15 minutes or until vegetables are tender. Add cream and seasonings, simmer for 1-2 minutes, and remove from heat. Let cool and store in an airtight container in the refrigerator. Makes six ¼ cup servings.

*Use two or more of the following vegetables: onion, carrot, mushroom, celery, green beans, bell peppers, okra, and asparagus.

Net carbs: 1 gram per ¼ cup serving.

Tomato Soup

1 cup (240 ml) water
½ cup (120 ml) tomato sauce
⅛ teaspoon celery seed
¼ teaspoon onion powder
⅛ teaspoon garlic powder
⅛ teaspoon paprika
1 teaspoon (5 ml) lemon juice
Salt and black pepper to taste

Combine first six ingredients into a saucepan, bring to a boil, reduce heat, and simmer for three minutes to blend flavors. Remove from heat and add lemon juice, salt, and pepper. Makes six ¼ cup servings.

Net carbs: 1.3 grams per ¼ cup serving.

Creamy Tomato

1 cup (240 ml) water
½ cup (120 ml) tomato sauce
⅛ teaspoon celery seed
¼ teaspoon onion powder
⅛ teaspoon garlic powder
⅛ teaspoon paprika
½ cup (120 ml) heavy cream
Salt and black pepper to taste

Combine first six ingredients in a saucepan, bring to a boil, reduce heat and simmer for three minutes to blend flavors. Remove from heat and add cream, salt, and pepper. Makes eight ¼ cup servings.

Net carbs: 1.3 grams per ¼ cup serving.

Tomato Beef Soup

¼ pound (120 g) ground beef
1 cup (120 ml) water
¼ cup (60 ml) tomato sauce
⅛ teaspoon celery seed
¼ teaspoon onion powder
⅛ teaspoon garlic powder
⅛ teaspoon paprika
¼ teaspoon salt
⅛ teaspoon black pepper
1 teaspoon (5 ml) lemon juice

Combine first nine ingredients into a saucepan, bring to a boil, reduce heat and simmer for 10 minutes. Remove from heat and add lemon juice. Makes seven ¼ cup servings.

Net carbs: 0.6 gram per ¼ cup serving.

Tomato Fish Soup

¼ pound (120 g) chopped fish*
1 cup (240 ml) water
¼ cup (60 ml) tomato sauce
⅛ teaspoon celery seed
¼ teaspoon onion powder
⅛ teaspoon paprika
⅛ teaspoon black pepper
2 teaspoons (10 ml) fish sauce

Combine all ingredients into a saucepan, bring to a boil, reduce heat and simmer for 5 minutes. Remove from heat and serve. Makes seven ¼ cup servings.

*Use any type of low-mercury fish such as sole, catfish, salmon, trout, flounder, haddock, mackerel, perch, whitefish, or tilapia. You can also use shellfish such as scallop, shrimp, or crab.

Net carbs: 0.5 gram per ¼ cup serving.

Cream of Asparagus

1 cup (240 ml) chicken broth
4 ounces (115 g) asparagus, chopped
½ cup (120 ml) heavy cream
¼ teaspoon basil
¼ teaspoon salt
⅛ teaspoon black pepper
½ teaspoon scallion, chopped

In a covered saucepan, simmer chicken broth and asparagus for 20 minutes until vegetables are soft. Remove from heat, put into a blender and blend until smooth. Add back to saucepan along with cream, basil, salt, and pepper. Heat to a simmer and cook 1 minute. Remove from heat. Serve with freshly chopped scallion sprinkled on top. Makes about six ¼ cup servings.

Net carbs: 1 gram per ¼ cup serving.

Cream of Broccoli with Cheese

1 cup (240 ml) chicken broth
1 cup (100 g) broccoli, chopped
½ cup (120 ml) heavy cream
¼ teaspoon salt
⅛ teaspoon black pepper
¼ cup (25 g) freshly grated Parmesan cheese
1 teaspoon scallion, chopped

In a covered saucepan, simmer chicken broth and broccoli for 20 minutes until vegetables are soft. Remove from heat, put into a blender and blend until smooth. Add back to saucepan along with cream, salt, pepper, and cheese. Heat to a simmer and cook 1 minute. Remove from heat. Serve with freshly chopped scallion sprinkled on top. Makes about six ¼ cup servings.

Net carbs: 1.3 grams per ¼ cup serving.

Cream of Spinach with Chicken

1 teaspoon (5 ml) butter
1 cup (120 g) uncooked chicken cut into bite size pieces
¼ cup (60 ml) water
¾ cup (180 ml) heavy cream
¼ teaspoon onion powder
⅛ teaspoon garlic powder
3 cups (80 g) spinach, chopped
Salt and black pepper to taste

Melt butter in sauté pan over medium heat. Add chicken and cook, stirring frequently, until it turns white, about 3 minutes. Add all remaining ingredients and simmer until spinach is tender. Makes seven ¼ cup servings.

Net carbs: 0.9 grams per ¼ cup serving.

Creamy Cinnamon Soup

1 cup (240 ml) heavy cream
½ cup (120 ml) water
1 teaspoon cinnamon
¼ teaspoon nutmeg
½ teaspoon (3 ml) vanilla extract

In a small saucepan heat cream, water, cinnamon, and nutmeg to a low simmer, stir frequently, do not boil. Cook for about 5 minutes. Heating draws the flavors of the spices into the cream. Add vanilla and remove from heat. Makes six ¼ cup servings.

Net carbs: 1.1 grams per ¼ cup serving.

Creamy Berry Soup

1 cup (240 ml) heavy cream
¾ cup (75 g) berries (blackberries, boysenberries, or raspberries)
½ cup (120 ml) water

Combine all ingredients into a blender and blend until smooth. Makes eight ¼ cup servings.

Net carbs: 1.5 grams per ¼ cup serving.

LOW-CARB SALAD DRESSINGS

I recommend eating at least one raw green salad daily. Tossed green salads are the most popular because a variety of ingredients can be used to create them. Don't limit yourself to the common iceberg lettuce—try butterhead lettuce, red leaf, romaine, and other varieties. Low-carb vegetables that go well with salads include cucumber, bell peppers, banana peppers, tomatoes, avocado, parsley, onion, shallots, scallions, radishes, jicama, parsley, cilantro, watercress, sprouts, celery, celery root (celeriac), bok choy (Chinese cabbage), napa cabbage, red and green cabbage, broccoli, cauliflower, spinach, chard, kale, carrots, Jerusalem artichoke, sauerkraut, chicory, endive, and snow peas. Salads don't always have to include lettuce. You can make a variety of lettuce-free salads with all these vegetables.

Toppings add spark to salads. Low-carb toppings include hard boiled eggs, ham, crumbled bacon, beef, chicken, turkey, pork, fish (salmon, sardines, etc.), crab, shrimp, nori, hard cheeses (cheddar, Monterey, Munster, etc.), soft cheeses (feta, cottage, etc.), nuts, olives, and pork rinds.

The dressing is perhaps the most important part of the salad. It is what makes the salad stand out and gives the other ingredients zing. Most commercially prepared dressings are made using a base of soybean or canola oils and often include sugar, high fructose corn syrup, MSG, and other undesirable additives. Many of them are promoted as low-calorie or low-fat, but few are low-carb. A better choice is a homemade low-carb salad dressing using healthier ingredients. The following are a few such recipes.

Mayonnaise

1 large egg yolk
2 teaspoons (10 ml) fresh lemon juice
1 teaspoon (5 ml) Dijon mustard
½ teaspoon salt
⅛ teaspoon black pepper
1 cup (240 ml) extra light olive oil

Have all ingredients at room temperature before beginning. Combine egg yolk, lemon juice, mustard, salt, pepper, and ¼ cup (60 ml) oil in blender or food processor. Blend for about 60 seconds. While machine is running, pour in the remaining oil *very slowly*, drop by drop at first and gradually building to a fine, steady stream. The secret to making good mayonnaise is to add the oil in slowly. Mayonnaise will thicken as oil is added. Taste and adjust seasonings as needed.

Net carbs: 0.2 grams per 1 tablespoon serving.

Coconut Mayonnaise

Make the Mayonnaise as directed but replace ½ cup of olive oil with ½ cup of coconut oil. Make sure coconut oil is at room temperature and liquid before using. Each tablespoon of coconut mayonnaise contains about ½ tablespoon of coconut oil.

Net carbs: 0.2 grams per 1 tablespoon serving.

Vinegar and Coconut Oil Dressing

¼ cup (60 ml) coconut oil
¼ cup (60 ml) extra light olive oil
2 tablespoons (30 ml) water
¼ cup (60 ml) apple cider vinegar
⅛ teaspoon salt
⅛ teaspoon white pepper

Put all ingredients into a Mason jar or similar container. Cover and shake vigorously until well blended. Let stand at room temperature until ready to use. May be stored in cupboard for several days without refrigeration. If the dressing is to be stored for more than a week, put it into the refrigerator. When chilled, the oil will tend to solidify. To liquefy, take it out of the refrigerator at least 1 hour before using. Each tablespoon of dressing contains about ¼ tablespoon of coconut oil.

Net carbs: 0 grams per 1 tablespoon serving.

Simple Vinegar Dressing

¼ cup (60 ml) apple cider vinegar

½ tablespoon (8 ml) water
Dash of salt
Dash of pepper

Mix all ingredients together. That's all there is to it—simple and easy.
Net carbs: 0 grams per 1 tablespoon serving.

Toasted Almond Dressing

½ cup (120 ml) coconut oil
¼ cup (25 g) slivered almonds
1 tablespoon (15 ml) extra light olive oil
2 tablespoons (30 ml) tamari sauce
1 tablespoon (15 ml) apple cider vinegar
¼ teaspoon ground ginger
¼ teaspoon salt

Put coconut oil in small saucepan. At medium to low heat, sauté slivered almonds until lightly browned. Remove from heat and let cool to room temperature. Stir in remaining ingredients. As the dressing sits, the oil will separate to the top and the almonds will sink to the bottom. Stir just before using. Spoon dressing onto salad, making sure to include the almonds. May be stored in cupboard for several days without refrigeration. If the dressing is to be stored for more than a week, put it into the refrigerator. Each tablespoon of dressing contains about ½ tablespoon of coconut oil.

Net carbs: 0.3 grams per 1 tablespoon serving.

Vinaigrette

¼ cup (60 ml) red or white wine vinegar
¼ teaspoon salt
⅛ teaspoon white pepper
¾ cup (180 ml) extra virgin olive oil

In a bowl, mix vinegar, salt, and pepper with a fork. Add oil and mix vigorously until well blended. Makes 1 cup.

Net carbs: 0 grams per ¼ cup serving.

Garlic Vinaigrette

Place 1 peeled, bruised clove of garlic into ¾ cup extra virgin olive oil and let stand 2-3 days at room temperature. Remove garlic and use oil to make the Vinaigrette recipe above.

Net carbs: 0 grams per ¼ cup serving.

Spanish Vinaigrette

Prepare Vinaigrette dressing as directed and place in a Mason jar with 1 tablespoon minced green olives and 1 teaspoon each minced chives, capers, parsley, and gherkin, and 1 sieved hard-boiled egg yolk. Shake, let stand at room temperature for 30 minutes; shake again before using.

Net carbs: 0.2 grams per ¼ cup serving.

Herb Vinegar

2 cups (200 g) fresh herbs*
2 cups (480 ml) apple cider or white wine vinegar, heated to boiling

Place herbs in a quart-size wide-mouth Mason jar and crush lightly with the handle of a wooden spoon. Pour in hot vinegar and cool to room temperature. Screw on lid and let stand in a cool spot (not the refrigerator) for 10-14 days. Once every day shake the jar to stir contents. Taste vinegar after 10 days and, if strong enough, strain through several thicknesses of cheesecloth into a fresh pint jar. If too weak, let stand for the full 14 days.

*Choose any of the following herbs: tarragon, chervil, dill, basil, or thyme.

Net carbs: 0 grams per ¼ cup serving.

Fresh Herb Dressing

½ cup (120 ml) extra virgin olive oil
1 tablespoon fresh dill, minced
1 tablespoon fresh chives, minced
1 tablespoon fresh parsley, minced
½ teaspoon salt
⅛ teaspoon black pepper
¼ cup (60 ml) tarragon vinegar*

Place oil, herbs, salt, and pepper in a Mason jar and let stand at room temperature 2-4 hours. Add vinegar and shake or stir well to blend.

*Use store bought tarragon vinegar or home-made (see Herb Vinegar recipe above).

Net carbs: 0 grams per ¼ cup serving.

Garlic Herb Dressing

1 clove garlic, peeled and crushed
½ teaspoon tarragon
½ teaspoon marjoram
½ teaspoon powdered mustard
¼ teaspoon salt
⅛ teaspoon black pepper
¼ cup (60 ml) extra virgin olive oil
2 tablespoons (30 ml) red or white wine vinegar

Put all ingredients in a pint Mason jar or similar container. Screw on lid and shake contents to mix. Let stand at room temperature at least 1 hour. Shake again just before using.

Net carbs: 0 grams per ¼ cup serving.

Buttermilk Dressing

½ cup (120 ml) apple cider vinegar
1 tablespoon (15 ml) extra virgin olive oil
1 teaspoon salt
⅛ teaspoon white pepper
1 tablespoon scallions, minced
1 cup (240 ml) buttermilk

Put all ingredients in a Mason jar or similar container. Screw on lid and shake contents to mix. Makes 1½ cups.

Net carbs: 2.2 grams per ¼ cup serving.

Sour Cream Dressing

1 cup (240 ml) sour cream
3 tablespoons (45 ml) white or apple cider vinegar
¼ teaspoon dill
½ teaspoon salt
⅛ teaspoon black pepper

Mix all ingredients, cover, and chill. Makes 1¼ cups.

Net carbs: 2 grams per ¼ cup serving.

Blue Cheese Dressing

½ cup (120 ml) heavy cream
½ cup (120 ml) sour cream
¼ cup (60 ml) mayonnaise
2 tablespoons (30 ml) lemon juice
6 ounces (170 g) blue cheese, crumbled
Salt and black pepper to taste

In a bowl whisk cream, sour cream, mayonnaise and lemon juice. Add cheese and put into a blender or food processor and blend for 1 minute. Makes about 1¾ cups.

Net carbs: 2.5 grams per ¼ cup serving.

Thousand Island Dressing

1 cup (240 ml) mayonnaise
¼ cup (60 ml) sour cream
2 tablespoons (30 g) dill pickle, chopped
6 black olives, chopped
¼ cup (60 ml) low-sugar ketchup or tomato sauce
2 tablespoons (30 ml) lemon juice

Combine all ingredients together and a bowl and mix thoroughly. Makes about 1¾ cups.

Net carbs: 1.5 grams per ¼ cup serving.

SAUCES

Sauces and gravies make excellent complements to vegetables and meats and can enhance their flavor and add variety to meals. Adding a little butter, salt, and black pepper to boiled, baked, sautéed, stir-fried, steamed, or mashed vegetables tastes great, but adding a sauce creates a whole new flavor sensation. Ordinary vegetables take on new life when combined with a sauce. The following recipes can be used with vegetables, meat, fish, poultry, and even eggs.

Tartar Sauce

1 cup (240 ml) mayonnaise
3 scallions, minced
1 tablespoon parsley, minced
¼ cup dill pickle, chopped
2 tablespoons capers
1 teaspoon (5 ml) prepared Dijon-style mustard
2 tablespoons (30 ml) red wine vinegar

Mix all ingredients, cover, and chill. Serve with seafood. Makes about 1¼ cups.

Net carbs: 0.1 grams per 1 tablespoon serving.

Creamy Cheese Sauce

2 tablespoons (30 ml) butter
½ cup (120 ml) heavy cream
1 cup (100 g) sharp cheddar cheese, shredded
⅛ teaspoon salt

In a saucepan, heat butter and cream until it begins to simmer and butter is melted. Turn off the heat, add cheese and salt stirring constantly until cheese is melted and mixture is thickened. Pour over cooked vegetables. Makes about 1 cup.

Net carbs: 1.2 grams per ¼ cup serving.

Shrimp Cheese Sauce

Make the Creamy Cheese Sauce as directed but delete the salt and add 1½ cups (150 g) precooked baby shrimp and 1 teaspoon of fish sauce. Makes an excellent topping for cooked vegetables.

Net carbs: 0.7 grams per ¼ cup serving.

Tex-Mex Cheese Sauce

Make the Creamy Cheese Sauce as directed and add ½ cup (120 ml) salsa.

Net carbs: 1.5 grams per ¼ cup serving.

Hot Pepper Cheese Sauce

Make the Creamy Cheese Sauce as directed and add ¼ cup (25 g) chopped jalapeño chili pepper.

Net carbs: 1.2 grams per ¼ cup serving.

White Sauce

2 tablespoons (30 ml) butter or coconut oil
½ cup 120 ml) heavy cream
1 cup (100 g) Monterey cheese, shredded*
⅛ teaspoon salt
¼ teaspoon onion powder

In a saucepan, heat butter and cream until it begins to simmer and butter is melted. Turn off the heat and add cheese, salt, and onion powder, stirring constantly until cheese is melted and mixture is thickened. Pour over cooked vegetables, eggs, or meat. Makes about 1 cup.

*May substitute Monterey Jack cheese if a spicier sauce is desired.

Net carbs: 0.9 gram per ¼ cup serving.

White Fish Sauce

2 tablespoons (30 ml) butter or coconut oil
½ cup 120 ml) heavy cream
1 cup (100 g) Monterey cheese, shredded
½ teaspoon (3 ml) fish sauce

In a saucepan, heat butter and cream until it begins to simmer and butter is melted. Turn off the heat and add cheese and fish sauce, stirring constantly until cheese is melted and mixture is thickened. Pour over cooked vegetables. Makes about 1 cup.

Net carbs: 0.9 gram per ¼ cup serving.

Sausage Cream Sauce

½ pound (240 g) ground pork sausage
2 cloves garlic, minced
½ cup (120 ml) heavy cream
¼ teaspoon onion powder
½ teaspoon dried sage
¼ teaspoon paprika
⅛ teaspoon salt
⅛ teaspoon black pepper
1 cup (100 g) Monterey cheese, shredded

In a saucepan, cook sausage and garlic until meat is browned and garlic is tender. Add cream and seasonings and bring to a simmer. Turn off the heat and add cheese, stirring constantly until cheese is melted and mixture is thickened. Pour over cooked vegetables, eggs, or meat.

Net carbs: 0.9 grams per ¼ cup serving.

Chicken Cream Sauce

2 tablespoons (30 ml) butter or coconut oil

1 cup (120 g) chopped cooked chicken
½ cup (120 ml) heavy cream
1 cup (100 g) Monterey cheese, shredded
¼ teaspoon dried sage
¼ teaspoon onion powder
⅛ teaspoon salt
⅛ teaspoon black pepper

Put butter, chicken, and cream in a saucepan and bring to a simmer. Turn off the heat and add cheese and seasonings, stirring constantly until cheese is melted and mixture is thickened. Pour over cooked vegetables, eggs, or meat.

Net carbs: 0.6 grams per ¼ cup serving.

Curry Sauce

2 tablespoons (30 ml) butter or coconut oil
½ cup (120 ml) heavy cream
1 cup (100 g) Monterey cheese, shredded
⅛ teaspoon salt
½ teaspoon curry powder or garam masala

In a saucepan, heat butter and cream until it begins to simmer and butter is melted. Turn off the heat and add cheese, salt, and curry powder, stirring constantly until cheese is melted and mixture is thickened. Pour over cooked vegetables, eggs, or meat. Makes about 1 cup.

Net carbs: 0.9 gram per ¼ cup serving.

MEALS FOR BREAKFAST, LUNCH, AND DINNER

For most people breakfast is the most difficult part of the low-carb diet. Traditionally, breakfast consists of high-carb foods such as hot or cold cereal, pancakes, waffles, French toast, hash brown potatoes, muffins, bagels, donuts, toaster pastries, toast and jelly, orange juice, cocoa, and such. The only traditional low-carb breakfast foods are eggs, bacon, ham, and sausage. You can do a lot with eggs. Serve them fried, scrambled, poached, hard or soft boiled, deviled, or as omelets and soufflés, and you already have a great variety. Adding meats and vegetables increases the serving possibilities further. One of the advantages of egg-based meals is that a full meal along with meat and vegetables generally contains fewer than 5 grams of carbohydrate. This allows for a larger amount of carbohydrate to be eaten at lunch and dinner. Several egg dishes are provided below.

As tasty and nutritious as eggs are, it is still nice to have variety for breakfast. Therefore, you should experiment with eating foods not generally considered a part of the traditional breakfast such as salads, soups, beef, chicken, fish, and vegetables. The following recipes can be used for breakfast, lunch, or dinner.

Most of the recipes below specify the use of coconut oil, but you may use butter, bacon drippings, red palm oil, or any other cooking oil you desire. You may also use a combination of oils. Coconut oil is specified in most recipes since this is one of the best ways to add coconut oil into the diet.

Oils are used in cooking primarily to prevent foods from sticking to the pans. The anti-sticking properties of oil vary from oil to oil. Lard has a very good anti-sticking character. By comparison, coconut oil has very modest anti-sticking properties. Coconut oil works very well when frying most vegetables and meats, but not as well with eggs and bread products (such as pancakes). The anti-sticking properties of coconut oil can be improved by mixing in a small portion of another oil, such as butter, bacon or sausage drippings, red palm oil, or olive oil. If an egg recipe calls for 1 tablespoon of coconut oil, for example, you may add an additional teaspoon (⅓ tablespoon) or so of butter or some other oil. This isn't required, but it will make removing the egg from the pan a little easier.

You don't have to be a gourmet chef to make delicious low-carb meals. Other than tossed salads, the easiest low-carb meals consist simply of a piece of cooked meat (roasted, fried, baked, grilled, poached, stir-fried) and a vegetable or two. The vegetables can be sautéed, steamed, roasted, poached, or raw. Easier still is to combine the meat and vegetables into a single skillet, crock pot, or baking dish and cook them together. The advantage to this is that it simplifies cooking, requires less cleanup, and, best of all, the meat drippings, especially when combined with seasoned salt or other spices, give the vegetables a wonderful taste. Below you will find several single skillet recipes to show you how simple and tasty this way of cooking can be.

In most of the recipes provided below you can use more oil than indicated. If you want to make sure you get your daily dose, include enough coconut oil so that your portion of the meal includes 1-2 full tablespoons of coconut oil. Calculate this so that you know exactly how much coconut oil is in the dish. When meat is cooked in coconut oil, the oil takes on the flavor of the meat drippings. Use the drippings like a sauce and pour it over your meat and vegetables. Fatty cuts of meat and chicken with the skins on produce the best-tasting drippings.

Easy Omelet

Omelets are easy to make and with different ingredients can be made into a dozen or more variations. Omelets made in the traditional French manner can be a bit complicated. This recipe is a simplified version that tastes just as good and allows for multiple variations. These directions are for a plain omelet.

2 tablespoons (30 ml) coconut oil
4 eggs
¼ teaspoon salt
⅛ teaspoon black pepper

Melt coconut oil in skillet over medium heat. Whisk together eggs, salt and pepper in a bowl. Pour mixture into the hot skillet, cover, and cook without stirring until the top of the omelet is set, about five minutes. Remove omelet from pan and serve hot. Serves two.

Net carbs: 1.2 grams per serving.

Cheese Omelet

Follow the directions for making the Easy Omelet, but after pouring the egg mixture into the hot skillet, sprinkle 1 cup of shredded cheese over the top. Cover and cook without stirring until the omelet is set and the cheese is melted. Serves two.

Net carbs: 2 grams per serving.

Sausage, Mushroom, and Tomato Omelet

This is a good example of how to prepare an omelet that is combined with meats and vegetables. See the many variations below.

1 tablespoon (15 ml) coconut oil
¼ pound (120 g) sausage
2 mushrooms, sliced
4 eggs
¼ teaspoon salt
½ cup (90 g) tomato, chopped

Heat coconut oil in a skillet. Add sausage and mushrooms and cook until browned. Whisk together eggs and salt in a bowl. Pour mixture into the hot skillet over the sausage and mushrooms, cover, and cook without stirring until the top of the omelet is set, about five minutes. Add tomato, cover, and cook 1 minute. Remove omelet from pan and serve hot. Serves two.

Net carbs: 2.8 grams per serving.

Variations: A variety of omelets can be made using many different ingredients including ham, bacon, chicken, sausage, ground beef, ground lamb, shrimp, crab, onions, eggplant, zucchini, garlic, sweet or hot peppers, tomatoes, avocado, asparagus, broccoli, cauliflower, spinach, and mushrooms. The meats and most of the vegetables are cooked before combining with the egg mixture. Tomato, avocado, and garnishes such as cilantro and chives are best used raw and added after cooking. Sour cream can be used as a garnish as well. Cheese can be melted on top during the cooking of the eggs. Any one or more of these ingredients can be combined. You need to make note of the quantities of each ingredient used so that you can calculate the net carbs.

Onion Frittata

This is an Italian omelet that is browned on both sides.

1 medium-size red onion, peeled and sliced very thin
2 tablespoons (30 ml) coconut oil
1 clove garlic, diced
4 eggs, lightly beaten
¾ teaspoon salt
⅛ teaspoon black pepper
1 teaspoon basil
2 tablespoons grated cheese
1 tablespoon (15 ml) extra virgin olive oil

Using a skillet, sauté onion in coconut oil over medium heat for about 5 minutes until limp, but not brown. Add garlic and cook an additional 1 minute. In a bowl mix together eggs, seasonings, and cheese. Add extra virgin olive oil to the onions and garlic in the skillet. Pour the egg mixture into the hot skillet. Cook without stirring 3-4 minutes until browned underneath and just set on top. Cut in quarters, turn, and brown flip side 2-3 minutes. Serves two.

Net carbs: 6.6 grams per serving.

Ham and Tomato Frittata

This is a variation of the traditional Italian omelet described above.

1 clove garlic, diced
2 tablespoons (30 ml) coconut oil
4 eggs, lightly beaten
½ cup ham, diced
¾ teaspoon salt
⅛ teaspoon black pepper
1 teaspoon basil
2 tablespoons grated fresh Parmesan cheese
1 medium tomato, chopped
1 tablespoon (15 ml) extra virgin olive oil

Using a skillet, sauté garlic in coconut oil over medium heat for 1-2 minutes, until lightly browned. In a bowl mix together eggs, ham, seasonings, cheese, and tomato. Add extra virgin olive oil to the garlic in the skillet. Pour the egg mixture into the hot skillet. Cook without stirring about 4 minutes until browned underneath and just set on top. Cut in quarters, turn, and brown flip side 2-3 minutes. Serves two.

Net carbs: 3.5 grams per serving.

Simple Soufflé

Soufflés are similar to omelets. This version starts on the stovetop like an omelet but is finished off in the oven, giving it a unique taste and texture. Use eggs at room temperature; this will give them better volume. It is important to use a pan that is both stovetop and oven safe.

4 eggs, separated
¼ teaspoon salt
⅛ teaspoon black pepper
2 tablespoons (30 ml) coconut oil

Preheat oven to 350 degree F (175 C). Beat egg yolks, salt, and pepper lightly with a fork. In a separate bowl beat egg whites until stiff peaks form. Gently mix one-fourth of the egg whites into the yolks. Fold remaining whites into the yolk mixture. Do not over mix. Heat oil in an oven safe pan on the stovetop. Pour egg mixture into hot pan and cook for 1 minute. Transfer pan to oven and cook uncovered for 15 minutes or until soufflé is puffy and delicately browned. Remove from oven, divide in half with a spatula, and serve. Serves two.

Net carbs: 1.2 grams per serving.

Cheese Soufflé

In this recipe you first make a cheese sauce which is then mixed into the egg whites. Use a pan that is both stovetop and oven safe.

2 tablespoons (30 ml) butter
½ cup (120 ml) heavy cream
1¼ cups (150 g) sharp cheddar cheese, shredded
3 eggs, separated
¼ teaspoon salt
⅛ teaspoon black pepper
2 tablespoons (30 ml) coconut oil

Melt butter in a saucepan over moderate heat. Add cream and cheese, stirring until cheese is melted. Beat egg yolks, salt, and pepper lightly with a fork. Blend about ¼ cup (60 ml) of hot cheese sauce into the yolks. Immediately stir the yolk mixture into the cheese sauce. Cook the sauce over low heat, stirring constantly, for 1-2 minutes. Remove from heat and let cool to room temperature. Meanwhile, preheat oven to 350 degree F (175 C). In a separate bowl, beat egg whites until stiff peaks form. Gently mix one-fourth of the egg whites into the sauce. Fold the remaining whites into the sauce. Do not over mix or your soufflé will become flat. Heat coconut oil in an oven safe pan on the stovetop. Pour egg mixture into hot pan and cook for 1 minute. Transfer pan to oven and cook uncovered for 18-20 minutes or until soufflé is puffy and delicately browned. Remove from oven, divide in half with a spatula, and serve. Serves two.

Net carbs: 3.2 grams per serving.

Variations: Prepare Cheese Soufflé as directed but before cooling cheese sauce, mix in any of the following: cooked ham or sausage, crisp crumbled bacon, minced sautéed chicken livers, deviled ham, minced sautéed mushrooms, minced cooked fish or shellfish, minced cooked vegetables (pimiento, asparagus, spinach, broccoli, cauliflower, cabbage, Brussels sprouts, or onions). Use ¼ to ½ cup (25-50 g) of any of these ingredients in the recipe. Adjust net carbs to account for additional ingredients.

Egg Foo Young

This egg dish is an interesting change from the traditional omelet or soufflé.

2 tablespoons (30 ml) coconut oil
2 eggs
½ cup (60 g) cooked meat (chicken, pork, or shrimp)
1 medium mushroom, sliced
½ cup (50 g) bean sprouts
1 scallion, chopped
¼ cup (25 g) shredded Chinese cabbage (or green cabbage)
2 teaspoons (10 ml) fish sauce

Heat coconut oil in skillet. In a bowl, beat eggs. Stir in remaining ingredients. Pour mixture into hot skillet, cover, cook until eggs are firm, turning once to lightly brown both sides. Remove from heat and serve. Makes two servings.

Net carbs: 2.4 grams per serving.

Fried Egg and Ham with White Sauce

1 tablespoon (15 ml) coconut oil
1 egg
3-5 ounces (80-140 g) sliced ham
¼ cup (60 ml) White Sauce (page 282)

Heat oil in a skillet. Fry egg and ham to desired doneness. Place ham on serving plate with egg on top, cover with White Sauce. Makes one serving.

Net carbs: 1.5 grams per serving.

Deviled Eggs

Deviled eggs can be made in advance and eaten as an on-the-go lunch or as a snack. Combined with a small salad or other raw vegetables, they can make an entire meal.

6 hard boiled eggs, peeled and halved lengthwise
¼ cup (60 ml) mayonnaise
2 teaspoons (10 ml) lemon juice
¼ teaspoon powdered mustard or 1 teaspoon (5 ml) Dijon mustard
1 teaspoon grated yellow onion
1 teaspoon (5 ml) Worcestershire sauce
Pinch white pepper

Suggested Garnishes:
Parsley, watercress, tarragon, dill, or chervil
Pimiento strips
Sliced green olive
Capers
Rolled anchovy fillets
Paprika

Mash yolks well, mix in remaining ingredients, mound into whites, and chill at least ½ hour. Add garnish as desired and serve. Makes 12 servings.

Net carbs: 0.5 grams per serving.

Zucchini Delight

While the eggs in this recipe may make this sound like a good breakfast meal, it is suitable for dinner as well.

2 tablespoons (30 ml) coconut oil (more may be added)
4 eggs
1 small zucchini, sliced
½ cup (50 g) onions, chopped
¼ cup (25 g) bell pepper, chopped
2 tablespoons (12 g) hot pepper (optional)
½ cup (60 g) cheese, shredded
½ cup 50 g) tomato, diced
Salt and pepper to taste

Heat oil in skillet and lightly sauté all vegetables except the tomatoes. In a bowl, beat eggs and pour over vegetables in the skillet. Cover and cook for about 5 minutes or until eggs are about half-cooked. Remove lid, sprinkle cheese on top, cover and cook until cheese is melted and eggs are thoroughly cooked. Uncover, sprinkle top with diced tomato, cover, and turn off heat. Let sit for 1-2 minutes to warm the tomato pieces without cooking them. Serves two.

Net carbs: 9.4 grams per serving.

Bratwurst and Cabbage

This delicious single skillet meal can be enjoyed for breakfast or for dinner.

2 tablespoons (30 ml) coconut oil (more may be added)
1 bratwurst
¼ cup (40 g) onion, chopped
¼ cup (40 g) bell pepper, chopped
1½ cups (125 g) cabbage, chopped
Salt and black pepper to taste

Heat coconut oil in skillet. Add bratwurst, onions, and bell pepper. Sauté until the vegetables are crisp and tender and bratwurst is lightly browned. Stir in cabbage, cover, and cook until tender. Add salt and black pepper to taste and serve. Pour meat drippings over vegetables. Serves one.

Net carbs: 9.2 grams per serving.

Rollups

Rollups can be prepared in advance and make an excellent lunch to go. They can also make tasty snacks or a quick breakfast.

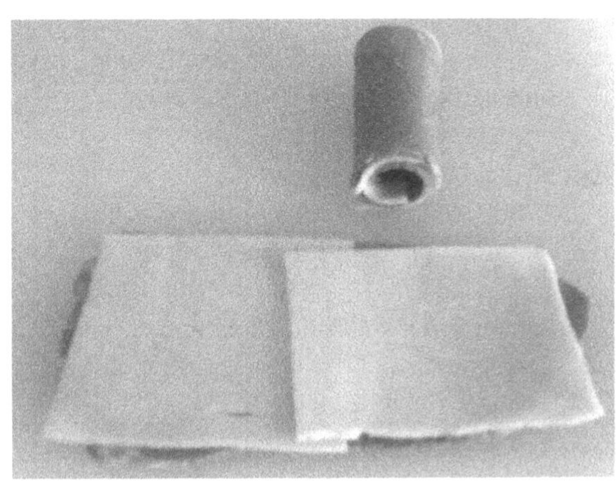

1 slice meat (1 oz)
1 slice cheese (1 oz)

You can use most any type of thinly sliced meat (ham, beef, corned beef, chicken, turkey) and thinly sliced hard cheese (cheddar, Colby, Edam, Monterey jack, Swiss, mozzarella, Muenster). To make the basic rollup, layer one thinly sliced piece of cheese on top of a thinly sliced piece of meat. Roll both slices into a log. Eat and enjoy.

Net carbs: about 0.5 gram depending on the type of cheese used, one rollup per serving.

Variations: A variety of rollups can be created by wrapping other ingredients in the center of the log. You can use any one or more of the following: mustard, mayonnaise, sprouts, cream cheese, guacamole, avocado, pickle, chopped eggs, cucumber, sauerkraut, sweet or hot peppers, scallions, and sprouts with Vinaigrette dressing (page 278).

Pork Chops and Green Beans

2 tablespoons (30 ml) coconut oil (more may be added)
2 pork chops
½ cup (50 g) onion, chopped
3 cups (300 g) green beans
4 mushrooms, sliced
Salt and black pepper to taste

Heat coconut oil in skillet. Add pork chops and cook until browned on one side. Turn pork chops over and add onion and green beans. Cover and cook until chops are browned on second side and vegetables are tender. Stir in mushrooms and cook until tender, about 2 minutes. Remove from heat. Add salt and pepper and serve. Pour meat drippings over vegetables. Serves two.

Net carbs; 10.5 grams per serving.

Hamburger Steak, Mushrooms, and Onions

Ground beef is cooked like a steak with mushrooms and onions. Tastes fantastic with White Sauce, see page 282.

1 tablespoon (15 ml) coconut oil (more may be added)
1 pound (450 g) ground beef
8 ounces (230 g) mushrooms, sliced
1 medium onion, sliced and separated
Salt and black pepper to taste

Heat the oil in a skillet. Divide ground beef into four patties and place in the hot skillet. Add the onions. Cook the meat until one side is browned and flip over. Add mushrooms and continue to cook until second side of beef patty is cooked and mushrooms are tender. Add salt and pepper to taste. Pour drippings over meat and vegetables. Two beef patties with half the vegetables constitute one serving.

Net carbs: 7.2 grams per serving.

Variation: Serve with White Sauce poured over the meat and vegetables.

Chicken and Broccoli

2 tablespoons (30 ml) coconut oil (more may be added)
1 pound (450 g) chicken parts (breast, thigh, or leg)
3 cups (200 g) broccoli, divided into stalks
Salt and black pepper to taste

Heat oil in a large skillet over medium heat. Place chicken, skin side down, in hot skillet, cover, and cook for 20-25 minutes. Turn chicken over, cover, and continue to cook for 15 minutes. Add broccoli, cover and cook another 10 minutes or until vegetables are tender and chicken is completely cooked. Add salt and pepper to taste. Pour meat drippings over broccoli. Divide chicken and broccoli into two servings.

Net carbs: 5.4 grams per serving.

Lamb Chops and Asparagus

2 tablespoons (30 ml) coconut oil (more may be added)
2 lamb chops (may also use pork chops or steak)
4 cups (400 g) asparagus
Salt and black pepper to taste

Heat oil in a skillet, add chops, cover, and cook until one side is browned. Flip chops and add asparagus, cover and cook until asparagus is tender and chops thoroughly cooked. Remove from heat and add salt and pepper to taste. Pour meat drippings over asparagus. Serves two.

Net carbs: 4.8 grams per serving.

Variation: Serve with White Sauce (page 282) poured over the vegetables.

Chicken Stir-Fry

2 tablespoons (30 ml) coconut oil (more may be added)
1 pound (450 g) chicken, cut into bite size pieces
½ cup (50 g) onion, chopped
½ cup (50 g) snow peas, cut in half
½ cup (50 g) bok choy, chopped
½ cup (50 g) bell pepper, chopped
4 mushrooms, sliced
1 cup (100 g) bean sprouts
½ cup (50 g) bamboo shoots
1-3 teaspoons (5-15 ml) rice vinegar
Salt to taste

Heat coconut oil in a skillet. Sauté chicken and vegetables until vegetables are tender and chicken is cooked. Turn off heat, add rice vinegar and salt to taste. Serves two.

Net carbs: 10.2 grams per serving.

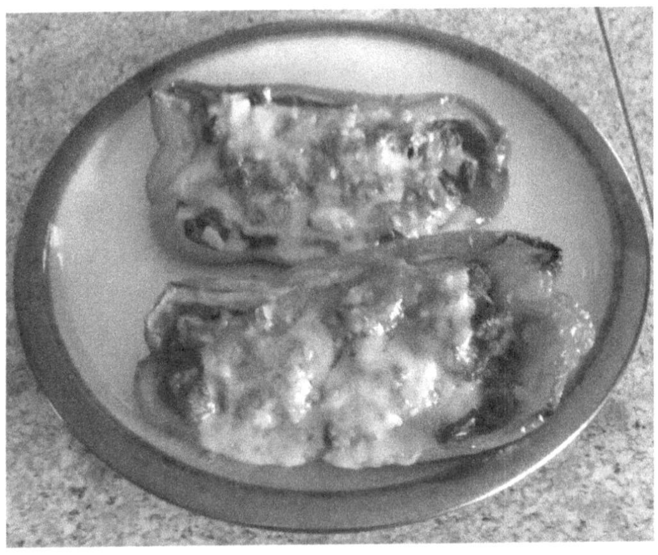

Stuffed Bell Peppers

1 bell pepper
½ pound (450 g) ground beef
¼ cup (25 g) onions, diced
2 mushrooms, chopped
1 tablespoon (15 ml) salsa
⅛ teaspoon salt
4 ounces (115 g) cheddar cheese

Preheat oven to 350 degrees F (175 C). Cut bell pepper in half lengthwise and remove stem, veins, and seeds. Place pepper halves aside. Mix together ground beef, onion, mushrooms, salsa, and salt. Fill each pepper shell with half of the mixture. Place the stuffed peppers on an oven safe pan or cookie sheet. Bake for 40 minutes. Divide the cheese in half and put half on each pepper. Cook another 10 minutes. Remove from the oven, cool, and enjoy. Makes two servings. Serve with a side salad or fresh vegetables.

Net carb: 6 grams per serving.

Fillet of Sole in Coconut Milk

2 tablespoons (30 ml) coconut oil (more may be added)
½ medium onion, chopped
½ cup bell pepper, chopped
2 cups (200 g) chopped cauliflower
2 cloves garlic, chopped
4 sole fillets*
1 teaspoon garam masala**
¾ cup (180 ml) coconut milk
Salt and black pepper to taste

Heat coconut oil in skillet and sauté onion, pepper, cauliflower, and garlic until tender. Push vegetable to side of skillet and add sole. Stir garam masala into coconut milk and add to skillet. Cover and simmer for about 8 minutes. Add salt and pepper. Makes four servings.

*You may use any type of fish in this recipe.

**Garam masala is a blend of spices commonly used in Indian cuisine and similar to curry powder. It's available in the spice section of most grocery stores. If you don't have garam masala, you can use curry powder.

Net carbs: 5.4 grams per serving.

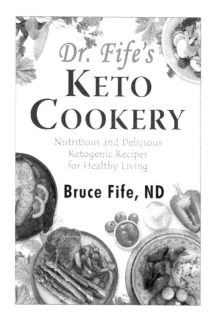

Appendix

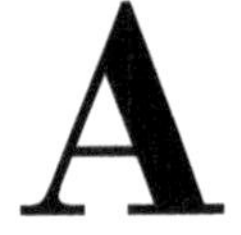

Mental Status Test

This test is similar to the Mini-Mental State Examination (MMSE) doctors use to evaluate cognitive function. It offers a quick and simple way to test memory, orientation, calculation, and language skills and to detect possible cognitive problems.

The MMSE is used to screen for cognitive impairment, determine severity of impairment, and is readministered periodically to monitor patient's response to treatment. This Mental Status Test can be used at home in a similar manner. It is a useful tool that anyone can use to evaluate for possible cognitive impairment. The test can be retaken periodically to monitor cognitive status.

Read the questions aloud to the person taking the test. If you want to take the test yourself, you may either have someone read it to you, or you may read it yourself. Do not time the test, but score it right away. Each answer is worth 1 point. To score, add the number of correct responses. The maximum score possible is 30 points.

	Correct	Incorrect
1. What is your age?	☐	☐
2. What is your date of birth?	☐	☐
3. What day of the week is it today?	☐	☐
4. What is the month?	☐	☐
5. What is the year?	☐	☐
6. What is your address (include street, house or apartment number, and zip/postal code)?	☐	☐
7. Whose home are you in at this time?	☐	☐
8. What city are you in?	☐	☐
9. What state (or county) are you in?	☐	☐
10. Write the following sentence: Good citizens always wear stout shoes.	☐	☐
Read the sentence again and try to remember it.		
11. Read or have someone say the followings words slowly and then repeat the words in order afterwards: hand, mirror, apple, shoe.	☐	☐
	Correct	Incorrect

12. Write the following sequence of numbers on a sheet of paper: 92537. Read it over and try to remember it. ☐ ☐
13. Name the current president/prime minister of the country in which you live. ☐ ☐
14. Count backwards from 20 to 1. ☐ ☐
15. Spell the word "SUNDAY" backwards (without looking at the word). ☐ ☐
16. On a blank piece of paper draw the following diagram. ☐ ☐

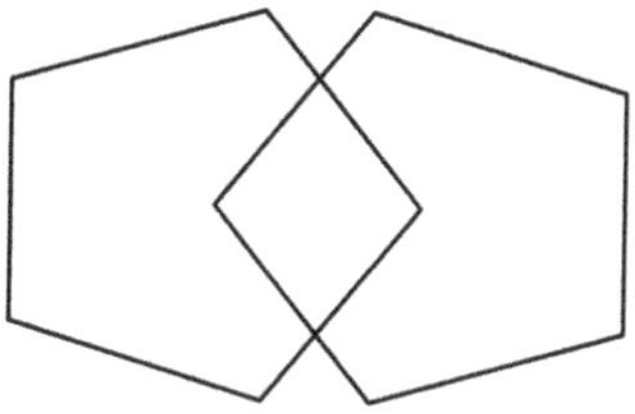

17-20. Earlier you were told to name four words in order, can you repeat those words without looking?

__________ ☐ ☐
__________ ☐ ☐
__________ ☐ ☐
__________ ☐ ☐

21-24. Name four fruits or vegetables that start with the letter C.

__________ ☐ ☐
__________ ☐ ☐
__________ ☐ ☐
__________ ☐ ☐

25-27. Calculate the sums for the following equations:

14 + 17 = _____ ☐ ☐
32 – 5 = _____ ☐ ☐
7 + 14 – 2 = _____ ☐ ☐

28. How is an apple like a turnip? ☐ ☐
29. Without going back to look, write down the sentence you wrote on a piece of paper earlier. ☐ ☐
30. Without going back to look, write down the sequence of numbers you wrote earlier. ☐ ☐

Total for each column ____ ____

Answers and Scoring

Score one point for each correct answer.

1-14. Answers are self evident.

15. YADNUS

16. All ten angles must be present and two must intersect.

17-20. Hand, mirror, apple, shoe. Score one point for each word recalled. The words need not be in order. Maximum score possible four points.

21-24. Score one point for each fruit or vegetable named. Some possible choices include cabbage, carrot, cauliflower, celery, chard, Chinese cabbage, corn, cucumber, cantaloupe, cherries, cranberries, and currants. Maximum score possible four points.

25-27. Answers are 31, 27, and 19.

28. Any sensible answer is permissible. For example: they come from plants, they are edible, they grow, they are living, they can fit in the palm of the hand, and so forth.

29. Good citizens always wear stout shoes.

30. Sequence is 92537.

A score of 25-30 points is considered normal. Any score below 25 suggests some cognitive impairment. A score of 21-24 points suggests mild impairment, 10-20 points moderate impairment, and 9 or fewer points severe impairment. Low scores correlate closely with the presence of dementia and should be confirmed by a more thorough medical examination.

This exam can be repeated periodically to monitor changes in cognitive function over time. Don't worry about using the same questions over again. Someone with cognitive difficulties will likely not remember the answers and anyone who can remember them apparently isn't troubled with cognitive problems.

Appendix B

Parkinson's Disease Rating Scale

This is a modified version of the Unified Parkinson's Disease Rating Scale (UPDRS), which is used to assess severity of Parkinson's symptoms and monitor therapy. The complete test, which is generally administered by a neurologist, is available online. You can find it by doing a search for "Unified Parkinson's Disease Rating Scale." This abbreviated version should be completed by someone who is in close daily contact with the patient or by someone who can ask such a person questions. Scores for performance are rated from 0 (normal) to 4 (severe). The higher the score, the greater the disability.

1. Speech
0 = Normal.
1 = Mildly affected. No difficulty being understood.
2 = Moderately affected. Sometimes asked to repeat statements.
3 = Severely affected. Frequently asked to repeat statements.
4 = Unintelligible most of the time.

2. Salivation
0 = Normal.
1 = Rare choking.
2 = Moderately excessive saliva; may have minimal drooling.
3 = Marked excess of saliva with some drooling.
4 = Marked drooling, requires constant tissue or handkerchief.

3. Swallowing
0 = Normal.
1 = Rare choking.
2 = Occasional choking.
3 = Requires soft food.
4 = Requires NG tube or gastrotomy feeding.

4. Handwriting
0 = Normal.
1 = Somewhat slow and clumsy, but no help needed.
2 = Moderately slow or small; all words are legible.
3 = Severely affected; not all words are legible.
4 = The majority of words are not legible.

5. Cutting food and handling utensils
0 = Normal.
1 = Somewhat slow, but no help needed.
2 = Can cut most foods, although clumsy and slow; some help needed.
3 = Food must be cut by someone, but can still feed slowly.
4 = Needs to be fed.

6. Dressing
0 = Normal.
1 = Somewhat slow, but no help needed.
2 = Occasional assistance with buttoning, getting arms in sleeves.
3 = Considerable help required, but can do some things alone.
4 = Helpless.

7. Hygiene
0 = Normal.
1 = Somewhat slow, but no help needed.
2 = Needs help to shower or bathe; or very slow in hygienic care.
3 = Requires assistance for washing, brushing teeth, combing hair, going to bathroom.
4 = Foley catheter or other mechanical aids.

8. Turning in bed and adjusting bed clothes
0 = Normal.
1 = Somewhat slow and clumsy, but no help needed.
2 = Can turn alone or adjust sheets, but with great difficulty.
3 = Can initiate, but not turn or adjust sheets alone.
4 = Helpless.

9. Falling (unrelated to freezing)
0 = None.
1 = Rare falling.
2 = Occasionally falls, less than once per day.
3 = Falls an average of once daily.
4 = Falls more than once daily.

10. Freezing when walking
0 = None.
1 = Rare freezing when walking; may have start hesitation.

2 = Occasional freezing when walking.
3 = Frequent freezing. Occasionally falls from freezing.
4 = Frequent falls from freezing.

11. Walking
0 = Normal.
1 = Mild difficulty. May not swing arms or may tend to drag leg.
2 = Moderate difficulty, but requires little or no assistance.
3 = Severe disturbance of walking, requiring assistance.
4 = Cannot walk at all, even with assistance.

12. Sensory complaints related to parkinsonism
0 = None.
1 = Occasionally has numbness, tingling, or mild aching.
2 = Frequently has numbness, tingling, or aching; not distressing.
3 = Frequent painful sensations.
4 = Excruciating pain.

13. Speaking
0 = Normal.
1 = Slight loss of expression, diction and/or volume.
2 = Monotone, slurred but understandable; moderately impaired.
3 = Marked impairment, difficult to understand.
4 = Unintelligible.

14. Tremor at rest (head, upper and lower extremities)
0 = Absent.
1 = Slight and infrequently present.
2 = Mild in amplitude and persistent. Or moderate in amplitude, but only intermittently present.
3 = Moderate in amplitude and present most of the time.
4 = Marked in amplitude and present most of the time.

15. Action or Postural Tremor of hands
0 = Absent.
1 = Slight; present with action.
2 = Moderate in amplitude, present with action.
3 = Moderate in amplitude with posture holding as well as action.
4 = Marked in amplitude; interferes with feeding.

16. Finger Taps
Have patient tap thumb with index finger in rapid succession.
0 = Normal.
1 = Mild slowing and/or reduction in amplitude.
2 = Moderately impaired. Definite and early fatiguing. May have occasional arrests in movement.

3 = Severely impaired. Frequent hesitation in initiating movements or arrests in ongoing movement.
4 = Can barely perform the task.

17. Hand Movements

Have patient open and close hands in rapid succession.
0 = Normal.
1 = Mild slowing and/or reduction in amplitude.
2 = Moderately impaired. Definite and early fatiguing. May have occasional arrests in movement.
3 = Severely impaired. Frequent hesitation in initiating movements or arrests in ongoing movement.
4 = Can barely perform the task.

18. Leg Agility

Have the patient tap his or her heel on the ground in rapid succession picking up entire leg. The foot should be lifted at least 3 inches off the ground.
0 = Normal.
1 = Mild slowing and/or reduction in amplitude.
2 = Moderately impaired. Definite and early fatiguing. May have occasional arrests in movement.
3 = Severely impaired. Frequent hesitation in initiating movements or arrests in ongoing movement.
4 = Can barely perform the task.

19. Arising from Chair

Have patient rise from a straight backed chair, with arms folded across chest.
0 = Normal.
1 = Slow or may need more than one attempt.
2 = Pushes self up from arms of seat.
3 = Tends to fall back and may have to try more than one time, but can get up without help.
4 = Unable to arise without help.

20. Posture

0 = Normal erect.
1 = Not quite erect, slightly stooped posture; could be normal for older person.
2 = Moderately stooped posture, definitely abnormal; can be slightly leaning to one side.
3 = Severely stooped posture with kyphosis (hunchback); can be moderately leaning to one side.
4 = Marked flexion with extreme abnormality of posture.

21. Gait

0 = Normal.
1 = Walks slowly, may shuffle with short steps, but no festination (hastening steps) or propulsion.
2 = Walks with difficulty, but requires little or no assistance; may have some festination, short steps, or propulsion.
3 = Severe disturbance of gait, requiring assistance.
4 = Cannot walk at all, even with assistance.

22. Postural Stability

Patient stands erect with eyes open and feet slightly apart. While patient is prepared, pull back on the patient's shoulders forcing him or her off balance.
0 = Normal.
1 = Steps backward or to the side, but recovers unaided.
2 = Absence of postural response; would fall if not caught by examiner.
3 = Very unstable, tends to lose balance spontaneously.
4 = Unable to stand without assistance.

Score

A score of 10 or less indicates the subject is essentially normal; 11-43 mild impairment; 44-65 moderate impairment; and 66-88 severe impairment. Although this is a subjective test that relies on the observations and opinions of the administrator, it can provide useful information for identifying problems and monitoring progress. The subject can be reevaluated periodically over time to assess changes in condition.

Source: Fahn, S. and Elton, R., Members of the UPDRS Development Committee. In: Fahn S., Marsden, C.D., Calne, D.B., Goldstein, M., eds. *Recent Developments in Parkinson's Disease, Vol 2*. Florham Park, NJ. Macmillan Health Care Information 1987, pp 15 3-163, 293-304.

Appendix C

Drugs Seniors Should Avoid

Drugs listed can cause or worsen brain disorders or lead to other serious health problems in older adults. This chart is arranged alphabetically by the drug's generic name, which is in bold letters. Brand names are listed under the generic name. This list contains many of the most common drugs that can have adverse effects on the central nervous system, however, it does not contain every such drug. Therefore, simply because a drug is not listed does not necessarily mean it is without risks.

Alprazolam
Benzodiazepine/tranquilizer
Alprazolam Intensol, Apo-Alpraz, Apo-Alpraz TS, Gen-Alprazolam, Novo-Alprazol, Nu-Alpraz, ratio-Alprazolam, Xanax, Xanax XR, Xanax TS, Niravam

Amitriptylin
Anticholinergic/antidepressant
Elavil, Amitriptyline, Apo-Amitriptyline, Levate, Novo-Triptyn, PMS-Amitriptyline

Amitriptyline/Perphenazine
Anticholinergic/antidepressant
Apo-Peram, Etrafon, PMS-Levazine, Duo-Vil 2-10

Amphetamine
Stimulant/antinarcoleptic
Adderall, Adderall XR, Dexedrin Spansule, Dexedrine

Atorvastatin
Statin/cholesterol reduction
Lipitor

Belladonna Alkaloids
Anticholinergic/antispasmodic/stomach disorders
Bentylol, Buscopan, Formulex, Gastrozepin, Levsin, Pro-Banthine, Propanthel, Robinul, Robinul Forte, Spasmoban, Transderm-V

Benztropine
Anticholinergic/treatment for Parkinson's
Cogentin, Apo-Benztropine

Biperiden
Anticholinergic/treatment for Parkinson's
Akineton

Bromocriptine
Dopamine agonist/treatment for Parkinson's
Parlodel, Cycloset, Apo-Bromocriptine, PMS-Bromocriptine

Butabarbital
Depressant/sedative
Butisol Sodium

Carisoprodol
Anticholinergic/muscle relaxant
Soma, Vanadom

Chlordiazepoxide
Benzodiazepine/tranquilizer
Librium, Limbitrol, Limbitrol DS, Apo-Chlordiazepoxide HCL, Apo-Chlorax, Librax

Chlorpheniramine
Anticholinergic/antihistamines/used in many cough and cold remedies
Ahist, Aller-Chlor, Allergy, Allergy Relief, Chlor-Trimeton, Chlor-Trimeton Allergy, Chlorpheniramine Maleate, Buckley's, Children's Nyquil Liquid, Children's Tylenol Cold, Chlor-Tripolon, Dimetapp, Dristan, Extra Strength Tylenol Allergy Sinus, Extra Strength Tylenol Cold Nighttime Caplet, Jack & Jill Children's Formula, Neo Citran, Polaramine, Sinutab, Triaminic, Vasofrinic, Vicks Formula 44m, Chlor-Tripolon

Chlorzoxazone
Anticholinergic/muscle relaxant
Paraflex, Parafon Forte DSC, Remular-S, Acetazone Forte C8, Acetazone Forte, Back-Aid Forte, Extra Strength Tylenol Aches and Strains

Cimetidine
Histamine blocker/antacid
Apo-Cimetidine, Cimetidine, Dom-Cimetidine, Gaviscon Prevent, Gen-Cimetidine, Novo-Cimetine, Nu-Cimet, Peptol, PMS-Cimetidine, Apo-Cimetidine, Tagamet, Tagamet HB

Clidinium
Anticholinergic/antacid
Quarzan

Climetidine
Histamine blocker/antacid
Tagamet, Tagamet HB, Apo-Cimetidine, Gen-Cimetidine, Nu-Cimet

Clonazepam
Benzodiazepine/psychiatric disorders/tranquilizer
Klonopin, Apo-Clonazepam, CO Clonazepam, Gen-Clonazepam, PMS-Clonazepam, ratio-Clonazepam, Rivotril, Sandoz Clonazepam

Clonidine
Antihypertensive
Iopidine, Apo-Clonidine, Catapres, Catapres-TTS-1, Catapres-TTS-2, Catapres-TTS-3, Clonidine HCL, Dixarit, Novo-Clonidine, Nu-Clonidine, Duracion

Clorazepate
Benzodiazepine/tranquilizer
Tranxene, Apo-Clorazepate, Novo-Clopate, Tranxene

Cyclobenzaprine
Anticholinergic/muscle relaxant
Amrix, Cyclobenzaprine Hydrochloride, Alti-Cyclobenzaprine, Apo-Cyclobenzaprine, Cyclobenzaprine-10, Dom-Cyclobenzaprine, Flexeril, Gen-Cyclobenzaprine, Novo-Cycloprine, Nu-Cyclobenzaprine-Tab, PMS-Cyclobenzaprine, PHL-Cyclobenzaprine, ratio-Cyclobenzaprine, Riva-Cycloprine

Cyproheptadine
Anticholinergic/antihistamine
Euro-Cyproheptadine, PMS-Cypro-heptadine HCL

Diazepam
Benzodiazepine/tranquilizer
Apo-Diazepam, Fio-Diazepam, Diazepam, Diazemuls, E Pam, Diastat, Novo-Dipam, PMS-Diazepam, Valium, Vivol, Diazepam Intensol, Valium Roche Oral

Dicyclomine
Anticholinergic/GI antispasmodic/stomach disorders
Bemote, Bentyl, Bentylol, Byclomine, Dibent, Dilomine, Di-Spaz, Or-Tyl, Dicyclomine HCL, Diclophen, Lomine, Formulex, Protylol, Riva-Dicyclomine

Diphenhydramine
Anticholinergic/antihistamine/sleep aid/used in many allergy and cold remedies

Aller Aide Plus, Allerdryl, Allergy Elixir, Allergy Formula, Allernix, Balminil Night-Time, Benadryl, Buckley's Bedtime, Calmex, Calmylin, Children's Tylenol Allergy, Contac, Contac Night Caplets, Diphenhydramine HCL Children's Liquid, Diphenist, DM Cough Syrup, Dormex Extra Fort, Dormiphen Comprime, Ergodryl, Insomnal, Jack And Jill Bedtime, Nadryl, Nytol Extra Strength, PMS-Diphenhydramine, Pulmorex DM, Scheinpharm Diphenhydramine, Simply Sleep, Sinutab N.T. Extra Strength, Sleep Aid, Sleep-Eze D, Sominex, Unisom Nighttime Sleep Aid, Anacin P.M. Aspirin Free, Coricidin Night Time Cold Relief, Excedrin PM, Excedrin PM Caplet, Headache Relief PM, Legatrin PM, Mapap PM, Midol PM, Percogesic Extra Strength, Tylenol Cold Relief Caplet, Tylenol Cold Relief Nighttime, Tylenol Cold Relief Nighttime Caplet, Tylenol Extra Strength PM, Tylenol Extra Strength PM Vanilla Caplet, Tylenol PM, Tylenol Severe Allergy Caplet, Tylenol Sore Throat Nighttime, Unisom with Pain Relief

Disopyramide
Anticholinergic/antiarrhythmic
Norpace, Norpace CR, Rythmodan, Rythmodan-LA

Doxazosin
Anticholinergic/antihypertensive
Apo-Doxazosin, Cardura, Cardura XL, Doxadura, Cascor, Carduran, Dom-Doxazosin, Doxazosin, Gen-Doxazosin, Novo-Doxazosin, PMS-Doxazosin, ratio-Doxazosin

Doxepin
Anticholinergic/antidepressant
Alti-Doxepin, Apo-Doxepin, Doxepine, Sinequan, Novo-Doxepin, Triadapin

Doxylamine
Anticholinergic/insomnia/sleep aid
Unisom, Aldex, Nighttime Sleep Aid, Vicks NyQuil Cold & Flu Relief, Vicks NyQuil Cold & Flu Symptom Relief Plus Vitamin C, Vicks NyQuil Cough, Vicks NyQuil D, Vicks NyQuil Sinus

Eszopiclone
Sedative/sleep aid
Lunesta

Famotidine
Histamine blocker/antacid
Pepcid, Pepcid AC, Pepcid RPD, Mylanta AR, Apo-Famotidine, Gen-Famotidine, Nu-Famotidine

Fluoxetine
Antidepressant
Prozac, FXT, Selfemra, Sarafem, Rapiflux, Apo-Fluoxetine, CO Fluoxetine, Gen-Flyoxetine, Novo-Fluoxetine, Nu-Fluoxetine, PMS-Fluoxetine, ratio-Fluoxetine, Sandoz Fluoxetine

Flurazepam
Benzodiazepine/tranquilizer
Apo-Flurazepam, Bio-Flurazepam, Dalmane, Flurazepam, Novo-Flupam, PMS-Flurazepam, Somnol, Som Pam

Fluvastatin
Statin/cholesterol reduction
Lescol

Glycopyrrolate
Anticholinergic/antispasmodic
Robinul, Robinul Forte

Haloperidol
Antipsychotic/psychiatric disorders
Haldol, Haldol Decanoate, Apo-Haloperidol, Haloperidol LA

Homatropine
Anticholinergic/cough suppressant
Hycodan, Tussigon, Hydromet, Hydrotropine, Hydromide, Hydropane

Hydroxyzine
Anticholinergic/antihistamine/tranquilizer
Hydroxyzine HCL, Apo-Hydroxyzine, PMS Hydroxyzine, Nu-Hydroxyzine, Novo-Hydroxyzin, Riva-Hydroxyzin, Atarax Syrup, Vistaril, Hyzine, Vistaject-50, Rezine, Vistacon, Vistacot, Vistasine

Hyoscyamine
Anticholinergic/antispasmodic/stomach disorders
Anaspaz, Cystospaz, Donnamar, ED-SPAZ, Gastrosed, HyoMax, HyoMax FT, Levbid, Levsin, Levsin/SL, Levsinex, NuLev, Hyoscyaminum, AD HP

Ibuprofen
NSAID/analgesic
Advil, Advil Migraine, Genpril, Ibu, Midol, Motrin, Nuprin, Ibutab, Junior Strength Motrin, Motrin Migraine Pain, PediaCare Fever, Apo-Ibuprofen, Motrin IB Extra Strength, Motrin IB Super Strength

Indomethacin
NSAID
Indocin, Indocin SR, Apo-Indomethacin, SAB-Indomethacin, ratio-Indomethacin, Indocid-P.D.A., Pro-Indo, Novo-Methacin, Rhodacine, Nu-Indo

Ipratropium
Anticholinergic/bronchodilator
Combivent, Atrovent HFA, Ipratropium Bromide, Apo-Ipravent, Gen-Ipratropium, ratio-Ipratropium, ratio-Ipratropium UDV

Ketorolac
NSAID/analgesic
Acular, Acular LS, Acuvail, A-Ketorolac, Ketorolac Tromethamine, Novo-Ketorolac, Nu-Ketorolac, Ratio-Ketorolac, Toradol, Apo-Ketorolac, ratio-Ketorolac, Toradol IM

Lorazepam
Benzodiazepine/tranquilizer
Ativan, Lorazepam Intensol, Apo-Lorazepam, Dom-Lorazepam, Novo-Lorazem, Nu-Loraz, PMS-Lorazepam, Pro-Lorazepam

Lovastatin
Statin/cholesterol reduction
Mevacor

Mepenzolate
Anticholinergic/antacid
Cantil

Meperidine
Narcotic analgesic
Demerol, Meperitab

Mephobarbital
Depressant/sedative
Mebaral

Meprobamate
Tranquilizer
Equanil, Miltown, MB-TAB, 282 Mep, Novo-Mepro, Apo-Meprobamate

Metaxalone
Anticholinergic/muscle relaxant
Skelaxin

Methocarbamol
Anticholinergic/muscle relaxant
Dodd's Back-Ease, Dodd's Extra Strength Back-Ease, Extra Strength Aspirin Backache, Extra Strength Muscle & Back Pain Relief, Methocarbamol, Methocarbamol Omega, Methoxacet, Methoxisal, Muscle and Back Pain Relief, Muscle Relaxant and Analgesic, PMS-Methocarbamol, Relaxophen, Robax Platinum, Robaximol, Robaxacet, Robaxin, Robaxisal, Spasmhalt

Methscopolamine
Anticholinergic/antacid
Pamine, Pamine Forte

Methyldopa
Benzodiazepine/antihypertensive
Apo-Methyldopa, Dopamet, Methyldopa, Novo-Medopa, Nu-Medopa

Methylphenidate
Stimulant/psychiatric disorders
Ritalin, Ritalin LA, Ritalin-SR, Concerta, Metadate CD, Metadate ER, Methylin, Methylin ER, Apo-Metoclop, Nu-Metoclopramide

Metoclopramide
GI stimulant/stomach disorders
Reglan, Metozolv, Octamide, Maxolon, Apo-Metoclop, Nu-Metoclopramide

Naproxen
NSAID
Aleve, Anaprox, EC-Naprosyn, Anaprox D.S., Apo-Napro-Na, Apo-Naproxen, Gen-Naproxen, Naprosyn, Novo-Naprox, Nu-Naprox, PMS-Naproxen Suppositories, Ratio-Naproxen, Riva-Naproxen, Sab-Naproxen, Synflex, Naproxen Sodium, Midol Extended Relief, Naprelan

Nifedipine
Anticholinergic/calcium channel blocker/antihypertensive
Adalat CC, Nifediac, Nifedical, Procardia, Procardia XL, Adalat XL, Apo-Nifed, Apo-Nifed PA

Nizatidine
Histamine blocker/antacid
Axid, Axid AR, Axid Pulvules, Nizatidine, Apo-Nizatidine, Gen-Nizatidine, PMS-Nizatidine

Orphenadrine
Anticholinergic/muscle relaxant
Norflex, Norgesic, Orphenadrine Citrate, Rhoxal-Orphenadrine, Orfenace, Sandoz Orphenadrine

Oxaprozin
NSAID
Daypro, Apo-Oxaprozin, Daypro, Rhoxal-Oxaprozin

Oxazepam
Benzodiazepine/tranquilizer
Oxazepam, Serax, Apo-Oxazepam, Bio-Oxazepam, Novoxapam, Oxpam, PMS-Oxazepam, Zapex

Oxybutynin
Anticholinergic/bladder antispasmodic
Apo-Oxybutynin, Ditropan, Ditropan XL, Oxytrol, Dom-Oxybutynin, Gen-Oxybutynin, Novo-Oxybutynin, Nu-Oxybutynin, Oxybutynine, Oxybutyn, Oxytrol, PHL-Oxybutynin, PMS-Oxybutynin, Riva-Oxybutynin, Apo-Oxybutynin, Uromax, Urotrol

Pentazocine
Narcotic analgesic
Talwin, Talacen, Talwin NX

Piroxicam
NSAID
Feldene, Apo-Piroxicam, Dom-Piroxicam, Gen-Piroxicam, Novo-Pirocam, Nu-Pirox, PMS-Piroxicam, Pro-Piroxicam, Alti-Piroxicam

Phenobarbital
Sedative/hypnotic
Phenobarbital Sodium, Solfoton, PMS-Phenobarbital

Pravastatin
(Statin/cholesterol reduction
Pravachol

Primidone
Anticonvulsant
Mysoline

Promethazine
Anticholinergic/antihistamine
Bioniche Promethazine, Histantil, Phenergan, PMS-Promethazine, Promethazine, Pentazine,

Propantheline
Anticholinergic/GI muscle relaxant
Propanthel, Pro-Banthine

Propoxyphene
Narcotic analgesic
Darvon, Darvon-N, Novo-Propoxyn, PP-Cap

Quetiapine
Antipsychotic
Seroquel

Ramelteon
Sedative/sleep aid
Rozerem

Ranitidine
Anticholinergic/histamine blocker/antacid
Zantac, Zantac EFFERdose, Apo-Ranitidine, CO Ranitidine, Gen-Ranitidine, Novo-Ranitidine, Novo-Ranidine, Nu-Ranit,

PMS-Ranitidine, ratio-Ranitidine, Sandoz Ranitidine, Taladine

Reserpine
Benzodiazepine/antihypertensive/tranquilizer
Harmonyl, Serpalan, Serpasil

Rosuvastatin
Statin/cholesterol reduction
Crestor

Scopolamine
Anticholinergic/motion sickness, antispasmodic
Scopace, Maldemar, Transderm Scop, Transderm-V

Secobarbital
Depressant/sedative
Seconal

Sertraline
Antidepressant/psychiatric disorders
Zoloft, Apo-Sertraline, Novo-Sertraline, ratio-Sertraline

Simvastatin
Statin/cholesterol reduction
Zocor

Temazepam
Benzodiazepine/sleep aid
Apo-Temazepam, Co Temazepam, Dom-Temazepam, Gen-Temazepam, Nu-Temazepam, Novo-Temazepam, PMS-Temazepam, ratio-Temazepam, Restoril

Thioridazine
Antipsychotic
Generic only. No brands available.

Tiotropium
Anticholinergic/bronchodilator
Spiriva

Tolterodine
Anticholinergic/GI antispasmodic
Detrol, Detrol LA, Unidet

Triazolam
Benzodiazepine/sleep aid
Triazolam, Gen-Triazolam, Apo-Triazo, Halcion, Novo-Triolam

Trihexyphenidyl
Anticholinergic/treatment for Parkinson's
Generic only. No brands available.

Trimethobenzamide
Anticholinergic/antiemetic
Tigan

Tripelennamine
Anticholinergic/antihistamine
Talacen, Talwin, Talwin NX, Vagin-X, PBZ, BPZ-SR

Valproate
Anticonvulsant
Depacon

Varenicline
Smoking cessation aid
Chantix

Zaleplon
Sedative/sleep aid
Sonata, Sotacor

Zolpidem
Sedative/sleep aid
Ambien, Ambien CR, Edluar, Zolpimist

Appendix

D Net Carbohydrate Counter

Units of Measure
1 tablespoon (tbsp) = ½ fl oz = 14.8 ml (approximately 15 ml)
3 teaspoons = 1 tbsp
4 tbsp = ¼ cup
16 tbsp = 1 cup
1 cup = 8 fl oz = 236.6 ml
1 inch (in) = 2.5 cm

Vegetables	Amount	Net Carbs (g)
Alfalfa sprouts	1 cup	0.4
Artichoke, boiled	1 medium	6.5
Arugula	1 cup	0.4
Asparagus, canned	1 cup	2.2
Asparagus, raw	1 cup	2.4
Asparagus, raw	5 in spear	0.2
Avocado (Haas)	1 each	3.5
Bamboo shoots, canned	1 cup	2.4
Beans, boiled		
black	1 cup	26.0
black-eyed peas	1 cup	25.0
garbanzo (chickpeas)	1 cup	32.0
great northern	1 cup	25.0
green beans	1 cup	4.1
kidney	1 cup	27.0
lentils	1 cup	24.0
lima	1 cup	24.0
navy	1 cup	36.0
pinto	1 cup	30.0
soybeans	1 cup	6.8
wax beans	1 cup	4.0

white beans	1 cup	34.0
Bean sprouts (mung)		
boiled	1 cup	4.2
raw	1 cup	4.4
Beets (sliced), raw	1 cup	9.3
Beet greens, boiled	1 cup	2.6
Broccoli, raw, chopped	1 cup	3.6
Brussels sprouts		
boiled	1 cup	7.0
raw	1 cup	4.6
Cabbage (green), shredded		
cooked	1 cup	3.2
raw	1 cup	2.2
Cabbage (red), shredded		
cooked	1 cup	4.0
raw	1 cup	2.8
Cabbage (savoy), shredded		
cooked	1 cup	3.8
raw	1 cup	2.0
Chinese cabbage (bok choy)		
cooked	1 cup	1.4
raw	1 cup	0.8
Carrot		
boiled, chopped	1 cup	10.5
raw, whole	1 medium	5.1
raw, shredded	1 cup	8.0
juice	1 cup	18.0
Cauliflower		
boiled	1 cup	1.6
raw, chopped	1 cup	2.8
Celery		
raw, whole	8 in long	0.8
raw, diced	1 cup	1.8
Chard		
boiled	1 cup	3.4
raw	1 cup	0.7
Chives, chopped	1 tbsp	<0.1
Collards		
boiled	1 cup	4.2
Cucumber, sliced		
raw with peel	1 cup	3.2
raw peeled	1 cup	1.8
Daikon, sliced	1 cup	2.0
Eggplant, raw	1 cup	3.0
Escarole, raw	1 cup	0.7
Garlic, raw	1 clove	0.9

Jerusalem artichokes, raw	1 cup	24.0
Jicama, raw	1 cup	5.0
Kale		
boiled, chopped	1 cup	3.0
raw, chopped	1 cup	2.0
Kohlrabi		
cooked, sliced	1 cup	7.0
raw, sliced	1 cup	9.0
Leeks,		
boiled	1 cup	6.8
raw	1 cup	11.0
Lettuce		
butterhead	1 leaf	0.1
iceberg	1 leaf	0.1
loose leaf, shredded	1 cup	0.6
Mushrooms (button)		
boiled	1 cup	4.0
raw, sliced	1 cup	2.4
raw	1 mushroom	0.4
Mustard greens, raw	1 cup	0.5
Okra, raw	1 cup	12.0
Onion		
raw, slice	¼ in thick	3.3
raw, chopped	1 tbsp	0.9
raw, chopped	1 cup	11.0
raw, whole medium	2½ in dia	9.6
Parsley		
raw, chopped	1 tbsp	0.1
Parsnips		
raw, chopped	1 cup	17.4
Peas		
edible-pod, cooked	1 cup	7.0
green, boiled	1 cup	7.0
split, boiled	1 cup	31.0
Peppers		
hot red chili, raw	1 cup	5.5
sweet (bell), raw	1 cup	4.4
sweet (bell), raw	1 medium	5.3
jalapeno, canned	1 pepper	0.4
Potatoes		
baked	1 small (4.9 oz)	26.0
baked	1 medium (6.1 oz)	33.0
baked	1 large (10.5 oz)	57.0
mashed, with milk	1 cup	34.0
hash brown	1 cup	41.0
Pumpkin, canned	1 cup	15.0

Radish, raw	1 medium	0.1
Rhubarb	1 cup	3.4
Rutabaga	1 cup	12.0
Sauerkraut	1 cup	6.0
Scallions,		
raw, chopped	1 tbsp	0.2
raw, chopped	4 in long	0.7
Shallots	1 tbsp	1.4
Spinach		
canned	1 cup	2.0
frozen, boiled	1 cup	4.6
raw	1 cup	0.4
Squash		
acorn, baked, mashed	1 cup	29.0
butternut, baked, mashed	1 cup	19.0
crookneck, raw sliced	1 cup	5.0
Hubbard, baked, mashed	1 cup	20
scallop, raw sliced	1 cup	3.0
spaghetti, baked	1 cup	6.0
zucchini, raw sliced	1 cup	3.0
Sweet potatoes		
baked	1 small (2.1 oz)	10.4
baked	1 medium (4.0 oz)	25.0
baked	1 large (6.3 oz)	31.4
Taro		
root, cooked, sliced	1 cup	24.0
leaves, steamed	1 cup	3.0
Tofu	½ cup	1.0
Tomato		
cooked	1 cup	10.0
raw, chopped	1 cup	5.0
raw, sliced	¼ in thick	1.0
raw	1 small (3.2 oz)	2.4
raw	1 medium (4.3 oz)	34.0
raw	1 large (6.4 oz)	5.0
cherry	1 medium (0.6 oz)	1.0
Italian	1 medium (2.2 oz)	2.0
juice	1 cup	8.0
sauce	½ cup	7.0
paste	½ cup	19.0
Turnips, raw cubed	1 cup	6.0
Turnip greens, raw	1 cup	1.4
Water chestnuts	1 cup	14
Watercress, raw chopped	1 cup	0.2
Yam, baked	1 cup	36.0

Fruit	Amount	Net Carbs (g)
Apples		
raw	1 each	18.0
juice	1 cup	29.0
applesauce, unsweetened	1 cup	24.0
Apricots		
raw	1 each	3.1
canned, in syrup	1 cup	51.0
Banana	1 each	25.0
Blackberries, fresh	1 cup	8.0
Blueberries, fresh	1 cup	17.0
Boysenberries, frozen	1 cup	9.1
Cantaloupe		
small	1 each (4¼ in dia)	34.8
medium	1 each (5 in dia)	43.6
large	1 each (6½ in dia)	64.3
cubes	1 cup	12.8
Cherries		
Sweet, raw	10 each	9.7
Cranberry		
Raw	1 cup	7.0
Sauce, whole berry canned	1 cup	102.0
Dates, raw		
whole without pits	1 each	5.2
chopped	1 cup	116.0
Elderberries, raw	1 cup	16.4
Figs	1 each	10.5
Gooseberries, raw	1 cup	8.8
Grapefruit, raw	1 half	7.0
Grapes		
Thompson seedless	1 each	0.9
American (slip skin)	1 each	0.4
juice, canned	1 cup	37.0
juice, frozen concentrate	1 cup	31.0
Honeydew		
small	1 each (5 ¼-in dia)	83.0
large	1 each (6-7 in dia)	106.3
balls	1 cup	14.7
Kiwi, raw	1 each	8.0
Lemon, raw	1 each	3.8
Lemon Juice	1 tbsp	1.3
Lime, raw	1 each	3.2
Lime Juice	1 tbsp	1.3

Loganberries, frozen	1 cup	11.0
Mandarin orange,		
canned, juice pack	1 cup	22.0
canned, light syrup	1 cup	39.2
Mango, raw	1 each	28.0
Mulberries, raw	1 cup	11.2
Nectarines, raw	1 each	13.0
Olives, black		
large	1 each	0.2
jumbo	1 each	0.3
Oranges, raw	1 each	12.0
Juice, fresh	1 cup	25.0
Juice, frozen concentrate	1 cup	27.0
Papayas, raw	1 each	12.0
Peaches		
raw, whole	1 each	8.0
raw sliced	1 cup	14.2
canned, light syrup	½ fruit	16.4
Pears		
raw	1 each	20.0
raw, sliced	1 cup	20.5
halves, canned	1 cup	15.1
Persimmon, raw	1 each	8.4
Pineapple,		
fresh, cubed	1 cup	17.2
canned unsweetened	1 cup	35.0
Plantains, cooked	1 cup	41.0
Plums, raw	1 each	7.6
Prunes		
dried	1 each	4.7
juice	1 cup	42.2
Raisins	1 cup	106.0
Raspberries, raw	1 cup	6.0
Strawberries		
raw, whole	1 small	0.4
raw, whole	1 medium	0.7
raw, whole	1 large	1.0
raw, halves	1 cup	8.7
raw, sliced	1 cup	9.5
Tangerines, fresh	1 each	7.5
Watermelon		
sliced	1 inch	33.0
balls	1 cup	11.1

Nuts and Seeds	Amount	Net Carbs (g)
Almonds		
sliced	1 cup	9.0
slivered	1 cup	9.0
whole	1 each	0.1
whole	22 kernels (1 oz)	2.2
almond butter	1 tbsp	2.0
Brazil nuts	7 each	1.4
Cashew		
halves and whole	1 cup (4.8 oz)	37.0
whole	18 nuts (1 oz)	8.4
whole	1 each	0.5
cashew butter	1 tbsp	3.0
Coconut		
fresh	1 piece (2 x 2 in)	2.0
fresh, shredded	1 cup	3.0
dried, unsweetened	1 cup	7.0
dried, sweetened	1 cup	35.0
coconut milk, canned	1 cup	6.6
coconut water	1 cup	6.3
Filberts (hazelnuts)		
whole	10 nuts	0.9
whole	1 each	0.1
whole	1 cup	11.0
Macadamia		
whole	7 nuts	1.5
whole	1 each	0.2
whole or halves	1 cup	7.0
Peanuts		
raw	1 cup	14.0
dry roasted	1 cup	19.5
dry roasted	30 nuts	3.8
peanut butter	1 tbsp	2.1
Pecans		
halves, raw	20 halves	1.2
halves, raw	1 cup	5.0
chopped, raw	1 cup	4.7
Pine nuts		
whole	10 nuts	0.1
whole	1 cup	12.7
Pistachio		
whole	1 each	0.1
whole	49 kernels	5.0
whole	1 cup	21.4

Pumpkin seeds		
whole	10 seeds	1.8
whole	1 cup	22.5
Sesame seeds		
whole	1 tbsp	1.0
sesame butter (tahini)	1 tbsp	2.5
Soy nuts, roasted	1 cup	42.3
Sunflower seeds		
whole, hulled	1 tbsp	1.0
Walnuts		
black, chopped	1 tbsp	0.3
black, chopped	1 cup	3.9
English, chopped	1 cup	8.4
English, halves	10 halves	1.4

Grains and Flours	**Amount**	**Net Carbs (g)**
Amaranth		
grain	1 cup	99.4
flour	1 cup	108.4
Arrowroot flour	1 tbsp	6.8
Barley		
pearled, cooked	1 cup	36.4
flour	1 cup	95.4
Buckwheat		
grain, roasted	1 cup	34.2
flour	1 cup	72.8
Bulgur, cooked	1 cup	25.6
Corn		
whole kernel	1 cup	25.1
ear, small	5½ - 6½ in long	11.9
ear, medium	6¾ - 7½ in long	14.7
ear, large	7¾ - 9 in long	23.3
grits, dry	1 cup	121.7
grits, cooked with water	1 cup	30.5
cornmeal, dry	1 cup	84.9
corn starch	1 tbsp	7.0
popcorn, air popped	1 cup	5.0
hominy, canned	1 cup	18.8
Millet, cooked	1 cup	25.8
Oats		
oatmeal, cooked	1 cup	21.3
oatmeal, dry	1 cup	46.4
oat bran, cooked	1 cup	19.3
oat bran, dry	1 cup	47.7
Quinoa, cooked	1 cup	43.0

Rice		
brown, cooked	1 cup	41.3
white, cooked	1 cup	43.9
instant, cooked	1 cup	40.4
wild rice, cooked	1 cup	32.0
brown rice flour	1 tbsp	7.1
white rice flour	1 tbsp	7.7
Rye flour, dark	1 cup	59.2
Semolina, enriched	1 cup	115.6
Soy flour	1 cup	21.6
Tapioca, pearl dry	1 tbsp	8.3
Wheat		
white, enriched	1 cup	92.0
white, enriched	1 tbsp	5.8
whole wheat	1 cup	72.4
whole wheat	1 tbsp	4.5
wheat bran	1 tbsp	0.8

Bread and Baked Goods	**Amount**	**Net Carbs (g)**
Bagels		
white enriched	1 each (3.7 oz)	57.0
whole grain	1 each (4.5 oz)	64.0
Bread		
rye	1 slice	13.0
whole wheat	1 slice	10.7
raisin bread	1 slice	12.5
hamburger bun	1 roll	20.4
hot dog bun	1 roll	20.4
hard/Kaiser roll	1 roll	28.7
Crackers		
saltine	1 each	2.2
multigrain	1 each	2.0
cheese	1 each (1 in square)	0.6
English muffin	1 each	24.0
Pancake	1 each (4 in dia)	13.4
Pita		
white	1 each	32.0
whole wheat	1 each	30.5
Tortilla		
corn	1 each (6 in)	11.0
flour	1 each (8 in)	22.0
flour	1 each (10½ in)	33.8
Wonton wrappers	1 each (3½ in)	4.5

Pasta	Amount	Net Carbs (grams)
Macaroni, cooked		
white, enriched	1 cup	37.9
whole wheat	1 cup	33.3
corn	1 cup	32.4
Noodles, cooked		
cellophane (mung bean)	1 cup	38.8
egg	1 cup	38.0
soba	1 cup	37.7
rice	1 cup	42.0
Spaghetti, cooked		
white, enriched	1 cup	37.3
whole wheat	1 cup	30.9
corn	1 cup	32.4

Dairy	Amount	Net Carbs (grams)
Butter	1 tbsp	0
Buttermilk	1 cup	11.7
Cheese (hard)		
American, sliced	1 oz	0.4
Cheddar, sliced	1 oz	0.4
Cheddar, shredded	1 cup	1.5
Colby, sliced	1 oz	0.7
Colby, shredded	1 cup	2.9
Edam, sliced	1 oz	0.4
Edam, shredded	1 cup	1.5
goat milk cheese	1 oz	0.6
Gruyere, sliced	1 oz	0.1
Gruyere, shredded	1 cup	0.4
Monterey, sliced	1 oz	0.2
Monterey, shredded	1 cup	0.8
mozzarella, sliced	1 oz	0.6
mozzarella, shredded	1 cup	2.5
Muenster, sliced	1 oz	0.3
Muenster, shredded	1 cup	1.2
Parmesan, sliced	1 oz	0.9
Parmesan, grated	1 tbsp	0.2
Parmesan, shredded	1 tbsp	2.0
Swiss, sliced	1 oz	1.5
Swiss, shredded	1 cup	5.8
Cheese (soft)		
cottage, non-fat	1 cup	9.7

cottage, 2% fat	1 cup	8.1
cream cheese, plain	1 tbsp	0.4
cream cheese, low-fat	1 tbsp	1.1
feta, crumbled	1 oz	1.2
feta, crumbled	1 cup	6.1
ricotta, whole milk	1 oz	0.9
ricotta, whole milk	1 cup	7.4
ricotta, part skim	1 oz	1.4
ricotta, part skim	1 cup	12.5
Cream		
heavy, whipping	1 cup	6.7
half and half	1 cup	10.6
sour	1 tbsp	0.5
Goat milk	1 cup	11.0
Milk		
skim, non-fat	1 cup	12.3
1%	1 cup	12.2
2%	1 cup	11.4
whole, 3.3% fat	1 cup	11.0
Soy milk, non-fat	1 cup	9.5
Soy milk, low-fat	1 cup	12.0
Yogurt		
plain, fat-free	1 cup	18.9
plain, whole milk	1 cup	12.0
vanilla, low-fat	1 cup	31.0
fruit added, low-fat	1 cup	43.0

Meat and Eggs	**Amount**	**Net Carbs (grams)**
Beef	3 oz	0
Buffalo	3 oz	0
Eggs	1 large	0.6
Egg yolk	1 large	0.3
Fish	3 oz	0
Lamb	3 oz	0
Poultry	3 oz	0
Pork	3 oz	0
bacon, cured	3 pieces	0.5
Canadian-style bacon	2 pieces	1
fresh side (natural bacon)	3 oz	0
ham	1 oz	0.7
Shellfish		
oysters	1 oz	1.4
crab	1 oz	0
clams, canned	1 oz	1.4

lobster, cooked	3 oz	1.1
mussels, cooked	1 oz	2.1
scallops	1 oz	0.5
shrimp, cooked	3 oz	0
Venison	3 oz	0

Miscellaneous	**Amount**	**Net Carbs (grams)**
Baking soda	1 tsp	0
Catsup		
regular	1 tbsp	3.8
low-carb	1 tbsp	1.0
Fats and oils	1 tbsp	0
Gelatin, dry	1 envelope	0
Gravy, canned or dry mix	½ cup	6.5 (average)
Fish sauce	1 tbsp	0.7
Herbs and spices	1 tbsp	1 (average)
Honey	1 tbsp	17.2
Horseradish, prepared	1 tbsp	1.4
Maple syrup	1 tbsp	13.4
Mayonnaise	1 tbsp	3.5
Molasses	1 tbsp	14.9
Molasses, blackstrap	1 tbsp	12.2
Mustard		
yellow	1 tbsp	0.3
Dijon	1 tbsp	0
Pancake syrup	1 tbsp	15.1
Pickles		
dill, medium	1 pickle	3.1
dill, slice	1 (0.2 oz)	0.2
sweet, medium	1 pickle	11.0
pickle relish, sweet	1 tbsp	5.3
Tartar sauce	1 tbsp	2.0
Salsa	1 tbsp	0.8
Soy sauce	1 tbsp	1.1
Sugar		
white, granulated	1 tbsp	12.0
brown	1 tbsp	13.0
powdered	1 tbsp	8.0
Vinegar		
apple cider	1 tbsp	0
balsamic	1 tbsp	2.0
red wine	1 tbsp	0
rice	1 tbsp	0
white wine	1 tbsp	0
Worcestershire sauce	1 tbsp	3.3

References

Chapter 1: Is There a Cure for Alzheimer's?

1. Vanitallie, T.B., et al. Treatment of Parkinson disease with diet-induced hyperketonemia: a feasibility study. *Neurology* 2005:64:728-730.
2. Roan, S. Dementia in one spouse increases risk in the other. *Los Angeles Times* May 5, 2010.

Chapter 2: The Human Brain

1. Gould, E., et al. Neurogenesis in the neocortex of adult primates. *Science* 1999;286:548-552.
2. Eriksson, P.S., et al. Neurogenesis in the adult human hippocampus. *Nat Med* 1998;4:1313-1317.

Chapter 3: The Many Faces of Neurodegeneration

1. Heron, M., et al. *National Vital Statistics Reports* 2009;57:9.
2. Beydoun, M.A., et al. Obesity and central obesity as risk factors for incident dementia and its subtypes: a systematic review and meta-analysis. *Obes Rev* 2008;9:204-218.
3. Hughes, T.F., et al. Association between late-life body mass index and dementia: The Kame Project. *Neurology* 2009;72:1741-1746.
4. Knopman, D.S., et al. Incident dementia in women is preceded by weight loss by at least a decade. *Neurology* 2007;69:739-746.
5. Ott, A., et al. Prevalence of Alzheimer's disease and vascular dementia: association with education. The Rotterdam study. *BMJ* 1995;310:970-973.
6. Aarsland, D., et al. Prevalence and characteristics of dementia in Parkinson disease: an 8-year prospective study. *Arch Neurol* 2003;60:387-392.
7. Friedman, J.H., et al. Monozygotic twins discordant for Huntington disease after 7 years. *Arch Neurol* 2005;62:995-997.
8. Hockly, E., et al. Environmental enrichment slows disease progression in R6/2 Huntington's disease mice. *Ann Neurol* 2002;51:235-242.
9. Wachterman, M., et al. Reporting dementia on the death certificates of nursing home residents dying with end-stage dementia. *JAMA* 2008;300:2608-2610.

Chapter 4: Premature Aging and Neurodegeneration

1. Sasaki, N., et al. Advanced glycation end products in Alzheimer's disease and other neurodegenerative diseases. *American Journal of Pathology* 1998;153:1149-1155.
2. Catellani, R., et al. Glycooxidation and oxidative stress in Parkinson's disease and diffuse Lewy body disease. *Brain Res* 1996;737:195-200.

3. Kato, S., et al. Astrocytic hyaline inclusions contain advanced glycation endproducts in familial amyotrophic lateral sclerosis with superoxide dismutase 1 gene mutation: immunohistochemical and immunoelectron microscopical analysis. *Aca Neuropathol* 1999;97:260-266.
4. Cai, W., et al. High levels of Dietary advanced glycation end products transform low-density lipoprotein into a potent redox-sensitive mitogen-activated protein kinase stimulant in diabetic patients. *Circulation* 2004;110:285-291.
5. Negrean, et al. Effects of low- and high-advanced glycation endproduct meals on macro- and microvascular endothelial function and oxidative stress in patients with type 2 diabetes mellitus. *Am J Clin Nutr* 2007:85:1236-1243.
6. Cai, W. et al. Reduced oxidant stress and extended lifespan in mice exposed to a low glycotoxin diet. *Am J Pathol* 2007;170:1893-1902.
7. Goldberg, T., et al. Advanced glycoxidation end products in commonly consumed foods. *J Am Diet Assoc* 2004;104:1287-1291.
8. Uribarri, J., et al. Circulating glycotoxins and dietary advanced glycation endproducts: two links to inflammatory response, oxidative stress, and aging. *J Gerontol Ser A: Biol Sci Med Sci* 2007;62:427-433.
9. Cerami, C., et al. Tobacco smoke is a source of toxic reactive glycation products. *Proc Natl Acad Sci USA* 1997;94:13915-13920.
10. Ahmed, N., et al. Assay of advanced glycation endproducts in selected beverages and food by liquid chromatography with tandem mass spectrometric detection. *Molecular Nutrition & Food Research* 2005;49:691-699.
11. Krajcovicová-Kudlacková, M., et al. Advanced glycation end products and nutrition. *Physiol Res* 2002;51:313-316.
12. Wu, C.H. and Yen, G.C. Inhibitory effect of naturally occurring flavonoids on the formation of advanced glycation endproducts. *J Agric Food Chem* 2005;53:3167-3173.
13. Kiho, T., et al. Tomato paste fraction inhibiting the formation of advanced glycation end-products. *Biosci Biotechnol Biochem* 2004;68:200-205.
14. Brackenridge, C.J. Relation of occupational stress to the age at onset of Huntington's disease. *Acta Neurologica Scandinavica* 2009;60:272-276.
15. Slow, E.J., et al. To be or not to be toxic: aggregations in Huntington and Alzheimer disease. *Trends in Genetics* 2006;22:408-411.
16. Davies, S.W., et al. Formation of neuronal intranuclear inclusions underlies the neurological dysfunction in mice transgenic for the HD mutation. *Cell* 1997;90:537-548.
17. Langley, K., et al. Effects of low birth weight, maternal smoking in pregnancy and social class on the phenotypic manifestation of attention deficit hyperactivity disorder and associated antisocial behaviour: investigation in a clinical sample. *BMC Psychiatry* 2007;7:26.
18. Conley, D. and Bennett, N.G. Is biology destiny? Birth weight and life chances. *American Sociological Review* 2000;65:458-467.
19. Jahoor, F., et al. Plasma apolipoprotein A1 and birthweight. *Lancet* 1997;350:1823-1824.
20. Franco, M.C.P., et al. Effects of low birth weight in 8- to 13-year-old children. Implications in endothelial function and uric acid levels. *Hypertension* 2006;48:45-50.
21. Valsmakis, G., et al. Causes of intrauterine growth restriction and the postnatal development of metabolic syndrome. *Annals of the New York Academy of Sciences* 2006;1092:138-147.
22. Barker, D.J.P. Type 2 (non-insulin-dependent) diabetes mellitus, hypertension and hyperlipidaemia (syndrome X): relation to reduced fetal growth. *Diabetologia* 1993;36:62-67.
23. Liem, J., et al. The risk of developing food allergy in premature/low birthweight children. *Journal of Allergy and Clinical Immunology* 2005;115:S242.
24. Raqib, R., et al. Low birth weight is associated with altered immune function in rural Bangladeshi children: a birth cohort study. *Am J Clin Nutr* 2007;85:845-852.

25. Moore, S.E. Nutrition, immunity and the fetal and infant origins of disease hypothesis in developing countries. *Proceedings of the Nutrition Society* 1998;57:241-247.
26. Falcone, D. Center for Neurodegenerative Disease Research, http://www.med.upenn.edu/cndr/TDP43androleonALS.shtml.
27. Yagi, H., et al. Amyloid fibril formation of alpha-synuclein is accelerated by performed amyloid seeds of other proteins. *Journal of Biological Chemistry* 2005;280:38609-38616.
28. Frank-Cannon, T.C., et al. Does neuroinflammation fan the flame in neurodegenerative diseases? *Molecular Neurodegeneration* 2009;4:47.
29. Reale, M., et al. Peripheral chemokine receptors, their ligands, cytokines and Alzheimer's disease. *J Alzheimers Dis* 2008;14:147-159.
30. Sawada, M., et al. Role of cytokines in inflammatory process in Parkinson's disease. *J Neural Transm Suppl* 2006;(70):373-381.
31.Bjorkqvist, M., et al. A novel pathogenic pathway of immune activation detectable before clinical onset in Huntington's disease. *J Exp Med* 2008;205:1869-1877.
32. Munch, G., et al. Advanced glycation end products in neurodegeneration: more than early markers of oxidative stress? *Ann Neurol* 1998;44 (3 Suppl 1):S85-S88.
33. Frank-Cannon, T.C., et al. Does neuroinflammation fan the flame in neurodegenerative diseases? *Molecular Neurodegeneration* 2009;4:47.

Chapter 5: Insulin Resistance and Neurodegeneration

1. de la Monte, S.M., et al. Impaired insulin and insulin-like growth factor expression and signaling mechanisms in Alzheimer's disease—is this type 3 diabetes? *J Alzheimers Dis* 2005;7:63-80.
2. Pavlovic, D.M. and Pavlovic, A.M. Dementia and diabetes mellitus. *Srp Arh Celok Lek* 2008;136:170-175.
3. Ristow, M. Neurodegenerative disorders associated with diabetes mellitus. *J Mol Med* 2004;82:510-529.
4. Craft, S. and Watson, G.S. Insulin and neurodegenerative disease: shared and specific mechanisms. *Lancet Neurol* 2004;3:169-178.
5. Morris, J.K., et al. Measures of striatal insulin resistance in a 6-hydroxydopamine model of Parkinson's disease. *Brain Res* 2008;1240:185-195.
6. Moroo, I., et al. Loss of insulin receptor immunoreactivity from the substantia nigra pars compacta neurons in Parkinson's disease. *Acta Neuropathol* 1994;87:343-348.
7. Sandyk, R. The relationship between diabetes mellitus and Parkinson's disease. *Int J Neurosci* 1993;69:125-130.
8. Hu, G., et al. Type 2 diabetes and the risk of Parkinson's disease. *Diabetes Care* 2007;30:842-847.
9. Farrer, L.A. Diabetes mellitus in Huntington's disease. *Clin Genet* 1985;27:62-67.
10. Podolsky, S., et al. Increased frequency of diabetes mellitus in patients with Huntington's chorea. *Lancet* 1972;1:1356-1358.
11. Warram, J.H., et al. Slow glucose removal rate and hyperinsulinemia precede the development of type 2 diabetes in the offspring of diabetic parents. *Ann Intern Med* 1990;113:909-915.
12. Whitney, E.N., et al. *Understanding Normal and Clinical Nutrition, Third Edition.* West Publishing Company, St. Paul, MN, 1991.
13. Whitmer, R.A. Type 2 diabetes and risk of cognitive impairment and dementia. *Curr Neurol Neurosci Rep* 2007;7:3730380.
14. Ott, A., et al. Diabetes and the risk of dementia: Rotterdam study. *Neurology* 1999;53:1937-1942.
15. Xu, W., et al. Mid- and late-life diabetes in relation to the risk of dementia: a population-based twin study. *Diabetes* 2009;58:71-77.

16. Roriz-Cruz, M., et al. (Pre)diabetes, brain aging, and cognition. *Biochim Biophys Acta* 2009;1792:432-443.
17. Sandyk, R. The relationship between diabetes mellitus and Parkinson's disease. *Int. J Neurosci* 1993;69:125-130.
18. Reyes, E.T., et al Insulin resistance in amyotrophic lateral sclerosis. *J Neurol Sci* 1984;63:317-324.
19. Hubbard, R.W., et al. Elevated plasma glucagon in amyotrophic lateral sclerosis. *Neurology* 1992;42:1532-1534.
20. Pradat, P.F., et al. Impaired glucose tolerance in patients with amyotrophic lateral sclerosis. *Amyotroph Lateral Scler* 2009;March 20:1-6.
21. Reger, M.A., et al. Intranasal insulin improves cognition and modulates beta-amyloid in early AD. *Neurology* 2008;70:440-448.

Chapter 6: Trauma

1. Uryu, K., et al. Repetitive mild brain trauma accelerates Abeta deposition, lipid peroxidation, and cognitive impairment in a transgenic mouse model of Alzheimer amyloidosis. *J Neurosci* 2002;15:446-454.
2. Friedman, J.H. Progressive Parkinsonism in boxers. *South Med J* 1989;82:543-546.
3. Strickland, D., et al. Physical activity, trauma, and ALS: a case-control study. *Acta Neurologica Scandinavica* 1996;94:45-50.
4. Piazza, O., et al. Soccer, neurotrauma and amyotrophic lateral sclerosis: is there a connection? *Curr Med Res Opin* 2004;20:505-508.
5. Gallagher, J.P. and Sanders, M. Trauma and amyotrophic lateral sclerosis: a report of 78 patients. *Acta Neurologica Scandinavica* 2009;75:145-150.
6. Chen, H., et al. Head injury and amyotrophic lateral sclerosis. *Am J Epidemiol* 2007;166:810-816.
7.Mortimer, J.A., et al. Head trauma as a risk factor for Alzheimer's disease: a collaborative re-analysis of case-control studies. EURODEM Risk Factors Research Group. *Int J Epidemiol* 1991;20 Suppl 2:S28-S35.
8. Kondo, K. and Tsubaki, T. Case-control studies of motor neuron disease: association with mechanical injuries. *Arch Neurol* 1981;38:220-226.
9. Rosso, S. M., et al. Medical and environmental risk factors for sporadic frontotemporal dementia: a retrospective case-control study. *J Neurol Neurosurg Psychiatry* 2003;74:1574-1576.
10. van Duijn, C.M., et al. Head trauma and the risk of Alzheimer's disease. *Am J Epidemiol* 1992;135:775-782.
11. Hebert, R., et al. Vascular dementia: incidence and risk factors in the Canadian study of health and aging. *Stroke* 2000;31:1487-1493.
12. Elkind, M.S., et al. Infectious burden and risk of stroke: the northern Manhattan study. *Arch Neurol* 2010;67:33-38.
13. Yamori, Y., et al. Pathogenesis and dietary prevention of cerebrovascular diseases in animal models and epidemiological evidence for the applicability in man, In: Yamori Y. and Lenfant C. (eds) *Prevention of Cardiovascular Diseases: An Approach to Active Long Life*. Elsevier Science Publishers, Amsterdam, the Netherlands, 1987.
14. Ikeda, K., et al. Effect of milk protein and fat intake on blood pressure and incidence of cerebrovascular disease in stroke-prone spontaneously hypertensive rats (SHRSP). *J Nutr Sci Vitaminol* 1987;33:31.
15. Kimura, N. Changing patterns of coronary heart disease, stroke, and nutrient intake in Japan. *Prev Med* 1985;12:222.

16. Omura, T., et al Geographical distribution of cerebrovascular disease mortality and food intakes in Japan. *Soc Sci Med* 1987;24:40.

Chapter 7: Drugs

1. Boustani, M., et al. The association between cognition and histamine-2 receptor antagonists in African Americans. *J Am Geriatr Soc* 2007;55:1248-1253.
2. Chen, X., et al. The recovery of cognitive function after general anesthesia in elderly patients: a comparison of desflurane and sevoflurane. *Anesth Analg* 2001;93:1489-1494.
3. Bohnen, N.I., et al. Alzheimer's disease and cumulative exposure to anesthesia: a case-control study. *J Am Geriatr Soc* 1994;42:198–201.
4. Muravchick, S. and Smith, D.S. Parkinsonian symptoms during emergence from general anesthesia. *Anesthesiology* 1995;82:305–307.
5. Xie, Z., et al. The inhalation anesthetic isoflurane induces a vicious cycle of apoptosis and amyloid beta-protein accumulation. *J Neurosci* 2007;27:1247-1254.
6. Xie, Z., et al. The common inhalation anesthetic isoflurane induces caspase activation and increases amyloid bets-protein level in vivo. *Ann Neurol* 2008;64:618-627.
7. Plassman, B.L., et al. Surgery using general anesthesia and risk of dementia in the Aging, Demographics and Memory Study. *Alzheimer's and Dementia* 2009;5:389.
8. Aisen, P.S., et al. Effects of rofecoxib or naproxen vs placebo on Alzheimer disease progression: a randomized controlled trial. *JAMA* 2003:289:2819-2826.
9. Martin, B.K., et al. Cognitive function over time in the Alzheimer's Disease Anti-inflammatory Prevention Trial (ADAPT): results of a randomized, controlled trial of naproxen and celecoxib. *Arch Neurol* 2008;65:895-905.
10. Breitner, J.C., et al. Risk of dementia and AD with prior exposure to NSAIDs in an elderly community-based cohort. *Neurology* 2009;72:1899-1905.
11. Carrière, I., et al. Drugs with anticholinergic properties, cognitive decline, and dementia in an elderly general population: the 3-city study. *Arch Intern Med* 2009;169:1317.
12. Hanlon, J.T., et al. Adverse drug events in high risk older outpatients. *J Am Geriatr Soc* 1997;45:945-948.
13. Cooper, J.W. Adverse drug reaction-related hospitalizations of nursing facility patients: a 4-year study. *South Med J* 1999;92:485-490.
14. Beers, M.H. Explicit criteria for determining potentially inappropriate medication use by the elderly. *Archives of Internal Medicine* 1997;157:1531-1536.
15. Fick, E.D., et al. Beers criteria for potentially inappropriate medication use in older adults. *Archives of Internal Medicine* 2003; 163: 2716-2724.
16. Eleven deaths during Aricept trial raises concern over FDA application to permit wider use of the drug. http://www.yourlawyer.com/articles/read/11516.
17. Golomb, B.A., et al. Statin adverse effects: a review of the literature and evidence for a mitochondrial mechanism. *Am J Cardiovasc Drugs* 2008;8:373-418.
18. Horner, H.C., et al. Glucocorticoids inhibit glucose transport in cultured hippocampal neurons and glia. *Neuroendocrinology* 1990;52:57-64.
19. Virgin, C.E., et al. Glucocorticoids inhibit glucose transport and glutamate uptake in hippocampal astrocytes: implications for glucocorticoid neurotoxicity. *J Neurochem* 1991;57:1422-1428.
20. Catania, C., et al. A steroid hormone-Alzheimer's disease connection? Upsides, downsides. *Molecular Bases of Neurodegeneration* 2005:21-42.
21. Sapolsky, R.M. Potential behavioral modification of glucocorticoid damage to the hippocampus. *Behav Brain Res* 1993;57:175-182.
22. Ehlenbach, W.J., et al. Association between acute care and critical illness hospitalization and cognitive function in older adults. *JAMA* 2010;303:763-770.

Chapter 8: Environmental Toxins

1. Costello, S., et al. Parkinson's disease and residential exposure to maneb and paraquat from agricultural applications in the Central Valley of California. *American Journal of Epidemiology* 2009;169:919-926.

2. Chen, H., et al. Consumption of dairy products and risk of Parkinson's disease. *Am J Epidemiol* 2007;165:998-1006.

3. Champy, P., et al. Annonacin, a lipophilic inhibitor of mitochondrial complex I, induces nigral and strata neurodegeneration in rats: possible relevance for atypical parkinsonism in Guadeloupe. *J Neurochem* 2004;88:63-69.

4. Lannuzel, A., et al. The mitochondrial complex I inhibitor annonacin is toxic to mesencephalic dopaminergic neurons by impairment of energy metabolism. *Neuroscience* 2003;121:287-296.

5. Champy, P., et al. Quantification of acetogenins in Annona muricata linked to atypical parkinsonism in Guadeloupe. *Mov Disord* 2005;20:1629-1633.

6. Cox, P.A., et al. Biomagnification of cyanobacterial neurotoxins and neurodegenerative disease among the Chamorro people of Guam. *Proc Natl Acad Sci USA* 2003;100:13380-13383.

7. Murch, S.J., et al. Occurrence of beta-methylamino-l-alanine (BMAA) in ALS/PDC patients from Guam. *Acta Neurol Scand* 2004;110:267-269.

8. Cox, P.A., et al. Biomagnification of cyanobacterial neurotoxins and neurodegenerative disease among the Chamorro people of Guam. *Proc Natl Acad Sci USA* 2003;100:13380-13383.

9. Pablo, J., et al. Cyanobacterial neurotoxin BMAA in ALS and Alzheimer's disease. *Acta Neurol Scand* 2009;120:216-225.

10. Cox, P.A., et al. Diverse taxa of cyanobacteria produce beta-N-methylamino-lalanine, a neurotoxic amino acid. *Proc Natl Acad Sci USA* 2005;102:5074-5078.

11. Choi, D. Glutamate neurotoxicity and diseases of the nervous system. *Neuron* 1988;1:623-34.

12. Lipton, S. and Rosenberg, P. Excitatory amino acids as a final common pathway for neurologic disorders. *N Engl J Med* 1994;330:613-22.

13. Whetsell, W. and Shapira, N. Biology of disease. Neuroexcitation, excitotoxicity and human neurological disease. *Lab Invest* 1993;68:372-387.

14. Olney, J. Glutamate, a neurotoxic transmitter. *J Child Neurol* 1989;4:218-26.

15. Olney, J., et al. Excitotoxic neurodegeneration in Alzheimer's disease. *Arch Neurol* 1997;54:1234-1240.

16. Hynd, M.R., et al. Glutamate-mediated excitotoxicity and neurodegeneration in Alzheimer's disease. *Neurochem Int* 2004;45:583-595.

17. Caudle, W.M. and Zhang, J. Glutamate, excitotoxicity, and programmed cell death in Parkinson disease. *Exp Neurol* 2009;220:230-233.

18. Morales, I., et al. Osmosensitive response of glutamate in the substantia nigra. *Exp Neurol* 2009;220:335-340.

19. Meredith, G.E., et al. Impaired glutamate homeostasis and programmed cell death in a chronic MPTP mouse model of Parkinson's disease. *Exp Neurol* 2009;219:334-340.

20. Shi, P., et al. Mitochondrial dysfunction in amyotrophic lateral sclerosis. *Biochim Biophys Acta* 2010;1802:45-51.

21. Brunet, N., et al. Excitotoxic motoneuron degeneration induced by glutamate receptor agonists and mitochondrial toxins in organotypic cultures of chick embryo spinal cord. *J Comp Neurol* 2009;516:277-290.

22. Foran, E. and Trotti, D. Glutamate transporters and the excitotoxic path to motor neuron degeneration in amyotrophic lateral sclerosis. *Antioxid Redox Signal* 2009;11:1587-1602

23. Kort, J.J. Impairment of excitatory amino acid transport in astroglial cells infected with human immunodeficiency virus type I AIDS. *Res Human Retroviruses* 1998;14:1329-1339.

24. Tritti, D. and Danbolt, N.C. Glutamate transporters are oxidant-vulnerable: a molecular link between oxidative and excitotoxic neurodegeneration. *TIPS* 1998;19:328-334.
25. Blanc, E.M., et al. 4-hydroxynonenal, a lipid peroxidation product, impairs glutamate transport in cortical astrocytes. *Glia* 1998;22:149-160.
26. Koenig, H., et al. Capillary NMDA receptors regulate blood-brain barrier function and breakdown. *Bran Res* 1992;588:297-303.
27. Van Westerlaak, M.G., et al. Chronic mitochondrial inhibition induces glutamate-mediated corticomotoneuron death in an organotypic culture model. *Exp Neurol* 2001;167:393-400.
28. Oddo, S., et al. Chronic nicotine administration exacerbates tau pathology in a transgenic model of Alzheimer's disease. *Proc Natl Acad Sci USA* 2005:102:3046-3051.
29. Jakszyn, P. and Gonzalez, C.A. Nitrosamine and related food intake and gastric and oesophageal cancer risk: a systematic review of the epidemiological evidence. *World J Gastroenterol* 2006;12:4296-4303.
30. Knekt, P., et al. Risk of colorectal and other gastro-intestinal cancers after exposure to nitrate, nitrite and N-nitroso compounds: a follow-up study. *Int J Cancer* 1999;80:852-856.
31. Larsson, S.C., et al. Processed meat consumption, dietary nitrosamines and stomach cancer risk in a cohort of Swedish women. *Int J Cancer* 2006;119:915-919.
32. Coss, A., et al. Pancreatic cancer and drinking water and dietary sources of nitrate and nitrite. *Am J Epidemiol* 2004;159:693-701.
33. del la Monte, S.M., et al. Epidemiological trends strongly suggest exposures as etiologic agents in the pathogenesis of sporadic Alzheimer's disease, diabetes mellitus, and non-alcoholic steatohepatitis. *J Alzheimers Dis* 2009;17:519-529.
34. de la Monte, S.M., et al. Nitrosamine exposure exacerbates high fat diet-mediated type 2 diabetes mellitus, non-alcoholic steatohepatitis, and neurodegeneration with cognitive impairment. *Molecular Neurodegeneration* 2009;4:54.
35. Tong, M., et al. Nitrosamine exposure causes insulin resistance diseases: relevance to type 2 diabetes mellitus, non-alcoholic steatohepatitis, and Alzheimer's disease. *J Alzheimers Dis* 2009;17:8270844.
36. Rossini, A.A., et al. Studies of streptozotocin-induced insulitis and diabetes. *Proc Natl Acad Sci USA* 1977;74:2485–2489.
37. Szkudelski T. The mechanism of alloxan and streptozotocin action in B cells of the rat pancreas. *Physiol Res* 2001;50:537–546.
38. Lester-Coll, N., et al. Intracerebral streptozotocin model of type 3 diabetes: relevance to sporadic Alzheimer's disease. *J Alzheimers Dis* 2006;9:13–33.

Chapter 9: Toxic Metals

1. Griffiths, P.D., et al. Iron in the basal ganglia in Parkinson's disease. *Brain* 1999;122:667-673.
2. Altamura, S. and Muckenthaler, M.U. Iron toxicity in diseases of aging: Alzheimer's disease, Parkinson's disease and atherosclerosis. *J Alzheimers Dis* 2009;16:879-895.
3. Yokel, R.A. Blood-brain barrier flux of aluminum, manganese, iron and other metals suspected to contribute to metal-induced neurodegeneration. *J Alzheimers Dis* 2006;10:223-253.
4. Pall, H.S., et al. Raised cerebrospinal-fluid copper concentration in Parkinson's disease. *Lancet* 1987;2:238-241.
5. Dantzig, P.I. Parkinson's disease, macular degeneration and cutaneous signs of mercury toxicity. *J Occup Environ Med* 2006;48:656.
6. Wu, J., et al. Alzheimer's disease (AD) like pathology in aged monkeys following infantile exposure to environmental metal lead (Pb): Evidence for a developmental origin and environmental link to AD. *J Neurosci* 2008;28:3-9.
7. Kamel, F., et al. Lead exposure as a risk factor for amyotrophic lateral sclerosis. *Neurodegenerative Diseases* 2005;2:195-201.

8. Coon, S., et al. Whole-body lifetime occupational lead exposure and risk of Parkinson's disease. *Environmental Health Perspectives* 2006;114:1872-1876.
9. Markesbery, W.R. and Ehmann, W.D. Brain trace elements in Alzheimer's disease. In: Terry, R.D., Katzman R., Bick, K.L., eds. Alzheimer's Disease, Raven Press, Ltd. New York, 1994.
10. Markesbery, W.R., et al. Brain trace element concentration in aging. *Neurobiol Aging* 1984;5:19-28.
11. Crapper, D.R., et al. Intranuclear aluminum content in Alzheimer's disease, dialysis encephalopathy and experimental aluminum encephalopathy *Acta Neuropath* 1980;50:19-24.
12. Crapper, D.R., et al. Brain aluminum distribution in Alzheimer's disease and experimental neurofibrillary degeneration. *Science* 1973;180:511-513.
13. Yoshida, S., et al. Bunina body formation in amyotrophic lateral sclerosis: a morphologic-statistical and trace element study featuring aluminum. *J Neurol Sci* 1995;30:88-94.
14. Bouras, C., et al. A laser microprobe mass analysis of the brain aluminum and iron in dementia pugilistica: a comparison with Alzheimer's disease. *Eur Neurol* 1997;38:53-58.
15. Campbell, A. The role of aluminum and copper on neuroinflammation and Alzheimer's disease. *J Alzheimers Dis* 2006;10:165-172.
16. Flaten, T.P. Aluminum as a risk factor in Alzheimer's disease, with emphasis on drinking water. *Brain Res Bull* 2001;55:187-196.
17. Michel, P.H., et al. Study of the relationship between Alzheimer's disease and aluminum in drinking water. *Neurobiol Aging* 1990;11:264.
18. Birchall, J.D. Dissolved silica and bioavailability of aluminum. *Lancet* 1993;342:299.
19. Yokel, R.A. and Florence, R.L. Aluminum bioavailability from the approved food additive leavening agent acidic sodium aluminum phosphate, incorporated into a baked good, is lower than from water. *Toxicology* 2006;227:86-93.
20. Flaten, T.P. Aluminium as a risk factor in Alzheimer's disease, with emphasis on drinking water. *Brain Res Bull* 2001;55:187-196.
21. Cosnes, A., et al. Inflammatory nodular reactions after hepatitis B vaccination due to aluminum sensitization. *Contact Dermatitis* 1990;23:65-67.
22. Nagore, E., et al. Subcutaneous nodules following treatment with aluminium-containing allergen extracts. *Eur J Dermatol* 2001;11:138-140.
23. McLaren, G.D., et al. Iron overload disorders: natural history, pathogenesis, diagnosis, and therapy. *Crit Rev Clin Lab Sci* 1983;19:205.
24. Gutteridge, J.M.C. and Halliwell, B. 1994. *Antioxidants in Nutrition, Health, and Disease.* Oxford University Press, Oxford, 1994.
25. McCord, J.M. Effects of positive iron status at a cellular level. *Nutrition Reviews* 1996;54:85.
26. Lauffer, R.B. *Iron and Your Heart.* St. Martin's Press, New York, 1991.
27. Powers, K.M., et al. Parkinson's disease risks associated with dietary iron, manganese, and other nutrient intakes. *Neurology* 2003:60:1761-1766.
28. Chapman, R.W., et al. Hepatic iron uptake in alcoholic liver disease. *Gastroenterology* 1983;84:143-147.
29. Friedman, I.M., et al. Elevated serum iron concentration in adolescent alcohol users. *Am J Dis Child* 1988;142:156-159.
30. Leong, C.C., et al. Retrograde degeneration of neurite membrane structural integrity of nerve growth cones following in vitro exposure to mercury. *Neuroreport* 2001;12:733-737.
31. Koehler, C.S.W. Heavy metal medicine. *American Chemical Society* 2001;10:61–65.
32. Monnet-Tschudi, F., et al. Involvement of environmental mercury and lead in the etiology of neurodegenerative diseases. *Rev Environ Health* 2006;21:105-117.
33. Pendergrass, J.C., et al. Mercury vapor inhalation inhibits binding of GTP to tubulin in rat brain: similarity to a molecular lesion in Alzheimer diseased brain. *Neurotoxicology* 1997;18:315-124.

34. Huggins, H.A. *Solving the MS Mystery: Help, Hope and Recovery*. Matrix, Inc., 2002.
35. FDA hearings/advisory panel rejects amalgam safety. www.mercurypoisoned.com/FDA_hearings/advisory_panel_rejects_amalgam_safety.html.
36. Echeverria, D., et al. Neurobehavioral effects from exposure to dental amalgam Hg(0): new distinctions between recent exposure and Hg body burden. *FASEB J* 1998;12:971-980.

Chapter 10: Infections

1. Mystery of the forgotten plague. http://news.bbc.co.uk/2/hi/health/3930727.stm.
2. Olanow, C.W., et al. Levodopa in the treatment of Parkinson's disease: current controversies. *Mov Disord* 2004;19:997-1005.
3. Solbrig, M.V. Acute Parkinsonism in suspected herpes simplex encephalitis movement disorder. *Movement Disorders* 1993;8:233-234.
4. Jang, H., et al. Highly pathogenic H5N1 influenza virus can enter the central nervous system and induce neuroinflammation and neurodegeneration. *Proc Natl Acad Sci USA* 2009;106:14063-14068.
5. Jang H., et al. Viral parkinsonism. *Biochim Biophys Acta.* 2008;1792:714–721.
6. Marttila, R.J., et al. Viral antibodies in the sera from patients with Parkinson disease. *Eur Neurol* 1977;15:25-33.
7. Kim, J.S., et al. Reversible parkinsonism and dystonia following probable mycoplasma pneumoniae infection. *Mov Disord* 1995;10:510-512.
8. Altschuler, E. Gastric Helicobacter pylori infection as a cause of idiopathic Parkinson's disease and non-arteric anterior optic ischemic neuropathy. *Med Hypotheses* 1996;47:413-414.
9. Epp, L.M. and Mravec, B. Chronic polysystemic candidiasis as a possible contributoer to onset of idiopathic Parkinson's disease. *Bratisl Lek Listy* 2006;107:227-230.
10. Martyn, C.N., et al Motoneuron disease and past poliomyelitis in England and Wales. *Lancet* 1988;1:1319-1322.
11. Hugan, J. ALS therapy: Targets for the future. *Neurology* 1996;47:S251-S254.
12. Nicolson, G.L., et al. High frequency of systemic mycoplasmal infections in Gulf War veterans and civilians with amyotrophic lateral sclerosis (ALS). *J Clin Neurosci* 2002;9:525-529.
13. MacDonald, A.B. Spirochetal cyst forms in neurodegenerative disorders…hiding in plain site. *Med Hypoth* 2006;67:819-832.
14. Halperin, J.J., et al. Immunologic reactivity against Borrelia burgdorferi in patients with motor neuron disease. *Arch Neurol* 1990;47:586-594.
15. Irkec, C., et al. the viral etiology of amyotrophic lateral sclerosis. *Mikrobivol Bul* 1989;23:102-109.
16. Ferri-De-Barros, J.E. and Moreira, M. Amyotrophic lateral sclerosis and herpes virus. Report of an unusual case: a cause of casual association? *Arg Neuropsiguiatr* 1998;56:307-311.
17. Maida, E. and Kristoferitsch, W. Amyotrophic Lateral Sclerosis following Herpes zoster infection in a patient with immunodeficiency. *Eur Neurol* 1981;20:330-333.
18. Auwaerter, P.G., et al. Lyme borreliosis (Lyme disease): molecular and cellular pathobiology and prospects for prevention, diagnosis and treatment. *Expert Rev Mol Med* 2004;6:1-22.
19.Hansel, Y., et al. ALS-like sequelae in chronic neuroborreliosis. *Wien Med Wochenschr* 1995;145:186-188.
20. Harvey, W.T. and Martz, D. Motor neuron disease recovery associated with IV ceftriaxonoe and anti-Babesia therapy. *Acta Neurol Scand* 2007;115:129-131.
21.Alotaibi, S., et al. Epstein-Barr virus in pediatric multiple sclerosis. *JAMA* 2004;291:1875-1879.
22. Haahr, S. and Hollsberg, P. Multiple sclerosis in linked to Epstein-Barr virus infection. *Rev Med Virol* 2006;16:297-310.
23. Levin, L.I., et al. Multiple sclerosis and Epstein-Barr virus. *JAMA* 2003;289:1533-1536.

24. Hayes, C.E. and Donald Acheson, E. A unifying multiple sclerosis etiology linking virus infection, sunlight, and vitamin D, through viral interleukin-10. *Med Hypotheses* 2008;71:85-90.
25. Volpi, A. Epstein-Barr virus and human herpesvirus type 8 infections of the central nervous system. *Herpes* 2004;11 Supple 2:120A-127A.
26. Honjo, K., et al. Alzheimer's disease and infection: do infectious agents contribute to progression of Alzheimer's disease? *Alzheimers Dement* 2009;5:348-360.
27. Meer-Scheerer, L., et al. Lyme disease associated with Alzheimer's disease. *Curr Microbiol* 2006;52:330-332.
28. Itzhaki, R.F., et al. Infiltration of the brain by pathogens causes Alzheimer's disease. *Neurobiol Aging* 2004;25:619-627.
29. Kountouras, J., et al. Association between Helicobacter pylori infection and mild cognitive impairment. *Eur J Neurol* 2007;14:976-982.
30. Miklossy, J., et al. Borrelia burgdorferi persists in the brain in chronic Lyme neuroborreliosis and may be associated with Alzheimer disease. *J Alzheimers Dis* 2004;6:639-649.
31. Wozniak, M.A., et al. Herpes simplex virus infection causes cellular beta-amyloid accumulation and secretase upregulation. *Neurosci Lett* 2007;429:95-100.
32. Wozniak, M.A., et al. Herpes simplex virus type 1 DNA is located within Alzheimer's disease amyloid plaques. *J Pathol* 2009;217:131-138.
33. Letenneur, L., et al. Seropositivity to herpes simplex virus antibodies and risk of Alzheimer's disease: a population-based cohort study. *PLoS One* 2008;3:e3637.
34. Jamieson, G.A., et al. Herpes simplex virus type 1 DNA is present in specific regions of brain from aged people with and without senile dementia of the Alzheimer type. *J Pathol* 1992:167:3665-368.
35. Itzhaki, R. Herpes simplex virus type 1, apolipoprotein E and Alzheimer's disease. *Herpes* 2004;11:77A-82A.
36. Mawhorter, S.D. and Lauer, M.A. Is atherosclerosis an infectious disease? *Cleve Clin J Med* 2001;68:449-458.
37. Elkind, M.S., et al. Infectious burden and risk of stroke: the northern Manhattan study. *Arch Neurol* 2010;67:33-38.
38. Ramirez, J.A. Isolation of Chlamydia pneumonia from the coronary artery of a patient with coronary atherosclerosis. The Chlamydia pneumonia/Atherosclerosis Study Group. *Ann Intern Med* 1996;125:979-982.
39. Danesh, J., et al. Chronic infections and coronary heart disease: is there a link? *Lancet* 1997;350:430-436.
40. Gura, T. Infections: a cause of artery-clogging plaques? *Science* 1998;281:35,37.
41. Gaydos, C.A., et al. Replication of Chlamydia pneumoniae in vitro in human macrophages, endothelial cells, and aortic artery smooth muscle cells. *Infect Immun* 1996;64:1614-1620.
42. Muhlestein, J.B. Chronic infection and coronary artery disease. *Med Clin North Am* 2000;84:123-148.
43. Balin, B.J., et al. Identification and localization of Chlamydia pneumonia in the Alzheimer's brain. *Med Microbiol Immunol* 1998;187:23-42.
44. Gerard, H.C., et al. Chlamydophila (Chlamydia) pneumonia in the Alzheimer's brain. *FEMS Immunol Med Microbiol* 2006;48:355-366.
45. Little, C.S., et al. Chlamydia pneumoniae induces Alzheimer-like amyloid plaques in brains of BALA/c mice. *Neurobiol Aging* 2004;25:419-429.
46. Volpi, A. Epstein-Barr virus and human herpesvirus type 8 infections of the central nervous system. *Herpes* 2004;11 Supple 2:120A-127A.
47. Zaiou, M. Multifunctional antimicrobial peptides: therapeutic targets in several human diseases. *J Mol Med* 2007;85:317-329.
48. Hammer, N.D., et al. Amyloids: friend or foe? *J Alzheimers Dis* 2008;13:407-419.

49. Nunomura, A., et al. Neurnoal death and survival under oxidative stress in Alzheimers and Parkinson diseases. *CNS Neurol Disord Drug Targets* 2007;6:411-423.
50. Soscia, S.J., et al. The Alzheimer's disease-associated amyloid beta-protein is an antimicrobial peptide. *PLoS One* 2010;5:e9505.
51. Dominguez, D., et al. Phenotypic and biochemical analyses of BACE1- and BACE2-deficient mice. *J Biol Chem* 2005;280:30797-30806.
52. Green, R.C., et al. Effect of tarenflurbil on cognitive decline and activities of daily living in patients with mild Alzheimer disease: a randomized controlled trial. *JAMA* 2009;302:2557-2564.
53. Itzhaki, R.F., et al. Infiltration of the brain by pathogens causes Alzheimer's disease. *Neurobiol Aging* 2004;25:619-627.
54. Miklossy, J., et al. Beta-amyloid deposition and Alzheimer's type changes induced by Borrelia spirochetes. *Neurobiol Aging* 2006;27:228-236.
55. Kountouras, J., et al. Relationship between Helicobacter pylori infection and Alzheimer disease. *Neurology* 2006;66:938-940.
56. Itzhaki, R.F., et al. Herpes simplex virus type 1 in brain and risk of Alzheimer's disease. *Lancet* 1997;349:241-244.
57. Roberts, G.W., et al. Beta A4 amyloid protein deposition in brain after head trauma. *Lancet* 1991;338:1422-1423.
58. Tesco, G., et al. Depletion of GGA3 stabilizes BACE and enhances beta-secretase activity. *Neuron* 2007;54:721-737.
59. Xie, Z., et al. Isoflurane-induced apoptosis: a potential pathogenic link between delirium and dementia. *J Gerontol A Biol Sci Med Sci* 2006;61:1300-1306.
60. Jang, H., et al. Highly pathogenic H5N1 influenza virus can enter the central nervous system and induce neuroinflammation and neurodegeneration. *Proc Natl Acad Sci USA* 2009;106:14063-14068.
61. Halperin, J.J., et al. Immunologic reactivity against Borrelia burgdorferi in patients with motor neuron disease. *Arch Neurol* 1990;47:586-594.
62. Konsman, J.P., et al. Cytokine-induced sickness behavior: mechanisms and implications. *Trends Neurosci* 2002;25:154-159.
63. Cunningham, C., et al. Systemic inflammation induces acute behavioral and cognitive changes and accelerates neurodegenerative disease. *Biol Psychiatry* 2009;65:304-312.
64. Holmes, C., et al. Systemic inflammation and disease progression in Alzheimer disease. *Neurology* 2009;73:768-774.
65. Aisen, P.S. the potential of anti-inflammatory drugs for the treatment of Alzheimer's disease. *Lancet Neurol* 2002;1:279-284.
66. McGeer, P.L. and McGeer, D.G. NSAIDs and Alzheimer disease: epidemiological, animal model and clinical studies. *Neurobiol Aging* 2007;28:639-647.

Chapter 11: The Dental Connection

1. Mylonas, A.I., et al. Cerebral abscess of odontogenic origin. *J Craniomaxillofac Surg* 2007;35:63-67.
2. Andersen, W.C. and Horton, H.L. Parietal lobe abscess after routine periodontal recall therapy. Report of a case. *J Periodontal* 1990;61:243-247.
3. Baddour, H.M., et al. Frontal lobe abscess of dental origin. Report of a case. *Oral Surg Oral Med Oral Pathol* 1979;47:303-306.
4. Marks, P.V., et al. Multiple brain abscesses secondary to dental caries and severe periodontal disease. *Br J Oral Maxillofac Surg* 1988;26:244-247.
5. Renton, T.F., et al. Cerebral abscess complicating dental treatment. Case report and review of the literature. *Aust Dent J* 1996;41:12-15.

6. Corson, M.A., et al. Are dental infections a cause of brain abscess? Case report and review of the literature. *Oral Dis* 2001;7:61-65.
7. Marques da Silva, R., et al. Characterization of Streptococcus constellatus strains recovered from a brain abscess and periodontal pockets in an immunocompromised patient. *J Periodontal* 2004;75:1720-1723.
8. Li, X., et al. Brain abscesses caused by oral infection. *Endod Dent Traumatol* 1999;15:95-101.
9. Zijlstra, E.E., et al. Pericarditis, pneumonia and brain abscess due to a combined Actinomyces-Actinobacillus actinomycetemcomitans infection. *J Infect* 1992;25:83-878.
10. Craig, R.G., et al. Periodontal diseases—a modifiable source of systemic inflammation for the end-stage renal disease patient on haemodialysis therapy? *Nephrol Dial Transplant* 2007;22:312-315.
11. Nibali, L., et al. Severe periodontitis is associated with systemic inflammation and a dysmetabolic status: a case-control study. *J Clin Periodontol* 2007;34:931-937.
12. Tonetti, M.S., et al. Treatment of periodontitis and endothelial function. *N Engl J Med* 2007;356:911-920.
13. US Department of Health and Human Services. Oral health in America: A report of the surgeon general. Rockville, MD: US and Department of Health and Human Services, National Institute of Dental and Craniofacial Research, National Institutes of Health; 2000. Available at: http://www2.nider.nih.gov/sgr/sgrohweb/home.htm.
14. Lucas, V. and Roberts, G.J. Odontogenic bacteremia following tooth cleaning procedures in children. *Pediatr Dent* 2000;22:96-100.
15. Rocas, I.N., et al. Oral treponemes in primary root canal infections as detected by nested PCR. *Int Endod J* 2003;36:20-26.
16. Miklossy, J. Chronic inflammation and amyloidogeneis in Alzheimer's disease—role of spirochetes. *Journal of Alzheimer's disease* 2008;13:381-391.
17. MacDonald, A.B. and Miranda, J.M. Concurrent neocortical borreliosis and Alzheimer's disease. *Hum Pathol* 1987;18:759-761.
18. Miklossy, J., et al. Borrelia burgdorferi persists in the brain in chronic Lyme neuroborreliosis and may be associated with Alzheimer disease. *J Alzheimer's Dis* 2004;6:1-11.
19. Miklossy, J., et al. Beta-amyloid deposition and Alzheimer's type changes induced by Borrelia spirochetes. *Neurobiol Aging* 2006;27:228-236.
20. Miklossy, J. Alzheimer's disease—a spirochetosis? *Neuroreport* 1993;4:841-848.
21. Miklossy, J. The spirochetal etiology of Alzheimer's disease: a putative therapeutic approach in: *Alzheimer Disease: Therapeutic Strategies. Proceedings of the Third International Springfield Alzheimer Symposium*, Part I. Giacobini, E., and Becker, R., eds. Birkhauser Boston, Inc., 1994, pp.41-48.
22. Miklossy, J., et al. Further morphological evidence for a spirochetal etiology of Alzheimer's disease. *Neuroreport* 1994;5:1201-1204.
23. Miklossy, J., et al. Senile plaques, neurofibrillary tangles and neuropil threads contain DNA? *J Spirochetal and Tick-borne Dis* 1995;2:1-5.
24. Miklossy, J., et al bacterial peptidoglycan in neuritic plaques in Alzheimer's disease. *Alzheimer's Res* 1996;2:95-100.
25. Miklossy, J. Chronic inflammation and amyloidogenesis in Alzheimer's disease: putative role of bacterial peptidoglycan, a potent inflammatory and amyloidogenic factor. *Alzheimer's Dis Rev* 1998;3:345-351.
26. Riviere, G.R., et al. Molecular and immunological evidence of oral Treponema in the human brain and their association with Alzheimer's disease. *Oral Microbiol Immunol* 2002;17:113-118.
27. Miklossy, J. Alzheimer's disease—a spirochetosis? *Neuroreport* 1993;4:841-848.
28. Itzhaki, R.F. and Wozniak, M.A. Herpes simplex virus type 1 in Alzheimer's disease: The enemy within. *Journal of Alzheimer's Disease* 2008;13:393-405.

29. Riviere, G.R., et al. Molecular and immunological evidence of oral Treponema in the human brain and their association with Alzheimer's disease. *Oral Microbial Immunol* 2002;17:113-118.
30. Balin, B.J., et al. Chlamydophila pneumoniae and the etiology of late-onset Alzheimer's disease. *Journal of Alzheimer's disease* 2008;13:371-380.
31.Nguyen, A.M., et al. Detection of Helicobacter pylori in dental plaque by reverse transcription-polymerase chain reaction. *J Clin Microbiol* 1993;31:783-787.
32. Kountouras, J., et al. Eradication of Helicobacter pylori may be beneficial in the management of Alzheimer's disease. *J Neurol* 2009;2556:758-767.
33. Kountouras, J., et al. Increased cerebrospinal fluid Helicobacter pylori antibody in Alzheimer's disease. *Int J Neurosci* 2009;119:765-777.
34. Miklossy, J. Chronic inflammation and amyloidogeneis in Alzheimer's disease—role of spirochetes. *Journal of Alzheimer's disease* 2008;13:381-391.
35. Shapira, L., et al. Effects of Porphyromonas gingivalis on the central nervous system: activation of glial cells and exacerbation of experimental autoimmune encephalomyelitis. *J Periodontal* 2002;73:511-516.
36. McGrother, C.W., et al. Multiple sclerosis, dental caries and fillings: a case-control study. *Br Dent J* 1999;187:261-264.
37. Jones, J.A., et al. Caries incidence in patients with dementia. *Gerodontology* 1993;10:76-82.
38. Comfort, A.O., et al. Dental health of Fiji institutionalized elderly (2003). *Pac Health Dialog* 2004;11:38-43.
39. Shimazaki, Y., et al. Influence of dentition status on physical disability, mental impairment, and mortality in institutionalized elderly people. *J Dent Res* 2001;80:340-345.
40. Stewart, R. and Hirani, V. Dental health and cognitive impairment in an English national survey population. *J Am Geriatr Soc* 2007;55:1410-1414.
41. Noble, J.M., et al. Periodontitis is associated with cognitive impairment among older adults: analysis of NHANES-III. *J Neurol Neurosurg Psychiatry* 2009;80:1206-1211.
42. Ellefsen, B., et al. Caries prevalence in older persons with and without dementia. *J Am Geriatr Soc* 2008;56:59-67.
43. Schwarz, J.H., et al. Increased periodontal pathology in Parkinson's disease. *Journal of Neurology* 2006;253:608-611.
44. Hanaoka, A. and Kashihara, K. Increased frequencies of caries, periodontal disease and tooth loss in patients with Parkinson's disease. *Journal of Clinical Neuroscience* 2009;16:1279-1282.
45. Galata, G. Results in a case of Parkinson's disease due to alveolar pyorrhea, treated with bismuth by parenteral route. *Policlinico Prat* 1964;71:220-223.
46. Stein, P.S., et al. Tooth loss, dementia and neuropathology in the Nun Study. *J Am Dent Assoc* 2007;138:1314-1322.
47. Kim, J.M., et al. Dental health, nutritional status and recent-onset dementia in a Korean community population. *Int J Geriatr Psychiatry* 2007;22:850-855.
48. Ogihara, R., et al. ADL and actual life styles of all Japanese centenarians as determined by a visitation interview survey. *Nippon Koshu Eisei Zasshi* 2000;47:275-283.
49. Kondo, K., et al. A case-control study of Alzheimer's disease in Japan—significance of life-styles. *Dementia* 1994;5:314-326.
50. Gatz, M., et al. Potentially modifiable risk factors for dementia in identical twins. *Alzheimer Dement* 2006;2:110-117.
51. Pihlstrom, B.L., et al. Periodontal diseases. *Lancet* 2005;366:1809-1820.
52. Kamer, A.R., et al. Inflammation and Alzheimer's disease: possible role of periodontal diseases. *Alzheimers Dement* 2008;4:242-250.
53. Pucher, J. and Stewart, J. Periodontal disease and diabetes mellitus. *Curr Diab Rep* 2004;4:46-50.

54. Iacopino, A.M. Periodontitis and diabetes interrelationships: role of inflammation. *Ann Periodontol* 2001;6:125-137.
55. Mealey, B.L. and Rose, L.F. Diabetes mellitus and inflammatory periodontal diseases. *Curr Opin Endocrinol Diabetes Obes* 2008;15:135-141.
56. Meining, G.E. *Root Canal Cover-Up*. Price-Pottenger Nutrition Foundation: La Mesa, CA, 1998.

Chapter 12: Cholesterol Is Good for You

1. White, P.D. Perspectives. *Prog Cardiovascular Dis* 1971;14:249.
2. Siri-Tarino, P.W., et al. Meta-analysis of prospective cohort studies evaluating the association of saturated fat with cardiovascular disease. *Am J Clin Nutr* 2010;91:535-546.
3. http://www.second-opinions.co.uk/cholesterol_myth_1.html.
4. Ravnskov, U. *The Cholesterol Myths: Exposing the Fallacy that Saturated Fat and Cholesterol Cause Heart Disease*. New Trends Publishing, Washington, DC 2000.
5. Krumholz, H.M. Lack of association between cholesterol and coronary heart disease and morbidity and all-cause mortality in persons older than 70 years. *JAMA* 1994;272:1335-1340.
6. Schatz, I.J., et al. Cholesterol and all-cause mortality in elderly people from the Honolulu Heart Program: a cohort study. *Lancet* 2001;358:351-355.
7. Anderson, K.M., et al. Cholesterol and mortality, 30 years of follow-up from the Framingham Study. *JAMA* 1987;257:2176-2180.
8. Garrett, H.E., et al. Serum cholesterol values in patients treated surgically for atherosclerosis. *JAMA* 1964;189:655-659.
9. Sachdeva, A., et al. Lipid levels in patients hospitalized with coronary artery disease: an analysis of 136,905 hospitalizations in Get With The Guidelines. *Am Heart J* 2009;157:111-117.
10. Al-Mallah, M.H., et al. Low admission LDL-cholesterol is associated with increased 3-year all-cause mortality in patients with non ST segment elevation myocardial infarction. *Cardio J* 2009;16:227-233.
11. Mehta, J.L., et al Interactive role of infection, inflammation and traditional risk factors in atherosclerosis and coronary artery disease. *J Am Coll Cardiol* 1998;31:1217-1225.
12. Koening, W. Atherosclerosis involves more than just lipids: focus on inflammation. *Eur Heart J* 1999;Suppl T:T19-T26.
13. Ross, R. Atherosclerosis—an inflammatory disease. *N Engl J Med* 1999;34:115-126.
14. Gutteridge, J.M.C. and Halliwell, B. *Antioxidants in Nutrition, Health, and Disease*. Oxford University Press, Oxford, 1994.
15. Addis, P.B. and Warner, G.J. Free Radicals and Food Additives. Aruoma, O.I. and Halliwell, B. eds. Taylor and Francis, London, 1991.
16. Muldoon, M.F., et al. Immune system differences in men with hypo- or hypercholesterolemia. *Clin Immunol Immunopathol* 1997;84:145-149.
17. Weinstock, C., et al. Low density lipoproteins inhibit endotoxin activation of monocytes. *Arterioscler Thromb Vasc Biol* 1992;12:341-347.
18. Feingold, K.R., et al. Role for circulating lipoproteins in protection from endotoxin toxicity. *Infect Immun* 1995;63:2041-2046.
19. Bhakdi, S., et al. Binding and partial inactivation of Staphylococcus aureus a-toxin by human plasma low density lipoprotein. *J Biol Chem* 1983;258:5899-5904.
20. Sivas, F., et al. Serum lipid profile: its relationship with osteoporotic vertebrae fractures and bone mineral density in Turkish post-menopausal women. *Rheumatol Int* 2009;29:885-890.
21. Pfrieger, F.W. Role of cholesterol in synapse formation and function *Biochem Biophy Acta* 2003;1610:271-280.
22. Tong, J., et al. A scissors mechanism for stimulation of SNARE-mediated lipid mixing by cholesterol. *Proc Natl Acad Sci USA* 2009;106:5141-5146.

23. Bjorkhem, I. and Meaney, S. Brain cholesterol: Long secret life behind a barrier. *Arteriosclerosis Thrombosis and Vascular Biology* 2004;24:806-815.
24. Wainwright, G., et al. Cholesterol-lowering therapy and cell membranes. Stable plaque at the expense of unstable membranes? *Arch Med Sci* 2009;5:289-295.
25. Klopfleisch, S., et al. Negative impact of statins on oligodendrocytes and myelin formation in vitro and in vivo. *J Neurosci* 2008;28:13609-13614.
26. Goritz, C., et al. Role of glia-derived cholesterol in synaptogenesis: new revelations in the synapse-gila affair. *J Physiol Paris* 2002;96:257-263.
27. Fan, Q.W., et al. Cholesterol-dependent modulation of tau phosphorylation in cultured neurons. *Journal of Neurochemistry* 2001;76:391-400.
28. Koudinov, A.R. and Koudinova, N.V. Cholesterol, synaptic function and Alzheimer's disease. *Pharmacopsychiatry* 2003;36:S107-S112.
29. Abad-Rodriguez, J., et al. Neuronal membrane cholesterol loss enhances amyloid peptide generation. *Journal of Cell Biology* 2004;167:953-960.
30. Dayton, S., et al. A controlled clinical trial of a diet high in unsaturated fat in preventing complications of atherosclerosis. *Circulation* 1969;40:1-63.
31. Dorr, A.E., et al. Colestipol hydrochloride in hypercholesterolemic patients—effect on serum cholesterol and mortality. *Journal of Chronic Disease* 1978;31:5-14.
32. Muldoon, M.F., et al. Lowering cholesterol concentrations and mortality: a quantitative review of primary prevention trials. *British Medical Journal* 1990;301:309-314.
33. Lindberg, G., et al. Low serum cholesterol concentration and short term mortality from injuries in men and women. *BMJ* 1992;305:277-279.
34. Muldoon, M.F., et al. Randomized trial of the effects of simvastatin on cognitive functioning in hypercholesterolemic adults. *Am J Med* 2004;117:823-829.
35. King, D.S., et al. Cognitive impairment associated with atorvastatin and simvastatin. *Pharmacotherapy* 2003;23:1663-1667.
36. Wagstaff, L.R., et al. Statin-associated memory loss: analysis of 60 case reports and review of the literature. *Pharmacotherapy* 2003;23:871-880.
37. Orsi, A., et al. Simvastatin-associated memory loss. *Pharmacotherapy* 2001;21:767-769.
38. Muldoon, M.F., et al. Effects of lovastatin on cognitive function and psychological well-being. *Am J Med* 2000;108:538-546.
39. Meske, V., et al. Blockade of HMG-CoA reductase activity causes changes in microtubule-stabilizing protein tau via suppression of geranylgeranylpyrophosphate formation: implications for Alzheimer's disease. *Eur J Neurosci* 2003;17:93-102.
40. McGuinness B., et al. Statins for the prevention of dementia. *Cochrane Database of Systematic Reviews* 2009, Apr 15;(2):CD003160.
41. Arvanitakis, Z., et al. Statins, incident Alzheimer disease, change in cognitive function, and neuropathology. *Neurology* 2008;70:1795-1802.
42. Szwast, S.J., Hendrie H.C., et al. Association of statin use with cognitive decline in elderly African Americans. *Neurology* 2007;69:1873-1880.
43. Edwards, I.R., et al. Statins, neuromuscular degenerative disease and an amyotrophic lateral sclerosis-like syndrome: an analysis of individual case safety reports from vigibase. *Drug Safety* 2007;30:515-525.
44. Huang, X., et al. Lower low-density lipoprotein cholesterol levels are associated with Parkinson's disease. *Mov Disord* 2007;22:377-381.
45. Sattar, N., et al. Statins and risk of incident diabetes: a collaborative meta-analysis of randomized statin trials. *Lancet* 2010;375:735-742.
46. Golomb, B.A. and Evans, M.A. Statin adverse effects: a review of the literature and evidence for a mitochondrial mechanism. *Am J Cardiovasc Drugs* 2008;8:373-418.

47. Amarenco, P., et al. Stroke Prevention by Aggressive Reduction in Cholesterol Levels (SPARCL) investigators. High-dose atorvastatin after stroke or transient ischemic attack. *N Engl J Med* 2006;355:549-559.
48. Vergouwen, M.D., et al. Statin treatment and the occurrence of hemorrhagic stroke in patients with a history of cerebrovascular disease. *Stroke* 2008;39:497-502.
49. Burger, M. *Altern und Krankheit, 3rd Ed.* Georg Thieme, Leipzig, 1957.
50. Corrigan F.M., et al. Dietary supplementation with zinc sulphate, sodium selenite and fatty acids in early dementia of Alzheimer's Type II: Effects on lipids. *J Nutr Med* 1991; 2: 265-71.
51. Elias PK, et al. Serum Cholesterol and Cognitive Performance in the Framingham Heart Study. *Psychosom Med* 2005; 67:24-30.
52. Lepara, O., et al. Decreased serum lipids in patients with probable Alzheimer's disease. *Bosn J Basic Med Sci* 2009;9:215-220.
53. Mason, R.P., et al. Evidence for changes in the Alzheimer's disease brain cortical membrane structure mediated by cholesterol. *Neurobiol Aging* 1992;13:413-419.
54. Ledesma, M.D., et al. Raft disorganization leads to reduced plasmin activity in Alzheimer's disease brains. *EMBO Rep* 2003;4:1190-1196.
55. Abad-Rodriguez, J., et al. Neuronal membrane cholesterol loss enhances amyloid peptide generation. *J Cell Biol* 2004;167:953-960.
56. Dupuis, L., et al. Dyslipidemia is a protective factor in amyotrophic lateral sclerosis. *Neurology* 2008;70:1004-1009.
57. Lamperti, E. Decreased concentration of low density lipoprotein cholesterol in patients with parkinson's disease. In: Musanti R, Rocca N, Ghiselli G, Parati E, editors. *Clinical Research* 1991;39:401A.
58. Huang, X., et al. Lower low-density lipoprotein cholesterol levels are associated with Parkinson's disease. *Mov Disord* 2007;22:377-381.
59. Huang, X., et al. Low LDL cholesterol and increased risk of Parkinson's disease: prospective results from Honolulu-Asia Aging Study. *Mov Disord* 2008;23:1013-1018.
60. Mielke, M.M., et al. High total cholesterol levels in late life associated with a reduced risk of dementia. *Neurology* 2005;64:1689-1695.
61. West, R., et al. Better memory functioning associated with higher total and low-density lipoprotein cholesterol levels in very elderly subjects without the apolipoprotein e4 allele. *Am J Geriatr Psychiatry* 2008;16:781-785.
62. Lee, D.Y., et al. Combination of clinical and neuropsychologic information as a better predictor of the progression of Alzheimer disease in questionable dementia individuals. *Am J Geriatr Psychiatry* 2006;14:130-138.
63. Howland, D.S., et al. Modulation of secreted beta-amyloid precursor protein and amyloid beta-peptide in brain by cholesterol. *J Biol Chem* 1998;273:16576-16582.

Chapter 13: The Ketone Miracle

1. Cahill, G.F. Jr. and Veech, R.L. Ketoacids? Good medicine? *Trans Am Clin Climatol Assoc* 2003;114:149-161.
2. Liu, Y.M., et al. A prospective study: growth and nutritional status of children treated with the ketogenic diet. *J Am Diet Assoc* 2003;103:707-712.
3. Sharman, M.J., et al. A ketogenic diet favorably affects serum biomarkers for cardiovascular disease in normal-weight men. *J Nutr* 2002;132:1879-1885.
4. Dashti, H.M., et al. Long term effects of ketogenic diet in obese subjects with high cholesterol level. *Mol Cell Biochem* 2006;286:1-9.
5. Patel, A., et al. Long-term outcomes of children treated with the ketogenic diet in the past. *Epilepsia* 2010; Feb 1, Epub ahead of print.

6. Kossoff, E.H., et al. Ketogenic diets: an update for child neurologists. *J Child Neurol* 2009;24:979-88.
7. Kinsman, S.L., et al. Efficacy of the ketogenic diet for intractable seizure disorders: review of 58 cases. *Epilepsia* 1992;33:1132-1136.
8. Nordli, D.R. Jr., et al. Experience with the ketogenic diet in infants. *Pediatrics* 2001;108:129-133.
9. Pulsifer, M.B., et al. Effects of ketogenic diet on development and behavior: preliminary report of a prospective study. *Developmental Medicine and Child Neurology* 2001;43:301-306.
10. Husain, A.M., et al. Diet therapy for narcolepsy. *Nuerology* 2004;62:2300-2302.
11. Nebeling, L.C., et al. Effects of a ketogenic diet on tumor metabolism and nutritional status in pediatric oncology patients: two case reports. *Journal of the American College of Nutrition* 1995;14:202-208.
12. Seyfried, T.N. and Mukherjee, P. Targeting energy metabolism in brain cancer: review and hypothesis. *Nutrition and Metabolism (London)* 2005;21:30.
13. Evangeliou, A., et al. Application of a ketogenic diet in children with autistic behavior: pilot study. *J Child Neurol* 2003;18:113-118.
14. Strahlman, R.S. Can ketosis help migraine sufferers? A case report. *Headache* 2006;46:182.
15. Murphy, P. et al. The antidepressant properties of the ketogenic diet. *Biological Psychiatry* 2004;56:981-983.
16. Kossoff, E.H., et al. Ketogenic diets: an update for child neurologists. *J Child Neurol* 2009;24:979-988.
17. Mavropoulos, J.C., et al. The effects of a low-carbohydrate, ketogenic diet on the polycystic ovary syndrome: a pilot study. *Nutrition and Metabolism (London)* 2005;2:35.
18. Yancy, W.S., et al. A low-carbohydrate, ketogenic diet to treat type 2 diabetes. *Nutrition and Metabolism (London) 2005*;2:34.
19.Minassian, B.A., et al. Mutations in a gene encoding a novel protein tyrosine phosphatase cause progressive myoclonic epilepsy. *Nat Genet* 1998;20:171-174.
20. Longo, N., et al. Progressive decline in insulin levels in Rabson-Mendenhall syndrome. *J Clin Endocrinol Metab* 1999;84:2623-2629.
21. Veech, R.L. The therapeutic implications of ketone bodies: the effects of ketone bodies in pathological conditions: ketosis, ketogenic diet, redox states, insulin resistance, and mitochondrial metabolism. *Prostaglandins, Leukotrienes and Essential Fatty Acids* 2004;70:309-319.
22. Lardy, H.A., et al. The metabolism of bovine epididymal spermatozoa. *Arch Biochem* 1945;6:41-51.
23. Beck, S.A. and Tisdale, M.J. Nitrogen excretion in cancer cachexia and its modification by a high fat diet in mice. *Cancer Res* 1989;49:3800-3804.
24. Nebeling, L.C. and Lerner, E. Implementing a ketogenic diet based on medium-chain triglyceride oil in pediatric patients with cancer. *J Am Diet Assoc* 1995;95:693-697.
25. Nebeling, L.C., et al. Effects of a ketogenic diet on tumor metabolism and nutritional status in pediatric oncology patients: two case reports. *J Am Coll Nutr* 1995;86:202-208.
26. Seyfried, T.N., et al. Role of glucose and ketone bodies in the metabolic control of experimental brain cancer. *British Journal of Cancer* 2003;89:1375-1382.
27. Mukherjee, P., et al. Dietary restriction reduces angiogenesis and growth in an orthotopic mouse brain tumour model. *Br J Cancer* 2002;86:1615-1621.
28. Fife, B. *Coconut Cures: Preventing and Treating Common Health Problems with Coconut.* Piccadilly Books, Ltd; Colorado Springs, CO, 2005.
29. Hasselbalch, S.G., et al. Changes in cerebral blood flow and carbohydrate metabolism during acute hyperketonemia. *Am J Physiol* 1996;270:E746-751.

30. Marie, C., et al. Fasting prior to transient cerebral ischemia reduces delayed neuronal necrosis. *Metab Bran Dis* 1990;5:65-75.
31. Prins, M.L., et al. Increased cerebral uptake and oxidation of exogenous βHB improves ATP following traumatic brain injury in adult rats. *J Neurochem* 2004;90:666-672.
32. Suzuki, M., et al. Effect of β-hydroxybutyrate, a cerebral function improving agent, on cerebral hypoxia, anoxia and ischemia in mice and rats. *Jpn J Pharmacol* 2001;87:143-150.
33. Twyman, D. Nutritional management of the critically ill neurologic patient. *Crit Care Clin* 1997;13:39-49.
34. Calon, B., et al. Long-chain versus medium and long-chain triglyceride-based fat emulsion in parental nutrition of severe head trauma patients. *Infusionstherapie* 1990;17:246-248.
35. Gasior, M., et al. Neuroprotective and disease-modifying effects of the ketogenic diet. *Behav Pharmacol* 2006;17:431-439.
36. Van der Auwera, I., et al. A ketogenic diet reduces amyloid beta 40 and 42 in mouse model of Alzheimer's disease. *Nutr Metab (london)* 2005;2:28.
37. Zhao, Z., et al. A ketogenic diet as a potential novel therapeutic intervention in amyotrophic lateral sclerosis. *BMC Neuroscience* 2006;7:29.
38. Duan, W., et al. Dietary restriction normalizes glucose metabolism and BDNF levels, slows disease progression, and increases survival in huntingtin mutant mice. *Proc Natl Acad Sci USA* 2003;100:2911-2916.
39. Kashiwaya, Y., et al. D-beta-hydroxybutyrate protects neurons in models of Alzheimer's and Parkinson's disease. *Proc Natl Acad Sci USA* 2000;97:5440-5444.
40. Tieu, K., et al. D-beta-hydroxybutyrate rescues mitochondrial respiration and mitigates features of Parkinson disease. *J Clin Invest* 2003;112:892-901.
41. VanItallie, T.B., et al. Treatment of Parkinson disease with diet-induced hyperketonemia: a feasibility study. *Neurology* 2005;64:728-730.
42. Van der Auwera, I., et al. A ketogenic diet reduces amyloid beta 40 and 42 in a mouse model of Alzheimer's disease. *Nutr Metab (London)* 2005;2:28.
43. Studzinski, C.M., et al. Induction of ketosis may improve mitochondrial function and decrease steady-state amyloid-beta precursor protein (AAPP) levels in the aged dog. *Brain Res* 2008;1226:209-217.
44. Costantini, L.C., et al. Hypometabolism as a therapeutic target in Alzheimer's disease. *BMC Neuroscience* 2008;9:S16.
45. Suzuki, M., et al. Beta-hydroxybutyrate, a cerebral function improving agent, protects rat brain against ischemic damage caused by permanent and transient focal cerebral ischemia. *Jpn J Phamacol* 2002;89:36-43.
46. Suzuki, M., et al. Effect of beta-hydroxybutyrate, a cerebral function improving agent, on cerebral hypoxia, anoxia and ischemia in mice and rats. *Jpn J Phamacol* 2001;87:143-150.
47. Imamura, K., et al. D-beta-hydroxybutyrate protects dopaminergic SH-SY5Y cells in a rotenone model of Parkinson's disease. *J Neuroscie Res* 2006;84:1376-1384.
48. Maalouf, M., et al. The neuroprotective properties of calorie restriction, the ketogenic diet, and ketone bodies. *Brain Res Rev* 2009; 59:293-315.
49. Koper, J.W., et al. Acetoacetate and glucose as substrates for lipid synthesis for rat brain oligodendrocytes and astrocytes in serum-free culture. *Biochim Biophys Acta* 1984;796:20-26.
50. Robinson, A.M. and Williamson, D.H. Physiological roles of ketone bodies as substrates and signals in mammalian tissues. *Physiol Rev* 1980;60:143-187.
51. Veech, R.L., et al. Ketone bodies, potential therapeutic uses. *IUBMB Life* 2001;51:241-247.
52. Kirsch, J.R., et al. Butanediol induced ketosis increases tolerance to hypoxia in the mouse. *Stroke* 1980;11:506-513.
53. Suzuki, M., et al. Effect of beta-hydroxybutyrate, a cerebral function improving agent, on cerebral hypoxia, anoxia, and ischemia in mice and rats. *Jpn J Pharmacol 2001*;87:143-150.

54. Chance, B., et al. Hydroperoxide metabolism in mammalian organs. *Physiol Rev* 1979;59:527-605.
55. Kashiways, Y., et al. D-β-hydroxybutyrate protects neurons in models of Alzheimer's and Parkinson's disease. *Proc Natl Acad Sci USA* 2000;97:5440-5444.
56. Schwartzkroin, P.A. Mechanisms underlying the anti-epileptic efficacy of the ketogenic diet. *Epilepsy Res* 1999;37:171-180.
57. Kossoff, E.H., et al. Efficacy of the ketogenic diet for infantile spasms. *Pediatrics* 2002;109:780-783.
58. Husain, A.M., et al. Diet therapy for narcolepsy. *Nuerology* 2004;62:2300-2302.
59. Evangeliou, A., et al. Application of a ketogenic diet in children with autistic behavior: pilot study. *J Child Neurol* 2003;18:113-118.
60. Strahlman, R.S. Can ketosis help migraine sufferers? A case report. *Headache* 2006;46:182.
61. Murphy, P. et al. The antidepressant properties of the ketogenic diet. *Biological Psychiatry* 2004;56:981-983.
62. Prins, M.L., et al. Increased cerebral uptake and oxidation of exogenous βHB improves ATP following traumatic brain injury in adult rats. *J Neurochem* 2004;90:666-672.
63. Reger, M.A., et al. Effects of beta-hydroxybutyrate on cognition in memory-impaired adults. *Neurobiol Aging* 2004;25:311-314.
64. VanItallie, T.B., et al. Treatment of Parkinson disease with diet-induced hyperketonemia: a feasibility study. *Neurology* 2005;64:728-730.
65. Duan, W., et al. Dietary restriction normalizes glucose metabolism and BDNF levels, slows disease progression, and increases survival in huntingtin mutant mice. *Proc Natl Acad Sci USA* 2003;100:2911-2916.
66. Zhao, Z., et al. A ketogenic diet as a potential novel therapeutic intervention in amyotrophic lateral sclerosis. *BMC Neuroscience* 2006;7:29.
67. Page, K.A., et al. Medium chain fatty acids improve cognitive function in intensively treated type 1 diabetic patients and support the in vitro synaptic transmission during acute hypoglycemia. *Diabetes* 2009;58:1237-1244.
68. Sokoloff, L. Metabolism of ketone bodies by the brain. *Ann Rev Med* 1973;24:271-280.
69. Yeh, Y.Y. and Zee, P. Relation of ketosis to metabolic changes induced by acute medium-chain triglyceride feeding in rats. *J Nutr* 1976;106:58-67.
70. Tantibhedhyangkul, P., et al. Effects of ingestion of long-chain and medium-chain triglycerides on glucose tolerance in man. *Diabetes* 1967;16:796-799.
71. Kashiwaya, Y., et al Substrate signaling by insulin: a ketone bodies ratio mimics insulin action in heart. *Am J Cardiol* 1997;80:50A-60A.
72. Seyfried, T.N., et al. Role of glucose and ketone bodies in the metabolic control of experimental brain cancer. *British Journal of Cancer* 2003;89:1375-1382.
73. Nebeling, L.C., et al. Effects of a ketogenic diet on tumor metabolism and nutritional status in pediatric oncology patients: two case reports. *J Am Coll Nutr* 1995;86:202-208.
74. Kashiwaya, Y., et al Substrate signaling by insulin: a ketone bodies ratio mimics insulin action in heart. *Am J Cardiol* 1997;80:50A-60A.
75. Suzuki, M., et al. Beta-hydroxybutyrate, a cerebral function improving agent, protects rat brain against ischemic damage caused by permanent and transient focal cerebral ischemia. *Jpn J Phamacol* 2002;89:36-43.
76. Alam, H.B., et al. Ketone Ringer's solution attenuates resuscitation induced apoptosis in rat lungs. *5th World Congress on Trauma, Shock, Inflammation, and Sepsis* 2000, pp63-66.
77. Hiraide, A., et al. Effect of 3-hydroxybutyrate on posttraumatic metabolism in man. *Surgery* 1991;109:176-181.
78. Mavropoulos, J.C., et al. The effects of a low-carbohydrate, ketogenic diet on the polycystic ovary syndrome: a pilot study. *Nutrition and Metabolism (London)* 2005;2:35.

79. Lardy, H.A. and Phillips, P.H. Studies of fat and carbohydrate oxidation in mammalian spermatozoa. *Arch Biochem* 1945;6:53-61.
80. Yancy, W.S., et al. A low-carbohydrate, ketogenic diet versus a low-fat diet to treat obesity and hyperlipidemia: a randomized, controlled trial. *Ann Intern Med* 2004;140:769-777.
81. Cahill, G.F. Jr. and Veech, R.L. Ketoacids? Good Medicine? *Transactions of the American Clinical and Climatological Association* 2003;114:149-163.
82. Fontana, L. Neuroendocrine factors in the regulation of inflammation: excessive adiposity and calorie restriction. *Exp Gerontol* 2009;44:41-45.
83. Kaunitz, H. and Johnson, R.E. Influence of dietary fats on disease and longevity. In: Chavez, A., Bourges, H., Basta, S., eds. Proceedings of the 9th International Congress on Nutrition, Mexico, 1972. Basel: Karger, 1975;1:362-373.
84. Costantini, L.C., et al. Hypometabolism as a therapeutic target in Alzheimer's disease. *BMC Neuroscience* 2008;9:S16.

Chapter 14: The Facts on Fats

1. Brunner, J., et al. Cholesterol, omega-3 fatty acids, and suicide risk: empirical evidence and pathophysiological hypotheses. *Fortschr Neurol Psychiatr* 2001;69:460-467.
2. Colin, A., et al. Lipids, depression and suicide. *Encephale* 2003;29:49-58.
3. Wells, A.S., et al. Alterations in mood after changing to a low-fat diet. *Br J Nutr* 1998;79:23-30.
4. http://en.wikipedia.org/wiki;Life_expectancy.
5. McGee, D., et al. The relationship of dietary fat and cholesterol to mortality in 10 years: the Honolulu Heart Program. *Int J Epidemiol* 1985;14:97-105.
6. Okamoto, K., et al. Nutritional status and risk of amyotrophic lateral sclerosis in Japan. *Amyotroph Lateral Scler* 2007;8:300-304.
7. Forsythe, C.E., et al. Comparison of low fat and low carbohydrate diets on circulating fatty acid composition and markers of inflammation. *Lipids* 2008;43:65-77.
8. Prior, I. A. Cholesterol, coconuts, and diet on Polynesian atolls: a natural experiment: the Pukapuka and Tokelau island studies. *Am J Clin Nutr* 1981;34:1552-1561.
9. Mendis, S., et al. Cardiovascular risk factors in a Melanesian population apparently free from stroke and ischaemic heart disease: the Kitava study. *J Intern Med* 1994;236:331-340.
10. Mendis, S. Coronary heart disease and coronary risk profile in a primitive population. *Trop Geogr Med* 1991;43:199-202.
11. Davis, G.P. and Park, E. *The Heart: The Living Pump.* Torstar Books, New York, 1983.
12. Aruoma, O.I. and Halliwell, B. eds. *Free Radicals and Food Additives.* Taylor and Francis, London, 1991.
13. Harman, D., et al. Free radical theory of aging: effect of dietary fat on central nervous system function. *J Am Geriatr Soc* 1976;24:301-307.
14. Seddon, J.M., et al. Dietary fat and risk for advanced age-related macular degeneration. *Arch Ophthalmol* 2001;119:1191-1199.
15. Ouchi, M., et al. A novel relation of fatty acid with age-related macular degeneration. *Ophthalmologica* 2002;216:363-367.
16. Sheddon, J.M., et al. Progression of age-related macular degeneration: association with dietary fat, transunsaturated fat, nuts, and fish intake. *Arch Ophthalmol* 2003;121:1728-1737.
17. Tewfik, I.H., et al. The effect of intermittent heating on some chemical parameters of refined oils used in Egypt. A public health nutrition concern. *Int J Food Sci Nutr* 1998;49:339-342.
18. Jurgens, G., et al. Immunostaining of human autopsy aortas with antibodies to modified apolipoprotein B and apoprotein(a). *Arterioscler Thromb* 1993;13:1689-1699.
19. Srivastava, S., et al. Identification of cardiac oxidoreductase(s) involved in the metabolism of the lipid peroxidation-derived aldehyde-4-hydroxynonenal. *Biochem J* 1998;329:469-475.

20. Nakamura, K., et al. Carvedilol decreases elevated oxidative stress in human failing myocardium. *Circulation* 2002;105:2867-2871.
21. Pratico, D. and Delanty, N. Oxidative injury in diseases of the central nervous system: focus on Alzheimer's disease. *The American Journal of Medicine* 2000;109:577-585.
22. Markesbery, W.R. and Carney, J.M. Oxidative alterations in Alzheimer's disease. *Brain Pathology* 1999;9;133-146.
23. Kritchevsky, D. and Tepper, S.A. Cholesterol vehicle in experimental atherosclerosis. 9. Comparison of heated corn oil and heated olive oil. *J Atheroscler Res* 1967;7:647-651.
24. Raloff, J. 1996. Unusual fats lose heart-friendly image. *Science News* 1996;150:87.
25. Mensink, R.P. and Katan, M.B. 1990. Effect of dietary trans fatty acids on high-density and low-density lipoprotein cholesterol levels in healthy subjects. *N Eng J Med* 323(7):439.
26. Willett, W.C., et al. 1993. Intake of trans fatty acids and risk of coronary heart disease among women. *Lancet* 341(8845):581.
27. Booyens, J. and Louwrens, C.C. The Eskimo diet. Prophylactic effects ascribed to the balanced presence of natural cis unsaturated fatty acids and to the absence of unnatural trans and cis isomers of unsaturated fatty acids. *Med Hypoth* 1986;21:387.
28. Grandgirard, A., et al. Incorporation of trans long-chain n-3 polyunsaturated fatty acids in rat brain structures and retina. *Lipids* 1994;29:251-258.
29. Pamplona, R., et al. Low fatty acid unsaturation: a mechanism for lowered lipoperoxidative modification of tissue proteins in mammalian species with long life spans. *J Gerontol A Biol Sci Med Sci* 2000;55:B286-B291.
30. Cha, Y.S. and Sachan, D.S. Oppostie effects of dietary saturated and unsaturated fatty acids on ethanol-pharmacokinetics, triglycerides and carnitines. *J Am Coll Nutr* 1994;13:338-343.
31. Siri-Tarino, P.W., et al. Meta-analysis of prospective cohort studies evaluating the association of saturated fat with cardiovascular disease. *American Journal of Clinical Nutrition* 2010;91:535-546.

Chapter 15: The Ultimate Brain Food

1. Turner, N., et al. Enhancement of muscle mitochondrial oxidative capacity and alterations in insulin action are lipid species dependent: potent tissue-specific effects of medium chain fatty acids. *Diabetes* 2009;58:2547-2554.
2. Isaacs, C.E. and Thormar, H. The role of milk-derived antimicrobial lipids as antiviral and antibacterial agents, in *Immunology of Milk and the Neonate* (Mestecky, J., et al., eds). Plenum Press, 1991.
3. Isaacs, C.E. and Thormar, H. The role of milk-derived antimicrobial lipids as antiviral and antibacterial agents. *Adv Exp Med Biol* 1991;310:159-165.
4. Isaacs, C.E., et al. Antiviral and antibacterial lipids in human milk and infant formula feeds. *Arch Dis Child* 1990;65:861-864.
5. Bergsson, G., et al. In vitro inactivation of Chlamydia trachomatis by fatty acids and monoglycerides. *Antimicrobial Agents and Chemotherapy* 1998;42:2290- 2292.
6. Petschow, B.W., et al. Susceptibility of Helicobacter pylori to bactericidal properties of medium-chain monoglycerides and free fatty acids. *Antimicrobial Agents and Chemotherapy* 1996;40;302-306.
7. Holland, K.T., et al. The effect of glycerol monolaurate on growth of, and production of toxic shock syndrome toxin-1 and lipase by, Staphylococcus aureus. *Journal of Antimicrobial Chemotherapy* 1994;33:41-55.
8. Sun, C.Q., et al. Antibacterial actions of fatty acids and monoglycerides against Helicobacter pylori. *FEMS Immunol Med Microbiol* 2003;36:9-17.
9. Bergsson, G., et al. Killing of Gram-positive cocci by fatty acids and monoglycerides. *APMIS* 2001;109:670-678.

10. Bergsson, G., et al. In vitro susceptibilities of Neisseria gonorrhoeae to fatty acids and monoglycerides. *Antimicrob Agents Chemother* 1999;43:2790-2792.
11. Ogbolu, D.O., et al. In vitro antimicrobial properties of coconut oil on Candida species in Ibadan, Nigeria. *J Med Food* 2007;10:384-387.
12. Bergsson, G., et al. In vitro killing of Candida albicans by fatty acids and monoglycerides. *Antimicrob Agents Chemother* 2001;45:3209-3212.
13. Chadeganipour, M, and Haims, A. Antifungal activities of pelargonic and capric acid on Miscrosporum gypseum. *Mycoses* 2001;44:109-112.
14. Isaacs, E.E., et al. Inactivation of enveloped viruses in human bodily fluids by purified lipid. *Annals of the New York Academy of Sciences* 1994;724:465-471.
15. Bartolotta, S., et al. Effect of fatty acids on arenavirus replication: inhibition of virus production by lauric acid. *Arch Virol* 2001;146:777-790.
16. Thormar, H., et al. Inactivation of visna virus and other enveloped viruses by free fatty acids and monoglycerides. *Ann NY Acad Sci* 1994;724:465-471.
17. Hornung, B., et al. Lauric acid inhibits the maturation of vesicular stomatitis virus. *J Gen Virol* 1994;75:353-361.
18. Thormar, H., et al. Inactivation of enveloped viruses and killing of cells by fatty acids and monoglycerides. *Antimicrob Agents Chemother* 1987;31:27-31.
19. Vazquez, C., et al. Eucaloric substitution of medium chain triglycerides for dietary long chain fatty acids improves body composition and lipid profile in a patient with human immunodeficiency virus lipodystrophy. *Nutr Hosp* 2006;21:552-555.
20. Wanke, C.A., et al. A medium chain triglyceride-based diet in patients with HIV and chronic diarrhea reduces diarrhea and malabsorption: a prospective, controlled trial. *Nutrition* 1996;12:766-771.
21. Thormar, H., et al. Hydrogels containing monocaprin have potent microbicidal activities against sexually transmitted viruses and bacteria in vitro. *Sex Transm Infect* 1999;75(3):181-185.
22. Kabara, J.J. *The Pharmacological Effect of Lipids.* Champaign, IL: The American Oil Chemists' Society, 1978.
23. Coconut Oil: A New Weapon Against AIDS, www.coconutresearchcenter.org/hwnl_5-5.htm.
24. Gordon, S. Coconut oil may help fight childhood pneumonia. *US News and World Report*, Oct 30, 2008.
25. Amith, H.V., et al. Effect of oil pulling on plaque and gingivitis. *JOHCD* 2007;1:12-18.
26. Tritten, C.B. and Armitage, G.C. Comparison of a sonic and a manual toothbrush for efficacy in supragingival plaque removal and reduction of gingivitis. *J Clin Periodontol* 1996;23:641-648.
27. Shadnia, S., et al. Successful treatment of acute aluminium phosphide poisoning: possible benefit of coconut oil. *Human & Experimental Toxicology* 2005;24:215-218.
28. Kono, H., et al. Medium-chain triglycerides enhance secretory IgA expression in rat intestine after administration of endotoxin. *Am J Physiol Gastrointest Liver Physiol* 2004;286:G1081-1089.
29. Medium-chain length fatty acids, glycerides and analogues as stimulators of erythropoiesis, http://www.wipo.int/pctdb/en/wo.jsp?IA=GB2004000457&DISPLAY=DESC.
30. Nolasco, N. A., et al. Effect of Coconut oil, trilaurin and tripalmitin on the promotion stage of carcinogenesis. *Philipp J Sci* 1994;123(1):161-169.
31. Reddy, B. S. and Maeura, Y. Tumor promotion by dietary fat in azoxymethane-induced colon carcinogenesis in female F344 rats: influence of amount and source of dietary fat. *J Natl Cancer Inst* 1984;72(3):745-750.
32. Cohen, L. A. and Thompson, D. O. The influence of dietary medium chain triglycerides on rat mammary tumor development. *Lipids* 1987;22(6):455-461.

33. Lim-Sylianco, C. Y., et al. A comparison of germ cell antigenotoxic activity of non-dietary and dietary coconut oil and soybean oil. *Phil J of Coconut Studies* 1992;2:1-5.
34. Lim-Sylianco, C. Y., et al. Antigenotoxic effects of bone marrow cells of coconut oil versus soybean oil. *Phil J of Coconut Studies* 1992;2:6-10.
35. Bulatao-Jayme, J., et al. Epdemiology of primary liver cancer in the Philippines with special consideration of a possible aflatoxin factor. *J Philipp Med Assoc* 1976;52:129-150.
36. Witcher, K. J, et al. Modulation of immune cell proliferation by glycerol monolaurate. *Clinical and Diagnostic Laboratory Immunology* 1996;3:10-13.
37. Projan, S. J., et al. Glyceryl monolaurate inhibits the production of β-lactamase, toxic shock syndrome toxin-1 and other Staphylococcal exoproteins by interfering with signal transduction. *J of Bacteriol* 1994;176:4204:4209.
38. Teo, T. C., et al. Long-term feeding with structured lipid composed of medium-chain and N-3 fatty acids ameliorates endotoxic shock in guinea pigs. *Metabolism* 1991;40(1):1152-1159.
39. Lim-Navarro, P. R. T. Protection effect of coconut oil against E coli endotoxin shock in rats. *Coconuts Today* 1994;11:90-91.
40. Dave, J. R., et al. Dodecylglycerol provides partial protection against glutamate toxicity in neuronal cultures derived from different regions of embryonic rat brain. *Mol Chem Neuropathol* 1997;30:1-13.

Chapter 16: Malnutrition and Neurodegeneration

1. Hu, F.B. and Malik, V.S. Sugar-sweetened beverages and risk of obesity and type 2 diabetes: epidemiologic evidence. *Physiol Behav* 2010;100:47-54.
2. Stranahan, A.M., et al. Diet-induced insulin resistance impairs hippocampal synaptic plasticity and cognition in middle-aged rats. *Hippocampus* 2008;18:1085-1088.
3. Cao, D., et al. Intake of sucrose-sweetened water induces insulin resistance and exacerbates memory deficits and amyloidosis in a transgenic mouse model of Alzheimer disease. *J Biol Chem* 2007;282:36275-36282.
4. Sanchez, A., et al. Role of sugars in human neutrophilic phagocytosis. *Am J Clin Nutr* 1973;26:1180-1184.
5. Higginbotham, S., et al. Dietary glycemic load and risk of colorectal cancer in the Women's Health Study. *Journal of the National Cancer Institute* 2004;96:229-233.
6. Corrada, M.M., et al. Reduced risk of Alzheimer's disease with high folate intake: the Baltimore Longitudinal Study of Aging. *Alzheimers Dement* 2005;1:11-18.
7. Smith, A.D., et al. Homocysteine-lowering by B vitamins slows the rate of accelerated brain atrophy in mild cognitive impairment: A randomized controlled trial *PLoS ONE* 2010;5:e12244.
8. Duan, W., et al. Dietary folate deficiency and elevated homocysteine levels endanger dopaminergic neurons in models of Parkinson's disease. *J Neurochem* 2002;80:101-110.
9. Moore, G.J., et al. Lithium-induced increase in human brain grey matter. *Lancet* 2000;356:1241-1242.
10. Nonaka, S., et al. Chronic lithium treatment robustly protects neurons in the central nervous system against excitotoxicity by inhibiting N-methyl-D-aspartate receptor-mediated calcium influx. *Proc natl Acad Sci USA* 1998;95:2642-2647.
11. Radesater, A., et al. Inhibition of GSK3 beta by lithium attenuates tau phosphoralation and degeneration. *Society for Neuroscience Abstracts* 2001;1:437.
12. Hullin, R. Zinc deficiency: can it cause dementia? *Therapaecia* 1983:26-30.
13. Harrison, F.E. and May, J.M. Vitamin C function in the brain: vital role of the ascorbate transporter SVCT2. *Free Radic Biol Med* 2009;46:719-730.
14. Goodwin, J.S., et al. Association between nutritional status and cognitive functioning in a healthy elderly population. *JAMA* 1983;249:2917-2921.

15. Herbert, V. Recommended dietary intakes (RDI) of vitamin B_{12} in humans. *American Journal of Clinical Nutrition1987*;45:671-678.
16. Halliwell, B. Reactive oxygen species and the central nervous system. *J Neurochem* 1992:59:1609-1623
17. Jiménez-Jiménez, F.J., et al. Serum levels of beta-carotene, alpha-carotene and vitamin A in patients with Alzheimer's disease. *Eur J Neurol* 1999;6:495-497.
18. Zaman, Z., et al. Plasma concentration of vitamin A and E and carotenoids in Alzheimer's disease. *Age Aging* 1992;21:91-94.
19. Okamoto, K., et al. Fruit and vegetable intake and risk of amyotrophic lateral sclerosis in Japan. *Neuroepidemiology* 2009;32:251-256.
20. Etminan, M., et al. Intake of vitamin E, vitamin C, and carotenoids and the risk of Parkinson's disease: a meta-analysis. *Lancet Neurol* 2005;4:362-365.
21. Morris, M.C., et al. Associations of vegetable and fruit consumption with age-related cognitive change. *Neurology* 2006;67:1370-1376.
22. Polidori, M.C., et al. High fruit and vegetable intake is positively correlated with antioxidant status and cognitive performance in healthy subjects. *J Alzheimers Dis* 2009;17:921-927.
23. Chan, A., et al. Apple juice concentrate maintains acetylcholine levels following dietary compromise. *J Alzheimers Dis* 2006;9:287-291.

Chapter 17: Brain Boosters

1. 2005 Dietary Guidelines for Americans. Center for Nutrition Policy and Promotion, U.S. Department of Agriculture. http://www.health.gov/DietaryGuidelines/dga2005/document/default.htm.
2. Bazzano, L.A., et al. Intake of fruit, vegetables, and fruit juices and risk of diabetes in women. *Diabetes Care* 2008;31:1311-1317.
3. Appel, L.J., et al. Effects of protein, monounsaturated fat, and carbohydrate intake on blood pressure and serum lipids: results of the OmniHeart randomized trial. *JAMA* 2005; 294:2455–64.
4. Llewellyn, D.J., et al. Serum 25-hydroxyvitamin D concentration and cognitive impairment. *J Geriatr Psychiatry Neurol* 2009;22:188-195.
5. Evatt, M.L., et al. Prevalence of vitamin D insufficiency in patients with Parkinson disease and Alzheimer disease. *Arch Neurol* 2008;65:1348-1352.
6. Wilkins, C.H., et al. Vitamin D deficiency is associated with worse cognitive performance and lower bone density in older African Americans. *J Natl Med Assoc* 2009;101:349-354.
7. Przybelski, R.J. and Binkley, N.C. Is vitamin D important for preserving cognition? A positive correlation of serum 25-hydroxyvitamin D concentration with cognitive function. *Arch Biochem Biophys* 2007;460:202-205.
8. Hayes, C.E. Vitamin D: a natural inhibitor of multiple sclerosis. *Proc Nutr Soc* 2000;59:531-535.
9. Hayes, C.E., et al. Vitamin D and multiple sclerosis. *Proc Soc Exp Biol Med* 1997;216:21-27.
10. www.vitamindcouncil.org.
11. Jang, S., et al. Luteolin reduces IL-6 produciton in microglia by inhibiting JNK phosphorylation and activation of AP-1. *Proc Nati Acad Sci USA* 2008;105:7534-7539.
12. Lim, G.P., et al. The curry spice curcumin reduces oxidative damage and amyloid pathology in an Alzheimer transgenic mouse. *J Neurosci* 2001;21:8370-8377.
13. Ng, T.P., et al. Curry consumption and cognitive function in the elderly. *Am J Epidemiology* 2006;164:898-906.
14. Chandra, V., et al. Incidence of Alzheimer's disease in a rural community in India: the Indo-US study. *Neurology* 2001;57:985-989.

15. Bousquet, M., et al. Beneficial effects of dietary omega-3 polyunsaturated fatty acid on toxin-induced neuronal degeneration in an animal model of Parkinson's disease. *FASEB J* 2008;22:1213-1225.
16. Morris, M.C., et al. Consumption of fish and n-3 fatty acids and risk of incident Alzheimer disease. *Arch Neurol* 2003;60:940-946.
17. Dell, C.A., et al. Lipid and fatty acid profiles in rats consuming different high-fat ketogenic diets. *Lipids* 2001;36:373-374.
18. Tomeo, A.C., et al. Antioxidant effects of tocotrienols in patients with hyperlipidemia and carotid stenosis. Lipids 1995;30:1179-1183.
19. Esterhuyse, A.J., et al. Dietary red palm oil supplementation protects against the consequences of global ischemia in the isolated perfused rat heart. *Asia Pac J Clin Nutr* 2005;14:340-347.
20. Yano, Y., et al. Induction of cytotoxicity in human lung adenocarcinoma cells by 6-0-carboxypropyl-alpha-tocotrienol, a redox-silent derivative of alpha-tocotrienol. *Int J Cancer* 2005;115:839-846.
21. Khanna, S., et al. Molecular basis of vitamin E action: tocotrienol modulates 12-lipoxygenase, a key moderator of glutamate-induced neurodegeneration. *J Biol Chem* 2003;278:43508-43515.
22. Walford, R.L. Calorie restriction: eat less, eat better, live longer. *Life Extension* 1998;Feb:19-22.
23. Bruce-Keller, A.J., et al. Food restriction reduces brain damage and improves behavioral outcome following excitotoxic and metabolic insults. *Ann Neurol* 1999;45:8-15.
24. Dubey, A., et al. Effect of age and caloric intake on protein oxidation in different brain regions and on behavioral functions of the mouse. *Arch Biochem Biophys* 1996;333:189-197.
25. Duan, W. and Mattson, M.P. Dietary restriction and 2-deoxyglucose administration improve behavioral outcome and reduce degeneration of dopaminergic neurons in models of Parkinson's disease. *J Neurosci Res* 1999;57:195-206.
26. Mattson, M.P. Neuroprotective signaling and the aging brain: take away my food and let me run. *Brain Res* 2000;886:47-53.
27. Boden, G., et al. Effect of a low-carbohydrate diet on appetite, blood glucose levels, and insulin resistance in obese patients with type 2 diabetes. *Ann Intern Med* 2005;142:403-411.
28. Volek, J.S., et al. Carbohydrate restriction has a more favorable impact on the metabolic syndrome than a low fat diet. *Lipids* 2009;44:297-309.
29. Halton, T.L., et al. Low-carbohydrate-diet score and risk of type 2 diabetes in women. *Am J Clin Nutr* 2008;87:339-346.
30. Sargrad, K.R., et al. Effect of high protein vs high carbohydrate intake on insulin sensitivity, body weight, hemoglobin A1c, and blood pressure in patients with type 2 diabetes mellitus. *J Am Diet Assoc* 2005;105:573-580.
31. Boden, G., et al. Effect of a low-carbohydrate diet on appetitie, blood glucose levels, and insulin resistance in obese patients with type 2 diabetes. *Ann Intern Med* 2005;142:403-411.
32. Volek, J.S. and Feinman, R.D. Carbohydrate restriction improves the features of metabolic syndrome. Metabolic syndrome may be defined by the response to carbohydrate restriction. *Nutrition & Metabolism* 2005;2:31.
33. Volek, J.S. and Sharman, M.J. Cardiovascular and hormonal aspects of very-low-carbohydrate ketogenic diets. *Obes Res* 2004;12:115S-1123S.
34. Rosedale, R., et al. Clinical experience of a diet designed to reduce aging. *J Appl Res* 2009;9:159-165.
35. Gaziano, J.M., et al. Fasting triglycerides, high-density lipoprotein, and risk of myocardial infarction. *Circulation* 1997;96:2520-2525.
36. Accurso, A., et al. Dietary carbohydrate restriction in type 2 diabetes mellitus and metabolic syndrome: time for a critical appraisal. *Nutrition & Metabolism* 2008;5:9.

37. Neilsen, J.V. and Joensson, E.A. Low-carbohydrate diet in type 2 diabetes: stable improvement of bodyweight and glycemic control during 44 months follow-up. *Nutrition & Metabolism* 2008;5:14.
38. Volek, J.S. and Feinman, R.D. Carbohydrate restriction improves the features of metabolic syndrome. Metabolic syndrome may be defined by the response to carbohydrate restriction. *Nutrition & Metabolism* 2005;2:31.
39. Forsythe, C.E., et al. Comparison of low fat and low carbohydrate diets on circulating fatty acid composition and markers of inflammation. *Lipids* 2008;43:65-77.
40. Volek, J.S., et al. Modification of lipoproteins by very low-carbohydrate diets. *J Nutr* 2005;135:1339-1342.
41. Craft, S. and Watson, G.S. Insulin and neurodegenerative disease: shared and specific mechanisms. *Lancet Neurology* 2004;3:169-178.
42. Colcombe, S.J., et al. Aerobic exercise training increases brain volume in aging humans. J Gerontol *A Biol Sci Med Sci* 2006;61:1166-1170.
43. Larson, E.B., et al. Exercise is associated with reduced risk for incident dementia among persons 65 years of age or older. *Ann Intern Med* 2006;144:73-81.
44. Lautenschlager, N.T., et al. Effect of physical activity on cognitive function in older adults at risk for Alzheimer disease: a randomized trial. *JAMA* 2008;300:1027-1037.
45. Honea, R.A., et al. Cardiorespiratory fitness and preserved medial temporal lobe volume in Alzheimer disease. *Alzheimer Dis Assoc Disord* 2009;23:188-197.
46. Faherty, C.J., et al. Environmental enrichment in adulthood eliminates neuronal death in experimental Parkinsonism. *Brain Res Mol Brain Res* 2005;134:170-179.
47. Liu-Ambrose, T., et al. Resistance training and executive functions: a 12-month randomized controlled trial. *Arch Intern Med* 2010;170:170-178.
48. Ravaglia, G., et al. Physical activity and dementia risk in the elderly: finding from a prospective Italian study. *Neurology* 2008;70:1786-1794.
49. Etgen, T., et al. Physical activity and incident cognitive impairment in elderly persons: the INVADE study. *Arch Intern Med* 2010;170:186-193.

Chapter 18: Low-Carb Therapy

1.Dell, C.A., et al. Lipid and fatty acid profiles in rats consuming different high-fat ketogenic diets. *Lipids* 2001;36:373-374.
2. Reger, M.A., et al. Effects of beta-hydroxybutyrate on cognition in memory-impaired adults. *Neurobiol Aging* 2004;25:311-314.
3. Likhodii, S.S., et al. Dietary fat, ketosis, and seizure resistance in rats on the ketogenic diet. *Epilepsia* 2000;41:1400-1410.
4. Gordon, N. and Newton, R.W. Glucose transporter type 1 (GLUT) deficiency. *Brain Dev* 2003;25:477-480.
5. Brighenti, F., et al. Effect of neutralized and native vinegar on blood glucose and acetate responses to a mixed meal in healthy subjects. *Eur J Clin Nutr* 1995;49:242-247.
6. Johnston, C.S., et al. Vinegar improves insulin sensitivity to a high-carbohydrate meal in subjects with insulin resistance or type 2 diabetes. *Diabetes Care 2004;27:281-282.*

Index

CPSIA information can be obtained
at www.ICGtesting.com
Printed in the USA
LVHW051328150223
739354LV00003B/145

9 781936 70912